Drama as Therapy

Volume 2

This book examines the many ways clients and therapists explore the therapeutic possibilities of drama. Whilst the first volume combined theory, practice and research in the field, this second volume concentrates on clinical material and practitioner research from a range of contexts, with thorough description and analysis of therapeutic work.

Bringing together international contributors, chapters explore work with various client groups in an array of contexts, including:

- work with clients with learning disabilities, dementia, HIV and cancer
- work with children, adolescents, adults, families and women's groups
- the justice system, education, family therapy and neuro-rehabilitation.

Drama as Therapy Volume 2: Clinical Work and Research into Practice is not only a welcome companion to the first volume, but is also an important stand alone work which will be of great interest to all those studying, practising or with an interest in dramatherapy.

Phil Jones lectures in Childhood Studies at the University of Leeds. He has lectured across Europe, Africa and North America and published widely on the arts therapies and on childhood. His books include *The Arts Therapies* (2005) and *Drama as Therapy: Theory, Practice and Research* (2007).

Drama as Therapy

Clinical Work and Research into Practice

Volume 2

Edited by Phil Jones

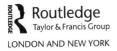
Routledge
Taylor & Francis Group

LONDON AND NEW YORK

First published 2010
by Routledge
2 Park Square, Milton Park, Abingdon, Oxon, OX14 4RN

Simultaneously published in the USA and Canada
by Routledge
711 Third Avenue, New York, NY 10017

Routledge is an imprint of the Taylor & Francis Group,
an informa business

Typeset in Times by RefineCatch Limited, Bungay, Suffolk
Paperback cover design by Andy Ward

British Library Cataloguing in Publication Data
A catalogue record for this book is available from the British Library

Library of Congress Cataloging-in-Publication Data
Jones, Phil, 1958–
    Drama as therapy : theory, practice, and research/Phil Jones.
  –Volume 2
    p.;cm.
    Includes bibliographical references and index
  1. Drama – Therapeutic use. I. Title.
  [DNLM: 1. Psychodrama. WM 430.5.P8 J78d 2007]
  RC489.P7J66 2007
  616.89′1523 – dc22

                                                    2007007576

ISBN: 978–0–415–47607–2 (hbk)
ISBN: 978–0–415–47608–9 (pbk)

This book is dedicated to the clients, students and colleagues from whom I have learned so much over the past 25 years.

Contents

Illustrations

Figures

Tables

Boxes

Vignettes

Contributors

Lindsay Chipman (CCC, RDT) has worked as programme and research coordinator/drama therapist providing oncology patients and their loved ones with free psychosocial services. She is a family consultant/drama therapist for a local school board, and works in private practice in the field of oncology through individual and group counselling. She is currently the Canadian representative to the National Association of Drama Therapy on their board of directors.

Ditty Dokter (PhD, RA'sT(D), SRDMT, UKCP) is Head of Arts Psychotherapies and professional lead at the Hertfordshire Partnership Foundation Trust. She has more than 25 years' experience of both teaching and of (inter)national practice with a variety of client groups and settings. She has published extensively including editing *Arts Therapists, Refugees And Migrants* (Jessica Kingsley) and *Supervision of Dramatherapy* (with Jones, Routledge).

Naomi Gardner-Hynd is a senior dramatherapist working with clients with learning disabilities and mental health problems in the National Health Service. She also works freelance with older adults with mental health problems. She is involved in lecturing and training in dramatherapy. She is also involved in the British Association of Dramatherapist's Employment and NHS Subcommittees.

Mario Guarnieri is a dramatherapist and supervisor with over ten years' full-time experience of working with offenders in high-secure and medium-secure NHS hospitals. Mario started his 'forensic career' with a performance and workshops of Kafka's *In The Penal Settlement* in HMP Norwich. He has worked with Geese Theatre Company (UK) and as a freelance dramatist using Boal's Forum Theatre in work with offenders on probation, ex-offenders and inner-city youth.

Eileen Haste, after qualifying as a dramatherapist, had a freelance practice in Cardiff, until 1999 when she left to travel and work overseas. On returning she made Bristol her base and developed work as a community artist.

She is now co-director of Tinker and Bloom, a company delivering participatory environmental arts projects.

Phil Jones (PhD) lectures in childhood studies at Leeds University. He is author of *Drama as Therapy* (Routledge), *The Arts Therapies* (Routledge), *Rethinking Childhood* (Continuum) and *Rethinking Children's Rights* (with Welch, Continuum). He is series editor for *New Childhoods* (Continuum); edited books include *Childhood* (with Moss, Tomlinson and Welch, Pearson), *Children's Rights in Practice* (with Walker, Sage) and *Supervision of Dramatherapy* (with Dokter, Routledge).

Athena Madan (CCC, PhD candidate) is a French-speaking arts therapist in Canada, researching social and geopolitical determinants of mental health. She also has experience as a part-time lecturer with the Faculty of Social Sciences at Brock University.

Pat McKenna is a clinical neuropsychologist who has worked in the NHS for the past 35 years, assessing and treating patients in neurology, neurosurgery and rehabilitation units. Throughout her career, she has been consistently involved in diverse research activities to improve assessment and treatment. Until retirement in 2008, she worked in neuro-rehabilitation unit for 19 years and it was here that she became interested in the potency of dramatherapy to aid patients' recovery.

Kirsten Meyer obtained her postgraduate diploma in dramatherapy from the University of Hertfordshire (UK) in 1999. She is co-founder and co-director of an NGO in South Africa and has run dramatherapy groups with diverse communities including: female offenders, children and adolescents living with HIV and AIDS and care workers. She currently works extensively throughout South Africa in various fields as therapist, facilitator and educator.

Christine Novy (MA, CCC) is a dramatherapist based in Canada. Her approach is to combine creativity with narrative practice and her special interest is to work with people to document and dramatise their narratives of change. Currently she collaborates with a variety of francophone and anglophone health care organisations to promote creative, narrative approaches to personal and community health. She is also a part-time lecturer with the creative arts therapies department at Concordia University.

Clare Powis has worked extensively as a freelance dramatherapist, mainly practising in special education. Over the years, freelance work has given way to employment in the National Health Service in work with clients with learning disabilities and in the field of child and adolescent mental health.

Emma Ramsden (PhD candidate) has a background as a dramatherapist in forensic psychiatry, education, homelessness and substance misuse. Emma has contributed to publications about her work in both forensic and educational settings. She is a doctoral research student at Leeds Metropolitan University for her study 'Children's Psychological Voices in Dramatherapy'.

Nisha Sajnani (RDT, PhD candidate) is a drama therapist with the Post Traumatic Stress Center in New Haven, CT and president-elect of the National Association for Drama Therapy (USA). She is a doctoral candidate at Concordia University where her research interests include critical theory, applied theatre, collective trauma and cultural intervention. Nisha is the director of Creative Alternatives, an applied arts network that provides continuing education on the role of the arts in health care, education and advocacy. Nisha is on the faculty of the Institute for the Arts in Psychotherapy in New York City.

Jay Vaughan is a dramatherapist who has been working with traumatised children in the care system since 1989 and has specialised in working with children who are long-term fostered or adopted since 1994. Jay currently manages Family Futures therapy service while continuing to work directly with children and families. Jay has a particular interest in somatic work with children and parents and is passionate about integrating different approaches to help traumatised children.

Preface

This book includes in-depth descriptions and analysis of practice from many perspectives. Given the enormous scope of dramatherapy work, any selection is bound to be partial; however, one of the aims of the book is to present a *range* of ideas and approaches. In a sense, it is a very personal selection as it draws on people I have met in my time as trainer and lecturer in the UK and Canada. It could have been four times its length: so I start with an apology to all those whose work could have made this book even more valuable, but who are not included this time. The book's range does not aim to be definitive in its extent. Its goal is to offer the reader an encounter with the diversity and versatility of the field, whilst, at the same time, giving an opportunity to review some of the parallels within the ways that dramatherapy works for clients. Volume 1 of Drama as Therapy introduced the field in the following way:

> During the twentieth century developments in a number of fields such as experimental theatre and psychology have resulted in new insights into the ways in which drama and theatre can be effective in bringing about change in people: emotional, psychological, political and spiritual change . . .
>
> (Jones 2007: 3)

This volume offers pictures of this developing insight. Different dramatherapists in Part 2 of the book take us into their work. The chapters give a real sense of the richness, potency and variety of how dramatherapy is being used and created by clients and therapists together.

Part 1 offers a number of frameworks within which to understand the chapters in Part 2. These include introductions to the idea of the professional context of dramatherapy and the practitioner-researcher (Chapter 1); political contexts as a way of understanding therapeutic practice (Chapter 2); and dialogues with key theorists to look at the theory behind the practice (Chapter 3). Each of these chapters contains direct, cited links to specific areas of Part 2, to help the reader link the preparatory chapters to the detailed edited collection of practice.

In Part 2 authors describe their work in detail. Contributors were asked to contextualise their practice, to give details of the way they work and to foreground how they gain insights into their clients' experiences of dramatherapy. An ethics statement about the therapy and research in this section can be found on page 66. The volume contains a wealth of inspired ideas and practices: interviews, focus groups, feedback from dramatic ways of evaluating how clients have experienced therapy, questionnaires, the use of mutually-analysed vignettes, non-participant observation, photographs and drawn images. The contributors were also asked to engage with the politics of the therapeutic encounter: most chapters in Part 2 look at the ways in which forces at work within the lives of clients, but often ignored within accounts of practice, can be understood within dramatherapy.

This second volume provides the field with a series of in-depth accounts and reflections on practice. As the book is completed, it is seventy years since Peter Slade's earliest documented use of the word 'dramatherapy' in a 1939 lecture to the British Medical Association (see Jones, 2007: 24). Drama as Therapy Volume 2 offers a compendium of the ways dramatherapists and clients together are advancing 'dramatherapy' as we approach the end of the first century since Slade's public launching of the term in his encounter with the British Medical Association.

Dr Phil Jones
Settle
North Yorkshire
21 February 2009

Acknowledgements

I would like to thank Sue Jennings, Robert Landy, Dorothy Langley, Adam Blatner, David Read Johnson and Helen Payne for the dialogues they have contributed to chapter three.

Part 1

Clinical practice: contexts, research and dialogues

1 The nature of practice and practitioner research

Phil Jones

Introduction: the emergence of the dramatherapy practitioner

Dramatherapy practice has emerged from a history of discoveries made by individuals and groups in many different contexts, as described in Volume 1. These included ideas and experiments in many countries prior to the established health systems of the twentieth century (Casson 1999; Jennings 1994; Jones 1996, 2007; Landy 2001). The term 'dramatherapy' developed as practices became more coherent: as individuals discovered each other's work occurring within health and care services, ranging from early psychiatric hospitals to special schools and units. From these early steps onwards, access to the therapeutic benefits of drama has expanded to meet an enormous range of client experiences, challenges, creativity and needs. The development of dramatherapy has been one of discovery within its own emergent methods and ideas, alongside dialogue and engagement with related disciplines from psychotherapy to Forum Theatre, from dance to neuroscience (Andersen-Warren and Grainger 2000; Langley 2006; Mitchell 1996; Pearson 1996). Volume 2 illustrates the ways in which this discovery and dialogue is still alive in contemporary dramatherapy. This chapter offers a context for the edited chapters, which cover a range of practice. It introduces the nature of enquiry in dramatherapy, and the frameworks within which dramatherapy occurs. The chapter will feature references to the chapters in Part 2, helping readers relate the issues it raises to the clinical practice and research contained in that section of the book.

In many countries, the way in which dramatherapy is practised is now framed by regulation and structures set in place by professional associations, recognised qualifications and by national or international health care systems or policies. The hard work undertaken by individuals and groups has created structures which aim to guarantee safety and assurance for the client entering into therapy concerning issues such as the level of training of their therapist, ethical procedures and the overseeing of the quality of the dramatherapy practice they experience. These systems also ensure the quality of training for those wishing to qualify in the field, and subsequent opportunities for them to follow a career which is structured within mainstream health care provision and to pursue career routes within different professional contexts. Though details vary, a standard approach is similar in many countries. This infrastructure consists of four interrelated components:

1   professional associations
2   trainings offered within agreed standards – usually set through a combination of the association with the education and health care systems
3   supervision and continuous professional development
4   research.

The role of the professional associations has been to bring practitioners together, to develop the field, to establish and carry a vision for the development of dramatherapy and to negotiate, and represent, its members in relation to standards, training and employment. The associations have also advanced the frontiers of research and enquiry. The pattern for most trainings to qualify as a dramatherapist is that they are set at postgraduate exit levels, with those entering study holding a relevant first degree in the art form or in a health-related subject such as psychology, nursing or social work. The trainings combine theoretical study with practical skills-based sessions, placement with training supervision and a sustained experience of dramatherapy as a training client. Supervision is seen as both an element of training, and as a process that supports, sustains and builds the professionalism of the practicing therapist. This process, distinct from managerial supervision, involves the dramatherapist meeting with a qualified professional to reflect on the processes at work within their practice. Some systems make supervision mandatory in practising as a professional within a period of time after qualification. Within recent UK research the experience of supervision was seen as essential to the continuous development of the therapist as a reflective practitioner and to understanding the nature and impact of dramatherapy (Tselikas-Portmann 1999; Jones and Dokter 2008).

The practice of research: researching practice

The fourth component of the infrastructure, research into dramatherapy practice and theory, involves developing insight into the field. It is engaged with by practitioners within the context of their work and also within the framework of academic institutions and health care providers. There are different perspectives on research, which reflect different directions in enquiry. Kellett (2005) has summarised three key values which are relevant to consider in relation to dramatherapy. She asserts that research is important because:

- its innovatory and exploratory character can bring about beneficial change
- its skeptical enquiry can result in poor or unethical practices being questioned

- its rigorous and systematic nature extends knowledge and promotes rigorous problem solving.

(Kellett 2005: 9)

She sees the broad canvas of research in a way that is useful for dramatherapy to work from:

> Research sets out ... to establish the 'truth' of something through a systematic and rigorous process of critical enquiry where even the most commonplace assumption is not readily accepted until it has been validated. Kerlinger (1986) refers to this skeptical form of enquiry as checking subjective belief against objective reality. Furthermore any 'truth' established by research also has a self-correcting process at work in the ongoing public scrutiny to which it is subjected (Cohen *et al.* 2000) and any research inaccuracies will ultimately be discovered and either corrected or discarded.

(Kellett 2005: 9)

Here Kellett draws together research's relationship to truth, skeptical enquiry, validity and its connection to both subjective and objective perspectives. In any research within the field of health and medical enquiry, particular elements of this relationship are drawn to the fore. These relate to the values Kellett identifies, concerning concepts of truth, validity and the relation between notions of the 'subjective' and 'objective'. As a discipline drawing both on the arts and on systems of health, dramatherapy engages with various, and often opposing, ideas about the validity of what is called subjective or objective, for example. In arts or theatre practice-based research, processes such as creativity, originality, innovation and the value of personal expression and richness of data are often foregrounded. Medical and health practice-related research is often concerned with a need to validate experiences and outcomes from a framework that values quantitative, objective or scientific criteria. These need not be oppositional, but can often be experienced as such within spaces that dramatherapy is practised in: for example, in hospitals or other health provision. Robson refers to a divide which reflects cultural and research traditions, and one which arts therapist practitioners and researchers will recognise:

> Differences fall within two main traditions which engage in sporadic warfare. One is labeled as positivistic, natural-science based, hypothetic-deductive, quantitative or even simply 'scientific'; the other as interpretive, ethnographic or qualitative – among several other labels . . .

(Robson 2002: 7)

Within many areas of contemporary cultural enquiry the fields of health and medicine and those of the arts are encountered in ways that emphasise their difference, even irreconcilability. The arts therapies enquirer can often experience this tension when it comes to research or concepts such as truth and validity. As I have said elsewhere (Jones 2005), the field of the arts therapies is responding to this cultural divide through a variety of responses:

> As the disciplines develop further, and as clients and therapists work together to discover more about both the potentials and ways of describing the methods and approaches, the nature and value of change in the arts therapies will become ever more established and articulate. This will not, and should not, happen by the arts therapies using one approach or framework: rather, as Grainger (1999: 143) says, 'we need to have several different languages at our command.'
>
> (Jones 2005: 246)

Practitioner research

The focus of recent work has reflected this variety in its approach to understanding dramatherapy practice. This book reflects the diversity of practitioner research: work within its chapters draws on qualitative and quantitative methods and is connected to systems that operate within medical care such as the notion of 'evidence based practice', whilst also engaging with other frameworks such as social models of health, and theatrical or sociological perspectives on change. The nature of enquiry is a broad one within the field and, as such, fits the different needs of an emergent discipline and a variety of contexts. One way of looking at this is in terms of a *necessary* diversity: from formal large scale research to informal research undertaken within day-to-day practice (Mahrer 1997). At one end of a scale is substantive, resourced formal research. An example of this would be an examination of efficacy within a national health service drawing on work undertaken in many settings, using models derived from a quantitative approach to evidence-based research often utilised within such a system. Another example of substantive research would be doctoral or postdoctoral enquiry drawing on extensive in-depth casework using qualitative methods in order to gain rich data and insight into the process and impact of the therapy. At the other end of this scale would be work which is not undertaken within such an intensive, resourced and supported framework. An example of this arena of research is that engaged with by a dramatherapist and client together within their everyday practice, as understood within what is often referred to as a 'practitioner researcher' framework. This acknowledges the 'correspondences between the reflective processes of qualitative analysis and the reflective processes' of the therapy itself (Clarkson and Angelo 1998: 20). Here the enquiry is undertaken by the therapist within their normal caseload, in reflection and supervision, as they explore the practice and develop insight within a structured framework of analysis.

This spectrum relates to the impetus and need behind the research into dramatherapy practice. A national health service's needs and those of a day centre, of a PhD student and a therapist and client working together in private practice are all related, but are also different. The design, goals and outcomes need to be fitted to the framework and available resources within which the research operates. This is not to say that the kinds of research tools and methods are necessarily different. Similar ways of examining efficacy, for example, might be used in the larger scale and the smaller scale work – the main difference can lie in the scope and extent of the enterprise and its claims. All are valid, but in different ways. Hence the formal large-scale framework may fit research within a national health service's resources and needs, whilst a practitioner researcher approach will fit the needs and resources of every-day work with clients. Dadds' descriptions of practitioner research fit the framework of many of the chapters in Part 2:

> Practitioner research . . . is not seeking generalisations in the way some large-scale forms of research attempt to do. Rather, it is seeking new understandings that will enable us to create the most intelligent and informed approach we can to improving our provision for those in our care. Stenhouse claimed that 'we are concerned with the development of a sensitive and self-critical subjective perspective and not with the aspir-ation to unattainable objectivity' (1975: 157). In accepting the mantle, as researchers, of professional communicators in a more public arena, there-fore, we seek to share our research stories with others so that colleagues can, if appropriate, engage with them and relate them to their own work . . . This is how the influence of the small-scale, particular project, shared across the profession, can work its way into the larger fabric.
>
> (Dadds 2008: 3)

This definition is one that many in the field might find of use, and it is a fitting definition for the enquiry and practice contained in Part 2. Within this book the research undertaken by the contributors reflects the different needs and possibilities within such a practitioner researcher framework.

A key aspect of many of the chapters concerns how to gain client perspec-tives on their experience of the therapy. This includes quantitative and quali-tative methods, narrative approaches to research, work with clients as co-researchers, the use of dramatic and other arts based methods as evaluation, questionnaires, structured and semi-structured interviews, focus groups, video and non-participant observation. The following excerpts from Part 2 give a sense of this range.

Novy, for example, in Chapter 4 uses narrative approaches to research in dramatherapy within vignette analysis of work involving clients as co-researchers:

> . . . Solange, Louise and Carole were interviewed all together about their experience during the project. I was curious to hear their evaluation of the methods that we worked with and, more specifically, their under-

standing of whether and how these were helpful. To begin the interview they were invited to choose a moment or moments that stood out in their experience of the project. I then asked each in turn to describe this moment and to reflect on its significance. The group interview was audio-recorded and later transcribed and translated into English. In the 'Reflection on theory and method' section that follows, I take the partici-pants' thoughts, meanings and language as a starting point for my theoretical reflections on the methods used in the second [*Narratives of Change*] project.

(Novy, Chapter 4, p. 77)

Guarnieri and Ramsden, in Chapter 8, use focus groups of fellow profes-sionals in their research into their practice:

... colleagues from other professions ... comment on implications for future practice. Our colleague reflections derive from a focus group, which ... enables a group of people to discuss and explore a theme or topic together, often within a defined open questions structure.

(Guarnieri and Ramsden, Chapter 8, p. 153)

This enabled them to gain the perceptions of colleagues who had experienced their work as co-facilitators within teams. These were drawn from other professions including psychology, nursing and music therapy. The research through focus group identifies issues that professionals perceived as important within their experience of the dramatherapy, for example:

The word power was mentioned many times during the discussion, in relation to the power of the drama. It was noted that 'there's something in dramatherapy that I've seen helps connect with the reality of the situ-ation in a much more powerful way than talking about it does ... there's something about scenarios ... actually you're in the room and you're feeling it, you're feeling what it would be like being in that situation. You're there and there's no hiding away that this is what that person did, and this is what it can make people feel like ... I think that's very powerful.'

(Guarnieri and Ramsden, Chapter 8, pp. 167–168)

Dokter uses a combination of questionnaires, interviews and focus group work in her approach to understanding clients' experiences of change in Chapter 11:

I had used evaluation questionnaires completed by clients and therapists at the end of each session, as well as individual semi-structured interviews and post-session focus groups to ascertain what clients and therapists found helpful and hindering in sessions.

(Dokter, Chapter 11, p. 211)

Haste and McKenna use a combination of qualitative and quantitative methods in their research:

> For the efficacy of gathering data for the study, feedback and observations of the programme were gathered in several ways. After each session the dramatherapist filled out 2 questionnaires. One devised by the neuropsychologist, helped to gauge the responsiveness of the participant. The other, devised by the dramatherapist, aimed to judge the appropriateness of the material for the particular individual. In the fourth session, a video camera was positioned in a corner of the room to allow later observation by the neuropsychologist. Only the neuropsychologist had access to the film. Following this fourth session, the neuropsychologist also filled in checklists after observing the session on video. Within a few days following the last session, the neuropsychologist carried out a semi-structured interview (with participants), which was tape-recorded ... The central questions were how enjoyable or worthwhile the course had been to them and what relationship this had, if any, to the rest of their experience in the hospital. They were also asked to rate the importance of the two main therapies, physiotherapy and occupational therapy as well as dramatherapy in their rehabilitation programme.
>
> (Haste and McKenna, Chapter 5, p. 88)

One way to look at this fascinating range is that they complete different parts of an ongoing, emerging picture of what occurs within dramatherapy, and examines how we understand what is effective from different viewpoints. This is not a fragmentary way of looking at research, but, rather, one that sees the appropriateness of diversity and relation. This book forms a part of this developing picture as it presents a variety of perspectives on how dramatherapy is seen and understood. Sandretto places practitioner research in relation to the development of theory, critical understanding of practice and to the impact of enquiry:

> According to Freire (1999), whose work focused on ways in which to support illiterate adults in reading in critical ways, praxis is 'reflection and action upon the world in order to transform it' (1999: 33). Praxis involves the careful consideration of our theories and our practices: 'Theory building and critical reflection inform our practice and our action, and our practice and action inform our theory building and critical reflection' (Wink 2000: 59). In addition, practice and the development of knowledge are inextricably linked: 'without practice there's no knowledge.' (Freire 1999: 33).
>
> (Sandretto 2008: 7)

As the above examples show, within the chapters in Part 2 we have practice that, in different ways, contributes to this emergent knowledge. The dramatherapist practitioner researchers contribute in ways devised to meet the questions their clients and contexts ask them: using single approaches and combinations of approaches, research that is engaged with through the client's voice; formal approaches, drawing on quantitative approaches and qualitative approaches. They are all acknowledging the richness and complexity of clients', therapists' and settings' needs.

The variety of dramatherapy practice

As this book will demonstrate, the ways in which dramatherapy is practised varies enormously, responding to the different situations that clients bring to therapy. Dramatherapy now exists in relation to many different health systems, works with many different client groups and has expanded into areas beyond the more traditional health settings of hospitals and clinics. The health systems range between those within the different cultural contexts of healing in many countries. Traditional paradigms of health often separate out physical illness from mental health, locate therapy in hospitals or clinics, but not in settings such as schools (Jennings 1994). The therapy contained within this book, as in much practice within the field, works against such divisions and separation. Dramatherapy is often practised in ways that do not separate out the physical from the mental, the spiritual from the bodily in its engagement with clients. Similarly, its practice is often working in ways that acknowledge the relevance and interdependence of health and creativity in an approach to space and healing that is interdisciplinary: working in schools, in arts settings and community settings as well as in clinics and hospitals. Different client groups and different reasons for coming to therapy are exemplified by this book. The chapters reflect work with people living with illnesses such as cancer, those within the justice system, in schools, in private practice, people with mental health problems and in prison. People dealing with different kinds of circumstances or different forms of social exclusion, from poverty to prejudice, are all shown to receive support within dramatherapy. As this variety indicates, the field has demonstrated its understanding of the way the therapy works for clients within theory and practice in an increasing range of contexts. When looking at accounts of practice it is possible to see similarity and divergence in the ways in which clients use dramatherapy. The next section will explore these parallels and differences.

The triangle in dramatherapy practice

The concept of a 'triangle' is often referred to in a number of arts therapies modalities as a way of describing a key aspect of what the arts therapies offer (Jones 2005). One way of looking at this triangle is to see it as concerning the ways the therapist, the client and the art form create the dramatherapy space together. This framework is useful in helping to differentiate the arts therapies from many other forms of therapy. The dramatherapy space, as discussed in theory and research literature, has some areas of constancy. These include the creation of boundaries, the use of the art form and the primacy of the art form as a means of expressing, exploring and resolving material over the use of words alone as the process and content of the therapy. My own writing has argued that basic processes are also present within all dramatherapy – though the ways they are drawn upon varies (Jones 2005, 2007). The following examples show parallels and differences between the ways in which therapist and client make use of dramatherapy together. They show how very diverse clients use the therapeutic space, relationship and form or language of dramatherapy in ways that are both similar and different. In the three examples the techniques, the space and their relationship with the therapist all concern objects and photography.

In Chapter 6 Chipman talks about how an individual client, coming to dramatherapy during her cancer treatment, uses photography and objects. The client, Gaïa, uses her own body and objects to stage a photograph that she takes of herself:

> Gaïa used props and costume to personify qualities and roles she wishes for herself in the future; her earrings the symbol of her creative self, the microphone as her artistic self, her dress as her femininity and sense of being a woman, a stuffed animal and baby to represent her hope for children and to be a mother, an engagement ring to signify marriage and partnership.
>
> (Chipman, Chapter 6, p. 118)

In Chapter 7 Meyer describes the uses of photography in her work with adolescents living with HIV and Aids:

> Each participant was given a camera to take home for the week and photograph themselves in as many different contexts as they liked. The photographs were then developed and the subject of which, formed part of one session through body sculptures. Here the participants were able to show each other their lives outside of the group. Some teens then decided they wanted to incorporate some of the photographs into their body maps.
>
> (Meyer, Chapter 7, p. 138)

In Chapter 4 Novy reflects on the uses her clients made of objects within her work with women who have come into conflict with the law:

> The toys' associations with childhood play seemed to make it easier for the participants to bring past events into the dramatic present. Louise used the small family dolls to tell the story of the abuse she experienced as a child. She said that when she saw the toys she felt like a child again and travelled back in time. Carole shared a similar experience of

transport: 'When I had the figurines in my hand, my story became clear: I was a child, I wasn't happy. I didn't feel loved or understood.'

(Novy, Chapter 4, p. 74)

On the one hand, parallel techniques are used: objects are introduced into the therapy space and used to capture, communicate and work therapeutically with experiences, feelings and relationships. The relationship between therapist and client are all, in part, mediated and expressed through this similar combination of objects, images and enactment. Here, though, we can also identify key differences in the way the space and process are used.

In the first, Gaïa uses dramatic projection with objects to create a self-image as an expression of herself within the session and then photographs them in front of the dramatherapist. She and Chipman situate this in a variety of different ways – a key part of it involves expressing her self-perceptions during her experience of cancer in a manner that words alone could not capture. Gaïa creates perspective: to try to witness, to see herself and to gain a sense of selfhood at a time when her well-being and identity is challenged. The taking of photographs is seen as an experience of empowerment at a time when she experiences the opposite. In Meyer's practice the photographic work operates differently in terms of the actual activity, in that it is used to create a connection between the clients' lives outside the session and the drama inside the therapy group – they do not take photographs within the session, but are bringing concrete images into the session. This, then, enables them to begin to express and explore their lives through the dramatic representation of the photographs and the creation of objects, role plays, improvisation and incorporation into image maps of their bodies. Here the use is as a way of supporting connection, the photographs take on the role of a script to help develop dramatic work and are used as objects to connect to images relating to the clients' experiences of their bodies and identities. Bringing issues about HIV into the therapy room is hard for the clients, and Meyer also notes the ways in which the group prefers to work in a concrete rather than symbolic way: so the use of photos here helps respond to this preference. The uses Novy and the clients she works with make of objects, have differences and similarities with the work of Chipman and Gaïa. The objects relate to the clients' sense of self, but whereas for Gaïa they are used primarily to project and explore aspects of her current self and situation, for Novy's group members they become allied with the past and past experiences. They become a language to connect with memories of experiences with which they are still unfinished. The objects become a means to express and examine the past as present in their current lives.

This illustrates the ways in which therapists and clients are sensitive to the different capabilities and issues brought to the space, language, processes and relationships within dramatherapy. They exemplify the flexibility of the medium of dramatherapy, and the way the therapist works to help the client maximise their personal needs in using dramatherapy. The language and process bear relationship to each other, but the potency of dramatherapy lies in the ways in which its variety is being tested and created by the live encounter between therapists and clients in different situations. As the next section will illustrate, the focus upon the client, the creative, client-centredness of drama-therapy means that definitions and practice have key components which are parallel, but dramatherapy's shape and impact is as varied as the people who work within the field.

Dramatherapy: practice, dialogues and research

The ways in which dramatherapy practice has been described and analysed reflect different kinds of attention. This attention often connects to the desire to articulate what dramatherapy has to offer as clearly as possible. One way this has happened is that broad attention is given to overall processes at work in dramatherapy sessions. This literature reflects this use as including the following ways:

• to have a framework to help the therapist develop structure and create practice
• for dramatherapists to articulate to themselves and others what occurs within dramatherapy sessions
• to evaluate how therapeutic work develops over time.
        (Andersen-Warren and Grainger 2000; Jones 2007; Langley 2006)

The following give examples of the ways dramatherapists in this book create relationships between overall processes, models and the specifics of their practice. Gardner-Hynd, in Chapter 9, shows how she used different frame-works for broad processes to underpin her approach and understanding, one from the arts therapies and one from the field of the arts and creativity:

> The creativity cycle influences the way my sessions are structured and provides insight into the therapeutic process. The following diagram represents the creativity cycle in relation to dramatherapy session structure which is based on a model by Payne (1993) used in dance movement therapy.
>   This process is cyclical and has four stages, which are, preparation (warm-up/games/relaxation), incubation (main activity e.g. free play/story/role play/mask work etc.), illumination (reflection and ending circle: use of words/movement/art or music to aid this process) and verification (can occur between sessions as material is processed conscious and subconsciously).
>   (Gardner-Hynd, Chapter 9, p. 177)

Access to theory and to models is used here by Gardner-Hynd to help her structure and understand the nature of her practice, and the way she sees change in her work with clients. She shows herself as a practitioner able to draw on connected fields of creativity and the arts therapies to meet the needs of her clinical situation. Broader perspectives are linked by her to support specific practice and client work.

The core processes (Jones 1996, 2005, 2007), as described in Chapter 3, are another example of an approach that looks at processes occurring in all forms of dramatherapy, rooted in creativity and theatre. Novy in Chapter 4 uses the core processes in the following way:

> The objects also made it possible for the participants to see their experience represented. Louise explained how creating and seeing the sculpture of a hanging person changed her ideas:
>
>> After I put together the hanging man, oh, it was like someone had stabbed me in the heart. Making it and seeing it really made me feel something. And then I said to myself 'my god' and I had goose bumps looking at it. I'm depressed but I mustn't let myself go that far.
>
> Louise's account fits with Jones' description of dramatic projection: 'the process by which clients project aspects of themselves or their experience into theatrical or dramatic materials . . . and thereby externalize inner conflicts' (2007: 84). Jones goes on to explain how 'the dramatic expression enables change through the creation of perspective.' For both Louise and Carole, externalising the problem in this way diminished its influence in their lives.
>
> (Novy, Chapter 4, pp. 78–79)

Whilst Vaughan, in Chapter 13, describes how the same core process of 'dramatic projection' featured within her practice, but in a different context:

> In Ruth's first session her dramatic projection was as extreme and potentially dangerous as her life had been. By the third session Ruth's dramatic projection, and the need for it to manage all her feelings, was minimal as she was able to use the art form to contain most of her feelings and not be activated into a 'fight, flight or freeze' response. Instead in this last session she was able to use her higher brain functioning to think about her bodily responses to the trauma and her feelings. Thus making sense of her experience in quite a different way. In this way the dramatic projection enabled her to gain a perspective on her life and so gain insights about her need to enact what had happened to her.
>
> (Vaughan, Chapter 13, p. 257)

In two very different situations Novy and Vaughan, as practitioner researchers, use the core processes to help articulate and evaluate the nature of how change is occurring, and to see how their therapy is effective for the client. Their access to broader concepts becomes a language to help assist in understanding the drivers of change, to identify what it is that enables and creates the therapy in dramatherapy. Gardner-Hynd's adaptation of Payne is similar, in that all try to encapsulate and understand the dynamics that fuel the dramatherapy. They draw on broader concepts and ideas about process but do not say that all practice is the same, rather giving practitioners a sense of how to see, and understand, change.

The advantages of this approach includes the use of a broad structural framework that is relevant to a range of contexts and approaches, along with the assertion that they are relevant and available to all practising therapists. The disadvantages include their broad-brush framework: some practitioners find the need to have an orientation within their work that either relates to a more specific identity or method: such as the 'Role method' (Landy 2001) or 'Sesame' (Pearson 1996). Others feel the need to relate to a specific therapeutic framework in dialogue with the wider field of therapy – such as CBT, family therapy or psychoanalysis.

As evidenced in the practice within this book, dramatherapists make use of such methods or models of ways of working. Chipman, in Chapter 6, draws on such a specific model in her assessment:

> Landy's (1993) taxonomy of roles is a standard method of assessment I use in my private practice. Having based much of my methodology on the Photo Theatre of the Self, work by Spence (1995) and role theory, my emphasis on the aspect of roles in identity formation was paramount. These roles would serve as the basis for later work using self-portrait photography in dramatherapy. I would also use this assessment throughout the therapeutic process in order to evaluate progress and change.
>
> (Chipman, Chapter 6, p. 110)

Here Chipman makes use of a specific model in a way that is judged, by her, to be relevant to the specific clinical practice she needs – an approach to assessment, drawing on role.

This relationship between specific clinical needs and the therapist creating dialogue with particular frameworks is reflective of dramatherapy's relationship with many fields and approaches. The practice described and analysed in this book often illustrates the ways in which such creative dialogue can occur. The client must remain the focus of all such attention – the question being: what can most benefit the client I am working with?

The different chapters reveal excellent practice where therapists naturally engage with this question. Their responses involve:

- the situation and the creativity brought by the client
- the ways clients respond within the therapy space and relationship including how they present the issues they are bringing to therapy
- the therapist's creativity and expertise

- dialogue with other professionals working in the same setting that the therapy is practised in
- dialogue with colleagues engaged in similar contexts nationally and internationally, including familiarity with research and evidence developed in parallel fields
- their encounter with the clinical situation through the reflective and exploratory process of supervision.

This combination brings together previous knowledge with the verve of spontaneous encounter: all lead to a diversity that represents a real engagement with the needs of the clients. The needs of the training and fledgling therapist can often seem to be different than those of the experienced dramatherapist, though the task is parallel. Often when training, or first-trained, the dramatherapist or student dramatherapist can, understandably, see such diversity as 'confusing' or as a lack in dramatherapy's identity. When practising, an experienced dramatherapist often naturally develops a route to practise reflecting a creative dialogue. This responds to the rich ground they are working within in terms of the clients' lives or issues, and the clinical context they are working within. As I have argued elsewhere, about the therapeutic relationship: 'the arts therapies have evolved in dialogue with other models of therapeutic relationship, and also with other disciplines such as teaching or arts practice . . . the arts therapies have (also) made unique discoveries about the relationship between client and therapist' (Jones 2005: 182).

The following gives two examples of this dialogue with other fields, such as therapeutic approaches or forms of theatre. Novy articulates a dialogue between dramatherapy, the framework of narrative approaches to therapy, thinking in her field and the experiences of the clients she works with:

> Several ideas about stories and their use in therapy informed the project's methodology. Among these, an idea shared by dramatherapists and narrative therapists alike: that our lives and identities can be represented in different ways and from varying perspectives; that life stories are, indeed, creations and, as such, they can be created or constructed differently. Often these more limiting narratives are created by others: people in positions of authority who hold the power of definition (Morgan 2000). One participant described her experience: 'Because I have a criminal record, the police don't take me seriously. I think in their eyes I am worthless. They see me as a liar, a thief, an addict.' During the project the participants were invited to step out of these, and other limiting stories, into a play space where their own knowledge about their lives was privileged.
>
> (Novy, Chapter 4, p. 68)

This illustrates the synergy between the therapist's knowledge of her field, dramatherapy; the knowledge in the literature of other practices concerning her client group; narrative approaches to therapy; the experiences of her clients as voiced by the participant; along with Novy's own creativity in response to the client's issues as brought to dramatherapy. This illustrates very effectively the nature and importance of the dialogue between different frameworks and understanding of change. It also reveals the therapist's natural, creative combination of a variety of perspectives – all focused on benefiting the individual client.

A parallel set of relationships, with a different focus, concerning dramatherapy and the field of theatre and change, is illustrated in Sajnani's perspective on dialogues in her work with a South Asian Women's Community Centre. She frames her work in the following manner:

> Boal has defined the central thesis of his performance pedagogy to be the active participation of the audience who bears witness to injustices embodied and staged; the transformation of the passive spectator to the 'spect-actor' who is complicit in the co-creation of the realities we as a society sustain and support . . . in their will to act upon injustice . . . ideas proposed by Brecht, Boal, and Kershaw are complemented by contemporary developments in ideas about social justice and social or cultural therapy. There is a growing trend in psychotherapy to challenge inequality and commit to social justice . . . and to redefine the role of the therapist to include outreach, prevention, and advocacy . . . enlarging the therapeutic space . . . usefully blurring the boundaries between the public and private . . . the purpose of therapy as facilitating an individual and/or group's capacities to identify, analyse and address the internalised, relational and systemic dynamics which limit the full arc of their desires.
>
> (Sajnani, Chapter 10, p. 194)

She goes on to illustrate the particular dialogues that shape their practice. As well as dramatherapy, Boal, Brecht and Kershaw, the facilitators draw on educational processes:

> Both of us also had an interest in expanding the frame of therapy to include an engagement with the social and political context, which shaped the lives of those with whom we worked. With this in mind, we chose to devote time to the development of a popular education process that would provide a scaffold for our group process, leading us and our group to a shared analysis of the relationship between intimate and structural violence and its psychological and social consequences . . . We hoped to share authority with participants in the group and create a performance that would communicate the relationship between psychological distress and intimate and systematic trauma.
>
> (Sajnani, Chapter 10, p. 195)

This way of working and thinking brings together ideas from education, theatre and therapy. This inter-relationship is key to Sajnani and Nadau finding an approach that serves the needs of their clients: how they, as workers, create or use dramatic exercises and processes. The use of scaffolding as described in the chapter, for example, influences their handling of their roles as facilitators with the group. Particular aspects of practice can also be seen in this way – as a dialogue with ideas and approaches (see Jennings 2009). The dramatherapist and client relationship can be developed and worked with in a variety of ways, for example, depending on such dialogues. It can be used differently depending upon the paradigm the dramatherapist works within. Hence the kinds of role relationship the client discovers within the therapy varies. The following examples from chapters in this book illustrate this aspect of the way a therapist handles their role: often referred to as a 'directive', or 'non-directive' approach. Dokter, for example, illustrates how a dialogue with psychodynamic understandings of group processes have influenced her thinking and approach to relationship and structure:

> Structuring connects to a therapist expectation of directive or non-directive interventions, often combined with a group process approach that aims to facilitate client independence. If the therapist keeps waiting for client initiatives while they feel very stuck, it can be counter-therapeutic. The findings of this research are that a more directive structure is useful to clients, if it leads to a sense of safety and containment. A non-directive approach can be experienced as empowering in being able to initiate and 'do your own thing.'
>
> (Dokter, Chapter 11, p. 222)

Guarnieri and Ramsden, in Chapter 8, propose the value of both non-directive and directive processes and relationship:

> This open, non-directive discussion, acts both as a grounding and a risk assessment, where we aim to identify both individual needs and group themes, expressed verbally and non-verbally. We are also noting the shape of the group, the needs of our support facilitators, and thinking of creative ideas based on the individual patient's narratives at this time. We aim to gain a sense of the individuals' process, psychologically and emotionally, at this point in the group's life. We can then respond spontaneously, attempting to meet the needs being presented in the here and now of each workshop session.
>
> (Guarnieri and Ramsden, Chapter 8, pp. 159–160)

Here the therapists create dialogue with psychodynamic ideas, and notions of non-directive approaches and relationship, but, as the detailed description and analysis in Chapter 8 shows, focus upon the needs of the clients they are working with, rather than adhering strictly to theory driven inflexible positions and create a dialogue with aspects of both.

The context of practice can also be a key determinant in the way such dialogues occur. Hence, a dramatherapist working in a family therapy setting will naturally develop a practice that, in both theory and activity, reflects a dialogue with the context they are working with and with the field of family therapy. They will combine *dialogue* with the *unique qualities* that they see dramatherapy as offering to the client. Examples of this dialogue can be seen in Chapter 13. A dramatherapist working in a forensic setting will, similarly, develop a relationship in their theoretical approaches and in the methods they use with the forensic setting, with the ideas and practices of forensic psychotherapy: again a combination of *dialogue* between other practices and ideas and the *unique voice* of dramatherapy. Examples of this dialogue can be seen in Chapter 8.

This kind of process is necessary for the client and for the healthy functioning of the therapist: a creative, diverse response. The effectively functioning dramatherapist holds many things in their creative encounter with clients. An essential 'holding' is their capacity to take their thinking and practice forward in dialogue with what the body of dramatherapy literature and experience has taught them – but, chiefly and importantly, to also stay fresh and alert to the evolving, new and unique situational encounter with their clients and colleagues in their setting. The practice within this book is rich in both aspects of this holding. The chapters will each demonstrate the individuality of the therapist's lively and creative encounter, whilst dialoguing with the body of knowledge within the field of dramatherapy.

The dramatherapy space

In clinical work the dramatherapy space is created by a number of different factors. These include the ways in which the therapy space is framed by the approach taken to change, the ways boundaries are created, the way the client arrives at the space through referral and the way the space is created in relation to the setting it is within. In addition, the space is created in relation to the rest of the client's life. It is not as if the dramatherapy space is something that is apart: it is different but related.

Meyer, for example, in Chapter 7, illustrates the way such an arena is created, showing how the space is not a fixed phenomenon but is reactive, with a dynamic relationship to the issues clients face in their lives:

> A therapeutic frame was clearly formulated with contract, time, space and group aims; however, this was a fragile group. This fragility manifested in illness, irregular attendance, ambivalence about the group, connection with each other and disconnection; speaking and silence; disruption and interruption.
>
> (Meyer, Chapter 7, p. 139)

The space is made by the therapist and client together. The therapist might bring their expertise and creativity in how to handle the creation of the space through the setting of boundaries, the ways they offer relationship and activities. The client brings themselves, their lives, their creativity and the complexity of the issues they need to work with. The dramatherapy space bears a symbolic relationship to many encounters within the lives of both parties. Therapist and client bring all this, and together make the dramatherapy space with it.

Conclusion

This chapter has reviewed the emergence of dramatherapy as a clinical practice. It has shown the different ways in which practice occurs, and the processes which support and develop clinical work. In particular, it has introduced the nature of practitioner research and the ways in which dramatherapists are discovering the impact of dramatherapy within many settings, in dialogue with different client groups and within different needs and frameworks for change. Mitchell has written of the need within the field of dramatherapy for 'forms of research' to be published which are rooted in 'practical studies which take place in the clinic, the studio, the community, the prison: work which grows from practice and the face-to-face encounter with clients' (Mitchell 1996: x). Part 2 of this book consists of such research: as this chapter has shown, it relates to the tradition of practitioner research. As Robson defines this area of enquiry, the role is crucial to the development of knowledge about efficacy and impact:

> The practitioner researcher is someone who holds down a job in a particular area and at the same time carries out systematic enquiry which is of relevance to the job. In education, this might be a teacher carrying out a study of a way of helping an individual child with a learning difficulty; or a project on delivering some aspect of the curriculum to a school class . . . corresponding foci of enquiry from individual to group . . . are not difficult to envisage for practitioners in other professions.
>
> (Robson 2002: 446)

Robson adds that such research has the advantage that it is located within a strong experience base: its concerns and findings are usually firmly located in the needs and concerns of professional practice. This is due to the research's origins and rationale being based in actual encounters which the practitioner has experienced within a field. In addition, his review of practitioner research concludes that the insights gathered from the practitioner's previous knowledge base and experience deepens the analysis of the findings. As the chapters in Part 2 reveal, these benefits of practitioner research are shown within the research being firmly linked to clinical needs, and to the rigour and richness brought by the experienced practitioners to their analysis.

2 The social and political contexts of dramatherapy

Phil Jones

Introduction: perspectives and contexts

This chapter will examine political and social issues concerning dramatherapy practice. It will consider the broader political context of factors such as poverty, inequality and the social divisions of society and how they relate to clients' and therapists' experiences of dramatherapy.

Within the research into practice within this book issues including mental health, disability and the experience of being a refugee, for example, will not merely be looked at in terms of clinical diagnosis, nor solely in terms of the ways clients 'present' in the therapy space. They will be contextualised within a wider framework. The different chapters will encourage the development of an understanding of the many ways in which factors, such as poverty, inequality and the system of health provision relate to what occurs in the therapy room. They will explore how dramatherapy relates to issues, including social justice, empowerment and a rights-based perspective on therapy. Other areas will include the ways in which the politics of health care provision impact on how the dramatherapy is offered to clients. This chapter will also feature references to examples within Part 2 of the book, helping readers relate the issues to the clinical practice and the contexts of work elsewhere in the book.

The idea of a political context for dramatherapy

Any act of therapy does not occur within a sealed environment. Boundaries are set to protect the space, but not to seal the therapy off from the world around it. Rather, the various activities and agreements aim to create a safe space within which to provide an alternate, or complementary, space to the one lived in by the clients in their everyday lives.

The ways that the space can be considered in a political context varies. On a macro, or large-scale level the beliefs, opinions and attitudes of national governments and political parties provide a key perspective. These are reflected in the ways in which movements and directions in national perspectives on health care provision are developed. In addition, the relationship between international agencies and bodies are often reflected in the ways national trends develop. The system of health care within which the therapy is primarily offered is part of a political landscape. This is created by policies set by a government and their agencies, such as health services, social or arts service providers, or by non-governmental agencies and client representative groups which are set alongside, or in contrast to, mainstream health services. The actions and attitudes of a government affect areas such as, the nature or extent of services; who can provide them; who can benefit from them; as well as those excluded or not considered within the provision. The ways that the policies and aims of settings that deliver at a micro, or local, level are also affected by such macro-perspectives on health care. Other voices, such as lobbying groups and representatives of user groups can also contribute to this level. Professional associations reflect and have input into the development of provision, and the ways in which policies that govern practitioners are interpreted, through the development of guidelines for practice. Issues, such as the relationship between different care or social services, or the ways in which priorities are given to certain kinds of approach, or the ways in which practice is evaluated or seen to be effective, also relate to these matters. This book will show how such forces relate to the direct work with clients. Much clinical description in the literature omits this area: different chapters will show how it is important to view clinical work from this perspective in order to create a fuller picture of how, and why, clinical work is provided. The next section illustrates why this angle on practice is important to consider in relation to clients' experiences of therapy.

The politics of provision: visible and invisible

Moss refers to disability activist and researcher Oliver's work on the relationship between attitudes towards disability and service provision: 'the patronising or hostile treatment of disabled people in society comes from deeply embedded ideologies . . . that disability is a personal tragedy and that individuals are afflicted by disabilities. In this way society denies responsibility for the conditions in which disabled people live. Disabled children have been historically segregated and isolated in separate schools and institutions' (Moss 2007: 47). She quotes Oliver's connection of attitude, political decision making and access to services:

> Not only do these definitions medicalise and individualise the problems of disability but they do the same to the solutions (policies) that are applied. Thus services too are based on individualised and medicalised views of disability and are designed by able-bodied people through a process over which disabled people have had little or no control.
> (Oliver 1990: 6 in Jones, Moss, Tomlinson and Welch 2007: 47)

Chapters 4 and 10, show the ways in which some sections of the population are 'seen' by policies and service provision, whilst others might be omitted or 'unseen,' or that the way they are seen is distorted due to the kinds of framing described by Moss and Oliver. Novy, for example, talks about therapy services being 'gender blind', whilst Meyer shows how children with HIV are silenced and unseen by policy and provision. These omissions, or distortions, are political in nature as they are reflected in the priorities set by national bodies, and reflect broad prejudices or tensions within society. Hence, one form of therapy might be prioritised over another or fashions in ways of accessing, assessing or evaluating work might be enforced through funding or policy making. Some client populations, more than others, have tended to be prioritised, or neglected, as a result of such national policies. Within a field such as dramatherapy, issues in the nature or availability of the discipline reflect political pressures from funding bodies and policies. Some kinds of approach, for example, might be deemed to be more likely to receive support within a service provider, or certain kinds of client might be seen to be more politically preferable for therapeutic attention, than others, as Chapter 10 discusses. The priorities and initiatives of national policies tend not to be couched in these terms, but a number of commentators have analysed the way provision is governed to show such an effect. The relationship between centrally funded provision and the availability of practice reflects this. The availability of therapy services within schools is clearly a matter of policy, funding priorities and political decision-making. So, for example, because children and young people in schools have less political power than other adult groups in society, some have argued that their emotional health needs, in the form of adequate support through therapy in schools, is often neglected by funding priorities being placed elsewhere (Kay, Tisdall, Davis, Hill and Prout 2006).

The politics of the client and the therapist

The position of the client is also a key area to be considered within a political framework. As will be discussed later, the macro forces of poverty, social exclusion and the social divisions of society are seen by some to be key issues in therapy. These concern the ways these forces relate to how clients see themselves, their experience of their lives and their relationship to the family, community and society they are within. Hence, prejudice may be a key reason why a client comes to therapy, or poverty may be a key force affecting a client's experience of their lives. Kay *et al.* (2006) refer to social exclusion relating to a variety of factors. It is seen as a process involving exclusion through poverty, oppression by majority groupings and discrimination: 'often crucially affected by membership of a particular status group based on personal characteristics, including gender, disability, ethnicity, age or appearance . . . These forms of differentiation are generally the product of informal, though powerful processes, but may be embodied in the law' (Kay *et al.* 2006: 3). White (1999) has described social exclusion in relation to different kinds of process affecting European ethnic minorities in a way that can be seen to be relevant to many other groupings within society:

- Exclusion though legal mechanisms: for example through the granting or denial of citizenship and political rights such as the right to vote, and access to certain kinds of employment – such as the civil service.
- Exclusion through the ideologies of 'othering' – the majority culture denies the rights of minority groups to access services and provision in ways that suit their needs or requirement – imposing those dictated by the majority's 'norms' and values.
- Exclusion through poverty and economic marginalisation – where patterns of economic disadvantage and exclusion occur.

(White 1999)

These processes are relevant to the way client and therapist work together. For example, the space and relationship between the client, the group and the therapist can be seen within this political framework. On one level, the boundaries and guidelines set within dramatherapy reflect the macro-levels of the society within which the group occurs, as discussed earlier in this chapter. They will, for example, reflect the global aims of a national service provider, the aims of the setting in the way they formulate client objectives and goals, as discussed in Chapters 5 and 9. Similarly, building on earlier points, the type of therapy offered and the people it can be offered to will be a reflection of the priorities of national and local services, as discussed in Chapters 4 and 7. The chapters will review, for example, how dramatherapy is offered in the light of White's comments about the majority culture denying minority groups, 'access to services and provision in ways that suit their needs or requirement – imposing those dictated by the majority's "norms" and values'.

The reasons people come to therapy and the response they are met with, vary according to the political, cultural and social context of the client's life and the systems of health care. This means that the client's understanding of what has happened to them, or their lack of well-being or health, vary within different cultural contexts. Similarly, the assumptions of health and ill health within health care systems within which they live vary. In addition, the act of seeking help, growth or change also varies. So, for example, a client who, within western systems, would be described as experiencing mental health problems might be seen differently within other cultural frameworks. The idea of tensions, or differences, within the issue of seeking help can also be experienced within the same cultural group or society. Diversity in attitude might be due to social divisions such as race, culture, gender, age or class. As Milioni states, the dramatherapist needs to be alert to such complex dynamics, by being aware of 'the meanings that people give to their experiences of living [that] are constitutive of their lives, as are the practices of self and practices of relationship that are associated with these meanings' (Milioni 2001: 14).

The literature often represents, and views, the client's reasons for coming to therapy as primarily within the discourse of a 'personal' realm: as if their need for therapy is solely to do with 'personal' problems, or that the way the need is seen is only to do with their intrapsychic experiences. Samuels argues that a review of the literature shows that the 'discourse' of therapy tends to speak as if it occurs in a social and political vacuum (Samuels 2006). Totton adds to this by observing that:

> If the client brings material from wider social and political situations the therapist might speak in such a way as to strip the material of this context – to reinterpret it as purely personal and autobiographical in meaning . . . although this kind of response can, on occasion, be bracing or even liberating . . . there is something rather mad, or at least dissoci- ated about its habitual use . . . it privileges one or two very specific frames (of which the therapist happens to be expert): that of the nuclear family, and that of individual agency. Like several other therapeutic strategies, it wrong foots and disempowers the client seemingly implying that political engagement itself is intrinsically mad, a misunderstanding of what, in the therapeutic context, matters.
>
> (2008: 146)

Another way of looking at this sees perspectives based on the nuclear family and intrapsychic approaches as an important part of the way a client can look at their experiences. However, it argues that it is crucial to look at, and engage with, a wider framework when understanding the client's need for therapy, and in exploring and resolving the issues the client brings. This sees it as vital for the therapist and client to look at the ways in which social and political factors may relate to the client's experiences. This looks at presenting problems, or needs, in terms of factors such as social exclusion, prejudice and the lived context of the client. Hence, a client's depression may in part be seen as a result of intrapsychic factors, or the immediate family context – but it might also be due to the ways in which they are treated within society or to the impact of issues concerning social exclusion. The literature argues that a richer engagement with the client's experiences can be reached if such factors are engaged with in the therapy. Therapists often ignore this, however. They are happy to ask questions about family dynamics, or intrapsychic factors, but often, because of training or the traditions they draw on in their work, choose not to ask questions about social or political factors. This could be seen to be a collusion with forces that work to oppress, marginalise and silence clients about their lives, or aspects of their lives.

One of the impacts of this way of approaching the act of therapy sees it as important within referral or in the assessment period to include socio- political issues as a focus. This might result in the setting or therapist deciding with the client, or clients, that a group that creates connection for people who are experiencing themselves and the society around them in similar ways.

Examples of this political stance can be found in Chapters 4, 7 and 10. The focus becomes not only on the individual's psyche but on connecting with others in similar situations in order to explore the forces at work in relation to themselves and each other. As Chapter 7 discusses, this can be seen to ally the act of therapy with a process of empowerment, connecting the individual's experiences with the potentials for growth and action in a group context. It also can result in the interconnection between therapeutic work, political awareness and the opportunities not only for individual actions for personal well-being, but also to share that with others as a political act as growth and for possible action together in challenging the forces and structures that oppress.

Within this approach it is clearly important that the politics of the therapist are not forced, projected onto or acted out by the therapist on the client. However, it is important to remember that the action of not looking at or acknowledging such forces is not neutral. If the therapist does not include these within the therapeutic space and exploration then this is as much a choice in the same way that it is a choice to include questions or suggestions about connecting the impact of the family upon the client's life. So, for example, a client might not introduce their father or mother into the therapeutic space. Many therapists would consider it appropriate to ask questions about the client's family members. However, in the same way, why should the therapist not ask about social and political forces such as the client's experience of social exclusion through or prejudice in relation to their experiences of gender? Neither is neutral, both are acts. If the therapist does not ask about a client's family context or dynamics, it could be argued that this might reflect a blind spot, or countertransference on the therapist's part. In a similar fashion, it could be argued that not paying attention to or asking about, socio-political issues affecting a client's life is a similar act of countertransference. It could, for example, be made to argue that such silence on the therapist's behalf is a colluding with a society that scapegoats people with the particular issues the client is encountering. By not asking, or exploring, such issues, it could be argued that the therapist is colluding with the silencing of this individual. This is done by making them feel as if they, individually, are 'to blame' for their feelings or issues, rather than seeing a part of the reason they are coming to therapy as rooted in society's attitudes and treatment: this is the unacknowledged elephant in the room. Totton summarises the importance of acknowledging these areas by identifying three frameworks:

> Firstly that therapy. . .[is]. . .tied firmly to the social and political context in which the therapy takes place; secondly that therapists and counsellors exercise political agency in their work, whether or not they are aware of it; and thirdly that, conscious or unconscious support from the therapist for mainstream cultural positions – at the expense of the positions of the client – can be both damaging and wounding.
>
> (Totton 2008: 145)

Such a position argues that because the therapist is, unconsciously, colluding with social attitudes, they may consider it inappropriate to engage with these areas as a therapist. In addition, it argues that therapists may not engage with these areas because they feel they do not know how to work with the client in this way. Within this book, the practice and research described reflects the variety and richness of how such issues are engaged with by dramatherapists and clients alike. The following material looks at the variety of ways in which these complex dynamics and issues can be engaged with by therapist and clients. There is not one answer to responding to the issues raised in the previous sections. However, the section will point to the chapters in Part 2 of the book to help contextualise the tensions and issues identified earlier in this chapter, to offer practical examples and to draw on research to gain insight into them. The aim is to assist dramatherapists to reflect upon, and gain insight into, their own work.

Opening understanding: examples of engaging with social and political contexts

The following examples are illustrations from the work within this book. They are offered as a way of developing insight into the different aspects of the approach to 'richness' discussed in the previous section.

Issues concerning the cultural background, class and gender factors that might influence client and therapist perception of the arts therapies groups are included within Dokter's chapter. Here, for example, she situates her practice in relation to the impact of cultural diversity. This includes the relationship between the urban and countryside catchment of the client and staff population. The monitoring and analysis within her research into practice looks at areas such as religious identity, socio-economic status and class. In her chapter the ways in which identity, experience and issues concerning social divisions of society – for both clients and staff – are examined in relation to their presence within the work. In her consideration of one of the client experiences, for example, we can see how this perspective is brought to the therapeutic encounter, broadening beyond a psychodynamic framework:

> Belle's sense of alienation and distrust can be psychodynamically explained by past experience, but it is interesting to note that she came from a mixed cultural background which remains unrecognised. She may be more comfortable as the daughter of a first-generation migrant with the first-generation migrant art therapist. A minority religion and lack of identification with one side of her cultural heritage, as a potential alternative to the abusive one, does not seem to have been open to her. Her sense of self-loathing diffusely connects to many factors that can not be causally linked, although culture as a contributing factor to a problematic identity formation could be argued.
>
> (Dokter, Chapter 11, p. 220)

This is an example of the importance to the therapy of this richness, of an awareness of the therapist and client relating to perspectives concerning ethnicity, discrimination, the effect of migration and class on the content and relationships within dramatherapy.

Gardner-Hynd, in Chapter 9, reflects on parallel issues from a particular perspective, looking at the issues of socio-economics, prejudice and ill health in relation to people with learning disabilities in her work:

> Society's view of individuals with learning difficulties can often be unhelpful which further undermines the creativity and independence of these individuals. Mindell, one of the few leading psychotherapists currently addressing social and political issues in their work, describes rank as 'the sum of a person's privileges' (Mindell 1995: 28). In this society very few differences are neutral with respect to power and rank. Gender, sexuality, class, ethnicity, income, age, disability – all carry with them enormous implications for perceived and experienced rank and . . . power. Rank is 'both perceived and experienced . . . the automatic . . . power and authority' that is within the therapeutic relationship, often unconsciously, but reflecting the social divisions and power relationships within society (Totton, 2008: 149–150).
>
> (Gardner-Hynd, Chapter 9, p. 174)

Here Gardner-Hynd brings different kinds of political awareness to her practice. From one angle she sees the issues brought by the clients within a framework of the ways in which prejudice, social exclusion and self-esteem are seen to be interrelated. This helps her as a therapist to achieve an alertness as to how factors within the client's life might relate to the presenting issues. She does not automatically assume that this arena is part of the causation: but her acknowledgement of its potential presence is something that is missing in much clinical discussion in dramatherapy. From another angle, she links the ways in which majority-culture attitudes towards disability can often take the form of negative treatment and views. This is part of the way she views the client's experiences of their own creativity, so this becomes a potential factor to help understand and frame how she works with her clients. It also forms a part of the way she understands the dynamics at work within the group in terms of her position as therapist. Issues concerning power and position to do with social exclusion are seen as part of the dynamics played out, consciously and unconsciously, within the dramatherapy sessions. In this way, part of the therapy comes to include an engagement with the macro forces at work within society, such as prejudice and social exclusion, as experienced in the micro-work within the therapy group. As her chapter shows, this political element and engagement with prejudice, clients' responses to exclusion and silencing become a part of the material within the group. If this kind of awareness were not given attention, the danger would be that key parts of the client's lived experience would not be engaged with in the sessions and would remain unworked with. This might have a counter-productive impact as key dynamics within the presenting issues might go unacknowledged.

In Chapter 8 Guarnieri and Ramsden identify the political tensions within the context their dramatherapy work occurs in and policies that are ambiguous concerning 'punishment' and 'treatment'. They show how such wider political and social issues extend into the therapy room:

> The three high-secure psychiatric hospitals that cover England and Wales are part of the National Health Service (NHS) rather than the prison system (HMP). '. . . prisons are not suitable places to treat people with serious mental disorders . . . we admit those who need in patient treatment to psychiatric units.' (Davison 2004: S19). The term high security relates to risk, perceived and actual, both legal and psychiatric and of harm being enacted by the individual offender towards self and other: 'the nature of the task of the high secure hospitals may be regarded as uniquely challenging. It concerns the confinement of individuals within a social context at once both sceptical about and unrealistic in their expectations of professional abilities to protect the public from harm . . . Their [patients] psychopathologies are such as to render the establishment of therapeutic alliances difficult and painful within the context of little hope of future change.' (Deacon 2004: 93).
>
> (Guarnieri and Ramsden, Chapter 8, p. 156)

Here Guarnieri and Ramsden are acknowledging the important political dimensions at work in relation to the nature of the dramatherapy space. The broader forces that dictate the identity and role of an organisation, or service, are shown here to reflect societal divisions and political tension between punishment, treatment and the act of therapy. This kind of awareness and analysis shows its value within the practice they discuss within their chapter: from the ways clients see themselves and the position of an organisation relating to 'confinement', 'protection' of the 'public' and 'hope of future change'. In a similar way to the framework brought by Gardner-Hynd to her relationships with her clients, Guarnieri and Ramsden show how the awareness of political and cultural attitudes is present within the therapy room and the dramatherapy encounter. As clients and therapists meet, they do so within a complex web of psychodynamic processes, but also processes that relate to the way in which the political and cultural 'work' and goals of the organisation are reflected. Hence, ambivalences about imprisonment and the nature of hope, possibilities of change and the nature of therapy become a part of how dramatherapy is experienced. Again, if this level of political awareness were not brought into the therapy, key forces would remain unacknowledged and would hinder the encounter. As the chapter shows in its work with clients and the focus-group work with staff such analysis is crucial to understanding the nature of the act of dramatherapy.

Meyer, in Chapter 7, also shows the importance of situating her work within a series of political and cultural forces. She comments on shifts and dynamics of national policies concerning health, children and HIV/Aids:

> According to the Department of Health (NSP 2007) South Africa has approximately seven million people in a population of 46 million who are HIV positive. Two million of these are said to be children and adolescents. However, South African social scientists are still struggling to accurately estimate the extent of the impact on children in the country (Higson-Smith *et al.* 2006). Gender also plays a role with women and girls being the most disproportionately affected: 55 per cent of HIV infected people (NSP 2007). In general much has been done since 1994 to address, at a policy level, the needs of children and young people in South Africa (Barbarin and Richter 2001). As with other HIV policies put into place, those concerning the policies around children have also not proven easy to implement.
>
> (Meyer, Chapter 7, p. 129)

Here the basic presence of any support for children is linked to broader forces that deny the existence of the disease, that make decisions that they are not a priority for treatment and therefore of therapy. She draws a framework that connects provision with forces such as medical treatment and government policy, poverty, denial, funding priorities and the exclusion of children. Her description and analysis of her work in Chapter 7 illustrates the necessity for the dramatherapist to situate their engagement with the ways the clients relate to the dramatherapy space within an understanding of such complex political and cultural forces.

In the Narratives of Change project described in Chapter 4, Novy considers the political dynamics of her work with women in conflict with the law in relation to inequalities such as the 'gender-blind treatment of women in prisons and within the criminal justice system'. This analysis looks at a variety of contributing factors:

> mental health systems continue to emphasise bio-medical over social factors in women's lives, and there seems to be little understanding of the context in which many women are criminalised (Pollock 2008). One of the purposes of the Narratives of Change project was to challenge the belief that the difficulties in the participants' lives were a reflection of their identities (White 2007). A cornerstone assumption in narrative therapy is that people are not their problems.
>
> (Novy, Chapter 4, p. 69)

Here Novy's understandings of her clients' situations involve a critical awareness of the ways in which divisions and inequality within society impact on the lives of her clients and upon their treatment within their country's services. Here, the consequences of a system that sees the women's situation primarily within a framework of criminalisation and the medical model are positioned by Novy as a contributing factor to the issues the women bring to work with in her groups. The therapeutic space becomes one where they can explore and develop their responses to the kinds of treatment and inequalities that have had a negative effect on their lives.

Dramatherapy, here, becomes a place to explore the political and social consequences of such experiences and to redress disempowerment and the exclusion of the voices and lives of women:

> Before I would always defer to others. I defined myself in relation to others. Now I have begun to define who I am myself. In short, I've taken a big step forward.
>
> (Carole in Novy, Chapter 4, p. 78)

This work approaches the potentials of dramatherapy to create different narratives for the women. As the chapter indicates this has a direct effect on the ways women experience themselves in relation to such silencing. It assists them in developing a new position on their identity, and this is directly taken into their lives outside the dramatherapy.

Sajnani's work in Chapter 10, 'Mind the gap: facilitating transformative witnessing amongst audiences', echoes this framework in a parallel way: identifying the social and political forces that impact on the women's experience of dramatherapy, by facilitating what she calls 'transformative witnessing'.

> In the project presented in this chapter, women who had recently migrated, by force or by choice, to Montreal lived with inconsistent access to health care and education as a result of their precarious legal status . . . This reality coupled with the racism, classism and sexism they would face outside their homes rendered them increasingly vulnerable to violence within their homes. Fundamentally, people continue to need reminders that they can effect change, have opportunities to debate and realise differing visions of change, and to see themselves as complicit in the struggles and victories of one another.
>
> (Sajnani, Chapter 10, p. 193)

Here the complexities of racism and discrimination faced by migrants are acknowledged, the impact on access to health systems and the interrelationship between the oppression they face in the community and in their home circle. The framework for the therapy the women undertake with Sajnani does not turn these into phenomena seen through a solely psychodynamic or intrapsychic lens, but allows a broader framework. In this way the women can work with aspects of their lives and address the forces that affect them. The following gives a sense of the ways in which they located their approach to this within their work:

> Immigrant women of colour also experience a lower social and economic status. Isolated and excluded through all these forms of structural violence and a lack of language skills in both English and/or French (in Quebec), the immigrant woman of colour is in a condition of higher risk of intimate forms of violence. In accordance with Razack (2008), these areas of exclusion and violence are the daily lived experience for these women of interlocking of racism, classism, and sexism . . . Another aspect of our approach was to stress the resilience and resistance of immigrant women of colour in the face of violence. Drawing on the work of Traci West (1999) we supported participants in the trainings to name the ways they survived and resisted violence, and in what ways their differing faith traditions had provided them with comfort if any, despite the suffering caused by forced migration and ongoing exclusion in Canada.
>
> (Sajnani, Chapter 10, pp. 199–200)

Vaughan, in Chapter 13, illustrates how a political perspective relates to the nine years' therapy programme in her account of work with Ruth:

> since the Children's Act (1989) it has been harder for local authorities to remove children and the tendency has been for children to be left for longer periods of time in neglectful and abusive families. It is sadly not unusual today for Family Futures to see children who were left for more than four years in neglectful and abusive situations. There is a belief around in the court system that children fare better if maintained in their birth families and lots of local authorities sadly still seem to be working on this principle. The consequence of this is that children are left in horrific situations for longer than they need to be and the cost to the child and society as a whole is huge as it is these children who without help end up populating our prisons and psychiatric hospitals. Ruth was at risk of being one such statistic.
>
> (Vaughan, Chapter 13, p. 249)

Here Vaughan indicates the ways in which government policies relate to her work with children. Hence, the experiences of social services, the justice system and the nature of interventions help Vaughan understand the position of her practice and to see how Ruth is presenting her past in relation to the therapeutic encounter.

Haste and McKenna also look at this perspective in relation to the different understandings present within a service provider:

> . . . the failure within the health setting of current practice and measures

of outcome to allow for this crucial stage in adjusting to physical disability. The medical model of care, which has characterised the health service for most of its existence, has viewed health mechanistically as a lack of physical infirmity . . . Unlike the social model of disability, which argues that it is society's social and physical constructs that disable individuals, the medical model focuses on the physical and neglects to acknowledge the part our emotional life plays in our well-being and quality of life. . . .

(Haste and McKenna, Chapter 5, p. 85)

In practice, there still remains the problem of how to redress the balance and nurture psychosocial well-being within the health care setting. This study reflected one attempt to consider the beneficial effects of dramatherapy within the traditional medical model within a regional neuro-rehabilitation unit.

In the examples analysed in this chapter the emphasis is upon the importance of the therapist not choosing to be blind to the social and political context of the lived experience of the client, nor to the way it is left out of the therapeutic space and relationship. The examples demonstrate the richness and crucial nature of this perspective, and offer an answer to the critique initially posed at the start of the chapter. The chapter shows how vital it is to engage with dramatherapy in a way that includes rather than excludes, and that recognises the bias that is present in much therapy which excludes the broader political issues that are very much present within the therapy room as well as in the streets and communities outside.

Conclusion

This chapter is not about proscription, it is about emphasising the importance of sensitivity and alertness to the broad range of perspectives possible within the room, and points to the variety of ways the therapist and client together can be actor or actress, director, witness and creative critic. All are crucial to successful therapy – there is not one answer to the interaction between the different roles and perspectives, but this framework is vital to alive, active engagement with the client and their lived situation. The danger is that elements are silenced within the therapy space. Haugh and Paul have described the changing attitude within training and practice:

Traditionally issues of diversity, power and anti-oppressive practice were not considered central to practice. At the very best, they were thought of as something that needed to be considered in addition to theory and practice training rather than being seen as pivotal to the counselling relationship. In the last five to ten years we are happy to note that this omission is being addressed. At least to some extent. Ironically, in our experience this has led some to assert, for example, that they do not physically see a person's colour/sex/physical abilities/age. In this example we have used physically obvious aspects of a person. This dynamic can also happen for those aspects of a person's lived experience that may not be so immediately obvious, such as ethnicity, sexuality or class. We believe that approaches to practice which ignore such dimensions are limited and counterproductive, adding to a person's [the client's] distress.

(Haugh and Paul 2008: 5)

The chapters in Part 2 of this book echo this position, and add to the idea that an acknowledgement of such areas are crucial to the richness and potency of the dramatherapy encounter.

3 The theory within the practice: dialogues with key theorists

Dialogues with Sue Jennings,
Robert Landy, Dorothy Langley,
Adam Blatner, David Read Johnson
and Helen Payne

Introduction

This chapter involves dialogues with key theorists whose work has influenced the discussion of theory and practice in *Drama as Therapy* Volumes 1 and 2. It aims to provide reflections on the relationships between different areas of theory. The authors are individuals whose work has influenced many, but in a way they are a personal choice for me in that their writing has played an especially important part in my own work. In a sense this reflects the ways in which dramatherapists make their own choices about theorists and theory which connects with their own developing practice. Authors exchanged samples of their writing with me, and discussed the relationship between their chosen extracts and the ideas in *Drama as Therapy*. Short excerpts are contained within this chapter, either when authors quote them, or in boxed extracts. The introduction to each dialogue links the areas that are discussed with the specific pieces of research and practice in Part 2 of this book. Hence, the coverage does not intend to be exhaustive, but represents key areas covered within the theory, research and clinical practice in this book.

Dialogue with Sue Jennings: 'Embodiment, projection, role: broad stages that contain many activities'

The first dialogue concerns the idea of a developmental approach within dramatherapy. This has been succinctly described by Langley as assuming 'a correspondence between what happens in dramatherapy and the way children learn to play . . . developmental psychology emphasises the sequence of the stages people go through during their lifetime. If there is a blockage at one stage, then this can become an issue in that person's life . . . The dramatherapist using this model aims to help the client locate the stage where an issue has arisen and to 'rework it dramatically' (Langley 2006: 26–27). The dialogue reflects on, and critiques, this approach with Sue Jennings who has proposed a much-used framework drawing on developmental ideas. The following dialogue also explores the nature and role of physical embodiment within dramatherapy.

Connections to practice and research in this book

Further discussion of a developmental perspective in dramatherapy or Sue Jennings' work regarding 'embodiment, projection, role' can be found on pages 107, 223 and 272. Other examples of clinical practice relating to embodiment can be found in the following:

- Chapter 6 Chipman: Expanding the frame: self-portrait photography in dramatherapy with a young adult living with cancer (pp. 109–118)
- Chapter 5 Haste and McKenna: Clinical effectiveness of dramatherapy in the recovery from severe neuro-trauma (pp. 88–95)
- Chapter 11 Dokter: Embodying difference – to join or not to join the dance (pp. 210–220).

Jones: One of the ways in which you have framed dramatherapy is through the notion of the processes of embodiment, projection, role (EPR). It has become widely used within the field: how do you view the way it has been engaged with by therapists, in retrospect?

Jennings: I think EPR is a useful developmental model – in broad terms – that is appropriate with all client groups – and it is possible to see when individuals – children and adults – have missed out on one or more stages. I believe it is possible to re-create them through dramatherapy and perhaps allow people to 'catch up'. It is important to note that they are the stages of 'dramatic development' that run in parallel process to other developmental stages (physical, social, emotional, cognitive, symbolic . . .), although dramatic development is of itself, it also makes an impact on the other stages – it is essential to fully function as a mature individual that the EPR stages have been navigated appropriately.

Jones: In the core processes I talk about embodiment not in a developmental way, but in terms of its functions within different aspects of drama in dramatherapy. Examples of this include clients developing the potentials of their own body, the benefits to clients of transforming their body to take on a different identity or role and work that explores the personal, social and political forces and influences that affect the body: dramatherapy offers the opportunity to explore areas such as body image or emotional traumas related to the body. How do you respond to these ideas about embodiment in dramatherapy and how do you relate your conceptualisation of embodiment in EPR in relation to them?

Jennings: I think in my writing I have inferred more the developmental approach, as you say, without intending it; what I become more

---

Box 3.1 **Excerpt: Sue Jennings: embodiment, projection, role**

Embodiment – Projection – Role are the markers of life changes that are ritualised through playing and drama from one stage to the next.

During the E (Embodiment) stage we can see how the child's early experiences are physicalised and are mainly expressed through bodily movement and the senses. These physical experiences are essential for the development of the 'body-self': we cannot have a body image until we have a body-self. . . . The changeover from the E stage to the P (Projection) stage is a time of transition, which is also a marker where Winnicott (1971) describes the 'transitional object' . . . During the P stage the child is responding to the world beyond the body, to things outside the body. . . . As the P stage develops children not only relate to different objects and substance, they also place them together in shapes and constellations. . . . Eventually the child starts to take on the roles, sometimes several in a scene, and we can observe the emergence of the R (Role) stage . . . It is as if the child has fully integrated E P and R as they create plays with movement, costumes and props and various characters. Usually the three stages of E and P and R are completed by the age of 7 years. However it does not stop there. We continue to visit these stages in pre-teen and teenage development, not always in the EPR sequence. Nevertheless they are experimented with, tried and tested as identity continues to develop. Finally we make choices as adults based on the stage that we have dominance in, and usually take up jobs and hobbies that have either an E or P or R focus.

(Jennings 2010)

---

and more aware of is what I term 'the unlived body'; that people with eating disorders do not 'live' in their own body (which poses the interesting question of whose body *do* they live in). One of my supervisors talks about how some people did not 'live behind their eyes'; this is extremely interesting as a physical experience and I have experimented with it when I am distracted – it is almost as if some people live with permanent distraction which is communicated physically. This I think links up clearly with one of your definitions of the core process of embodiment:

> The first area involves clients in developing the potential of their own body. Here the body is focused upon in terms of dramatic skill. Dramatic work focuses upon aiding the client to inhabit or use their body more effectively. This might, for

example, concern communicating with others more effi-
ciently. This is related to the area described by Jennings concerning people who have difficulty in using their bodies in
positive, effective and creative ways.

(Jones 2007: 27)

Jones: I think that sometimes people seem to use your EPR in the literature purely or mainly as a developmental framework. As you
commented, I don't think you intended it *only* in that way at all
– though, clearly, your concepts draw from a developmental
approach?

Jennings: These are broad stages that contain many activities – I do wonder
whether I should differentiate more in the projective stage, for
example, between construction play (with bricks or puzzles) and
drawing and painting; but they are all form-making activities.
Each stage has a transition that I have noticed more and more:
at one time I thought for the infant the transition was literally
Winnicott's 'object' – however that is one thing that in a sense
conceptualises EP and R – i.e. – it is sensory and 'out there' and
has a role function of being 'the other'; however I have also been
looking at other transitionary material: for example a lot of sensory play (although it also occurs very early) comes shortly around
1–18 months: messy play and finger painting – I always put it
under projection but it is also under embodiment because of the
very physicality of it. There is also a transition between projection
and role stages – as the projective play becomes more and more
'dramatic in nature'; the stories are told/recounted as dramas;
the dolls house of the puppets become characters in the dramas
too – and often the child/adult is very involved with the roles that
the characters take on. I have also been spending more time on
looking at attachment and the very early child development – last
three months of pregnancy and first six months of living – and
noticed how sensory play and dramatic play are crucial: attachment is creative and playful and the dramatic play seems an essential process here (I am sure you know that babies start to imitate
their mothers' expressions within hours of birth and imitation is
an act of drama). My notion of neuro-dramatic play encapsulates
almost a miniature EPR that happen with babies in these early
months pre/post birth.

Jones: Can you say a little more about your concept of neuro-dramatic
play – is this concept mainly relevant to the 'miniature EPR'
for babies?

Jennings: This has been a whole revelation of wonder for me – realising
how blind I was in not seeing certain things – especially this
early 'imitation' of facial expression within hours of birth – that
although I see 'role' as a developed activity happening much

Box 3.2 **Excerpt: Sue Jennings: neuro-dramatic play**

Most infants pass through the stages of sensory and dramatic play within the family that provides 'good enough' attachment (Bowlby 1969) and parenting. These two playful processes commence during pregnancy and continue in their most intense form until the infant is 6 months old. The dynamic quality of interaction between a mother and a young baby can be predictive of the emotional attachment relationship between them many months later (Trevarthen 2005). Neuro-dramatic play (NDP) is the term given to this play process because it makes an impact on the neural pathways and developing brain of the infant.

(Jennings 2010)

---

later – nevertheless dramatic play is happening from birth – the idea that we are 'born dramatic' goes further than an EPR in miniature – the overwhelming idea that healthy attachment is dramatic in nature – and then much parenting is needed to change away from the functional and incorporate the sensory and symbolic; the ingredients 'sensory play and dramatic play' I see as the core (that word again!) of NDP and healthy attachment. It is also where empathy starts to develop, and one of the concerns now is that we have a generation of teenagers who are unable to empathise with their victims. The very early experience of 'being the other' is what goes on in dramatic play between significant carer and baby. I am really sticking my colours on the mast in saying that humans are based in dramatic exchange – rather than linguistic. I guess any framework – whether EPR or the core processes – is reductive in that it takes lively, varied, wild, unpredictable phenomenon such as emotions, art forms, interactions between people, representations of lived experiences, change (to name a few!!) – and tries to account or help find a way to accurately help see and communicate what is going on. I guess both EPR and core processes at least try to root their ways of accounting to dramatherapy itself? Would you agree? I guess if I think of the ways the core processes talk about dramatic projection, for example, the description is based directly on what occurs in dramatherapy. Your paragraph: 'The third concerns work which explores the personal, social and political forces and influences that affect the body. Here dramatherapy offers the opportunity to explore areas such as body image or emotional traumas related to the body' (Jones 2007: 27) is very important especially in relation to what I term 'body messaging'

– when we receive conflicting messages about our bodies about what is appropriate or not – the personal, social and political and the 'distorted social' (sexual or physical abuse) and political (rituals of violence); somewhere in our body intelligence is a message that knows certain activities are inappropriate, but unfortunately 'brain washing' from someone more powerful than ourselves can override what we know. The impact of trauma/abuse on the body is extraordinary and so often not addressed in a tranformational way in therapy – especially through 'mere words'.

Jones: Absolutely – and I feel that so often accounts of practice are still over-influenced by Freudian notions of what 'matters' within therapy, focusing almost exclusively on the family within the encounter. Dramatherapy can explore the much wider influences present within the material brought into the room. I feel that there has been a reluctance to do this – to explore the client's relationship to the impact of the social divisions within society – the ways that social exclusion affects their lives, past and present. Comments in the core process try and reflect this, such as:

> By physically participating in a dramatic activity the body and mind are engaged together in discovery. Issues are encountered and realised through physical embodiment – they are made and encountered through the body. In dramatherapy this physicalised knowing and being within a dramatic representation of a problem or issue makes a crucial difference to the verbal recounting or description of a client's material.
>
> (Jones 2007: 27)

This is important to consider within the therapy from a perspective that examines the client's response to the ways society's positions on gender, race and class are 'written on the body' and psyche – to reclaim or respond to those and look at how the client wishes to engage with them. I guess this aspect of looking at practice relates to your input in the field from the perspective of anthropology.

Jennings: To me this sums up a lot of the important core of what we are all trying to do – I like your expression 'physicalised knowing' – and the fact that it has an integrative function; the physical expression can make an impact on the brain itself. Of course 'physicalised knowing' is also crucial in therapy when the body memories stay locked. Unfortunately that potential can also be misused, for example in false memory situations; we have moved a long way with understanding more about emotional intelligence and social intelligence – but have a long way to go to reach bodily intelligence.

Dialogue with Robert Landy: 'Healing occurs through the ability to live within the paradoxical realities of actor/role, world/stage'

The following dialogue concerns the idea of a role orientated approach within dramatherapy. Meldrum has described this framework as based in the assumption 'that the individual's personality is made up of a number of different roles, which he or she plays in different contexts and with various groups . . .' (1994: 75). Landy has talked about this perspective as rooted in an understanding that 'healthy development concerned one's ability to integrate contradictory tendencies, which I conceptuaized as role and counterrole, a dialectical notion' (2008: 3). There is an emphasis upon the relationship between the roles played in life and the encounter with roles within the dramatherapy space. Despite 'the archetypal, dramatic, social and genetic determining factors, human beings are still creators of their own identities, at least in part . . . each act of role taking and role playing is creative in the sense that one is building a piece of one's identity' (2008: 10). This dialogue reflects on and critiques ideas and practice within dramatherapy that are connected to role and to ideas of the client and therapist working with notions of audience and witnessing.

Connections to practice and research in this book

Further discussions drawing on role and witnessing in practice, or Landy's work regarding role can be found on pages 110 and 187. Other examples of clinical practice relating to role and witnessing can be found in the following:

- Chapter 4 Novy: The Narratives of Change project: dramatherapy and women in conflict with the law (pp. 69–82)
- Chapter 8 Guarnieri and Ramsden: Dramatherapy and victim empathy: a workshop approach in a forensic setting (pp. 157–166)
- Chapter 12 Powis: Cinderella – the role fights back (pp. 227–240).

Jones:	You've written much on the nature of role in dramatherapy and the relationship with ideas such as the self. In *Role Theory and the Role Method of Drama Therapy* you critique the concept of self, for example (Landy 2009: 5).
Landy:	What I write in the referenced chapter is: 'I argued that the Self was a problematic, tired term too easily linked to modern, humanistic models and that role theory offered a more post-modern understanding of human existence as multidimensional.' When I wrote about the need to move beyond a notion of Self as a central core construct (Landy 1993), I did so in support of my burgeoning notion of role theory, informed by post-modernist thought and the therapeutic goal of helping people recognise their multiplicity. My intention was to offer a critique of the reigning humanist

and modern perspective held by many in the field of drama therapy.

Jones: I wonder how you view the process I've described as witnessing in relation to this idea that there is no 'observing ego'? I guess I'm wondering also about the work of role, counter role and guide – for example when you talk about the client 'internalising' the guide (Landy 2009: 9) in relation to the idea of witnessing?

Landy: I accept your definition of witnessing as 'the act of being an audience to others and to oneself within dramatherapy' (Jones 2007: 101). I certainly do not deny the existence of a witness or even of an observing ego. Witness is one of the roles within my taxonomy and role profiles assessment. For me, however, the function of witnessing is part of the concept that I call the guide. One function of the guide is to witness the interplay of role and counter role, protagonist and antagonist. The guide is more of a spiritual concept, a figure that holds things together even as it stands outside any dialogue, containing it. The guide as witness is similar to your concept of witnessing. My unique take on this, however, is that the guide is a role in itself, and a property of any one specific role, such as hero, villain and victim. These three and all others can be guides that stand outside an action and hold together contradictory roles.

Box 3.3 **Excerpt: Robert Landy: role, counter role and guide**

In theatrical terms, the role is the protagonist in the client's drama, even though this figure might not yet be aware of the struggles it will undergo in its search for awareness and connection. The counter role (CR) is the figure that lurks on the other side of the role, the antagonist. It is not necessarily the opposite of the role as evil is to good, but rather other sides of the role that may be denied or avoided or ignored in the ongoing attempt to discover effective ways to play a single role. CR is not necessarily a dark or negative figure. If one plays the social role of mother, the CR might be brother or daughter or father. Or it might be something more particular to a client's issues, like helper. The guide is the final part of the role trinity. The guide is a transitional figure that stands between role and CR and is used by either one as a bridge to the other. One primary function of the guide is integration. Another is to help clients find their own way. As such, the guide is a helmsman, pilot and pathfinder; a helper who leads individuals along the paths they need to follow. In its most basic form the guide is the therapist. One comes to therapy because there is no effective guide figure available in one's social or intrapsychic world.

(Landy 2009: 7–8)

So, too, can they witness roles in dialogue as they are being played out. As such, the function of witness serves to contain.

Landy: The simplistic argument of the death of the self is no longer of great interest to me. What is more interesting is speaking about the complexity of existence and the ability of people to discover their complexities and learn to live within their many contradictions. Witnessing is one process that further marks that complexity. I think that both the witness and the guide are in many ways synonymous. When playing witness or guide of oneself, certainly the element of surprise can arise. It is often surprising to view oneself from the outside and to see parts of oneself as if for the first time, especially those aspects that have remained unconscious. The ability to look and see in different ways is the key here. The dream offers images of the unconscious. How does one see what one purposefully consigns to a place of unseeing? One answer is to simultaneously play the dual roles of actor and witness, taking on roles in the dream and witnessing oneself doing so at the same time, aware of the paradox, as much as an actor is on stage. The process is not really sequential – where first George plays the roles and then reflects upon them – but rather a confluent process of living in the paradox of actor and witness. That is the source, I think, of the surprise. Surprise, as an artefact of witnessing, comes also from living in the paradoxical moment of actor, the one who takes on a fictional persona, and role, the fiction that is taken on. This paradoxical moment of surprise and wonder is that which propels human beings

---

Box 3.4 **Excerpt: Robert Landy: George**

George, a visual artist in his late fifties, came to therapy because he felt like a professional failure. I pointed out that failure was more of a quality than a role and helped George discover that the failed role was that of artist. We worked with the artist role through stories and dreamwork and role play. Soon we discovered that it was not the artist part of George that felt like a failure, but its counterpart whom George first named the bank and then the businessman.

In identifying his problematic role as the businessman, George did not appear to be exploring a sub role of the artist but in fact discovering a counter role. When George acknowledged his feelings of incompetence concerning the sale of art, he was able to reclaim the artist on the other side of the businessman and work toward integrating the two with the help of several guide figures whom he identified and named.

(Landy 2009: 22)

to both create and witness theatre, and to experience the healing properties of all dramatic activities.

Jones: You've said that 'aesthetic distance can be seen as closely related to the playspace' (Landy 2009: 16) – can you say why the connection between distance and play and the idea of a 'play space' is important to you as a therapist? I'm also wondering about your response to Vaughan's comments about the play space in our research conversation when she analyses her perceptions of the core processes occurring within her work and says that the play space offers the opportunity to step out of the daily life and try something different with enough distance to allow them to feel safe (Vaughan cited in Jones 2007: 92–93)

Landy: My work, like that of most all drama therapists, is about working within a frame. That frame is an aesthetic one, shared by all creative arts therapists. The distance created by working within the frame is the essential element that marks both the creative process and the healing potential of an applied art from. When you remove the distance, you no longer are within a representational space. Therefore, drama and play lose their essential aesthetic and healing properties. Play and the play space are frames marked by their degree of distance from reality. When very close to reality, they appear to be real, with potential tragic implications. When very far from reality, they appear stylised and comedic, at the extreme bordering on the absurd and farcical. When balanced between the two poles of reality and fantasy, tragedy and comedy, they serve important functions: to please or enlighten an audience, to heal people who are in pain, for example. Vaughan's comment is about working within the balanced place where thought and action are possible, where the reality of a family's history can exist in relationship to its possibilities of future change. When I look at your core processes, I notice that several concern this issue of distance and play, what I have called above the aesthetic frame: dramatic projection, dramatherapeutic empathy and distancing, role playing and personification, witnessing dramatising the body, playing, and especially, life–drama connection. I wonder if you also see that there is an essential concept that links all of these processes?

Jones: Your concept of aesthetic distance was one that deeply influenced my thinking and writing about core processes. You've talked about aesthetic distance as being 'characterised by emotional expression that is clarifying and relieving, rather than obscuring and overwhelming and that invites an engagement of the rational, reflective capacities' (Landy 2001: 58), for example. That connects, for me, with the idea that the basis of dramatherapy is not, nor should be, psychotherapy with enactment, or CBT with role play – but an enabling of the potentials of theatre and drama to heal. The bringing together of the fictive and the real; the creation of helpful perspective and bringing the emotional and the rational into particular kinds of relationship are key to how drama is therapeutic. I suppose one way of looking at the core processes is that they try to say how those qualities can be engaged with by therapist and client together in dramatherapy.

Landy: I agree that the healing occurs through the ability to live within the paradoxical realities of actor/role, world/stage. Non-dramatic forms of healing can also help clients locate a place of aesthetic distance, but only if the therapists accept the notion of a post-Cartesian human being, who, despite many splits, seeks integration in mind and body, affect and spirit. I believe that the best therapists, despite their orientation, attempt to help people discover integrations and do so in whatever ways are required by the clients. I remember, for example, many years ago lying on a psychoanalyst's couch, freely associating. I found myself devoid of words, but instead focusing upon a vase of flowers in front of me, marvelling at the forms and subsequent stories that emerged from my imagination. My analyst was happy to encourage my imaginal experience. Likewise, I think it would be highly useful for those who practice CBT or client-centred therapy to be knowledgeable of the core processes and to have them handy as a guide to understanding the client's process and need for negotiating the fictional and actual realms of existence and seeking the necessary integrations. The concept of role has been most basic to my theory of drama therapy, because it is the one indivisible concept in all forms of theatre – that is, one can remove setting, audience, language, narrative, and many other theatrical devices and still have theatre – as in forms of theatrical venues created by Beckett, Brook and many postmodern theatre and performance artists. But in all forms of theatre, that I am aware of, role persists and defines an event as theatrical. Remove role and there is no theatre. Role in everyday life, based in the theatrical metaphor, doesn't necessarily codify one's way of thinking, feeling or behaving. Rather it points to certain archetypal qualities of role, both in theatre and in everyday life; qualities repeated over time and across cultures. So by saying that role suggests a particular way of thinking, feeling or acting I am saying that any given role is measured against its archetype, but does not necessarily match it. So that when one plays a clown in theatre, there is the suggestion or implication of a standard way of thinking, feeling and acting defined by theatrical tradition, but that any particular clown is nuanced and unique in these attributes. This is also the case in everyday life when one plays a clown in New Guinea or London. Clowning suggests certain behaviours, but these behaviours can be highly nuanced and relative to aspects of personality and culture.

Jones: You ask the question – is there a connection between what an actor does on stage and what a human being does in everyday life (Landy 2006: 5–6)? You discuss metaphor, and move quickly from this to the 'dramatic assessment of behaviour in everyday life' – do you see this as the key role metaphor has to play in dramatherapy?

Landy: I am fascinated with the ways that artists and everyday human beings wrestle with issues of identity. Artists are unique in that they are aware, usually, that their art is representational. Many play on the edge of fiction and reality, putting a frame around, for example, an everyday object, such as a urinal or a can of soup and calling it art. The connection between drama and everyday life is, to my way of thinking, also active in the mind, certainly as represented by the brain. In the discovery of mirror neurons, for example, Gallese and his colleagues have empirically demonstrated a connection between action and observation. Under certain circumstances, when one watches a play and identifies with the pain of a protagonist, the mirror neurons are activated in the same way as when one has a similar experience of that pain in everyday life. As in your core processes of projection, role playing and personification, playing, and life–drama connection, there is a continuity between drama and everyday life, one that shifts according to specific circumstances. As for the metaphor of world as stage, life as drama, person as persona – I find it everywhere I look. What intrigues me are the moments when I observe (witness) people attempting to be real and authentic, only to recognise how very human they really are. I recall my orthodox Jewish grandfather hard at prayer in the morning. When I came into the room as a small child, he would not stop praying but would add to his chant something about remembering to brush my teeth. Goffman says: 'All the world is not, of course, a stage, but . . . crucial ways in which it isn't are not easy to specify' (Goffman 1959: 72).

Dialogue with Dorothy Langley: 'The dramatherapist is actor, audience, director and interpreter'

The following dialogue further concerns the idea of a role-orientated approach within dramatherapy however it looks at the way therapeutic change is seen. Langley proposes that a key aspect of the client's experience of change concerns reflection and discussion. This is seen as a time for clients to 'search for some sort of cognitive order from the experience . . . reflecting on the enaction and the roles. It is in this period of reflection that clients are likely to give expression to the connections they have made between the activity and their personal material' (Langley 2006: 100). Authors such as James (1996) have pointed out that verbal ways of encountering, and accounting for, change are not the sole means of identifying the effects of dramatherapy.

She acknowledges the value of the non-verbal within dramatherapy. James talks of work that 'aims to uncover the value of non-verbal communication through the use of music, movement and touch as integral aspects of the dramatic medium . . . quality of contact can deepen profoundly when making relationships without words, and I have found that there is such a depth of human experience which cannot be spoken. To talk without words involves sensory awareness, emotional literacy and intuition, qualities that have perhaps been devalued in our particularly logocentric culture' (1996: 22–23). This dialogue reflects on, and critiques, ideas and practice within dramatherapy that are connected to how change is perceived and experienced by the client and by the therapist.

Connections to practice and research in this book

Discussion drawing on the nature of reflection and issues concerning the nature of insight and change which Langley talks about can be found on pages 121 and 184. Other examples of clinical practice relating to the act of reflection and the nature of change can be found in the following:

- Chapter 5 Haste and McKenna: Clinical effectiveness of dramatherapy in the recovery from severe neuro-trauma (pp. 89–95)
- Chapter 8 Guarnieri and Ramsden: Dramatherapy and victim empathy: a workshop approach in a forensic setting (pp. 157–166)
- Chapter 9 Gardner-Hynd: Dramatherapy, learning disabilities and acute mental health (pp. 175–185).

Langley: The dramatherapy space assists the development of role and of the client seeing the impact of the drama. This may also happen outside the dramatherapy session. The drama helps clients to see the advantages of change and encourages development. Role in dramatherapy can assist understanding of real-life roles and the two understandings can fuse to enrich real roles. I wonder if this can happen if the client is resistant to change or in denial?

Jones: You put an emphasis here, it seems to me, on 'understanding' – so are you saying here that a client 'sees' something in their own ways of using role within the dramatherapy session, and then this *thinking* is taken by them into their life outside? This 'seeing' you talk about – the client seeing 'the advantages of change' as you put it: what, in your experience, does this involve – is it primarily a cognitive learning, is it an insight which they adopt from the session? Or would you say is it primarily an emotional release or shift in old ways of feeling and being that emerges in the session, and that this changes them in whatever context they are in? Is it a combination or something else entirely?

Langley: I think it is an insight from the session which may or may not

---

Box 3.5 Excerpt: Dorothy Langley: action, reflection and healing

By enacting role . . . clients can experience and reflect on a range of qualities contained in these roles. When a role is understood and appreciated, it is possible to experiment with different ways of performing it in diverse situations . . . Reflection on the various scenarios enacted can help clients to understand their behaviours as it has been revealed by the role play (Langley 2006: 86–87)

De-roling is in some ways the antithesis of warming up – a cooling off from the involvement with dramatic work. It may lead to reflection. When dealing with vulnerable clients it is sometimes better to leave the metaphor un-interpreted and allow the revelations to remain unconscious and clients to assimilate their insight in their own time and at their own pace . . . belief in the advantages of working with metaphor and therapeutic distance is fundamental to dramatherapy, and is in fact the substance of its being . . . Reflection on the dramatherapy experience facilitates healing. It is in this reflective phase that group members consider the relevance of the action they have just experienced to their own lives and understanding.

(Langley 2006: 99–100)

---

become cognitive – for example in work with children it may not do so. If adults can verbalise it I think there is a much stronger possibility that cognitive learning that may come from the experience.

Jones: I'm very interested in what you seem to be saying here about 'insight' that 'may not become cognitive', Dorothy. My own connection with that is the idea of the dramatic body and the non-verbal – that in dramatherapy bodily communication and expression is crucial to much work, that the self can take on a different bodily identity and that this can lead to exploration, perspective even release. However, you seem to be adding to this? Are you saying that insight needn't be cognitive?

Langley: I think the image of self is fashioned by the 'witness' of others and the way we interpret the speech and body language of the 'witness'. This is internalised and becomes part of one's self regardless of the right or wrong of interpretation.

Jones: So are you also implying here that part of what can happen in dramatherapy is that experiences and 'fashioning' of being witnessed in a 'wrong' way can be identified and re-worked in dramatherapy through finding 'right' experiences of witnessing? Also how would you describe this 'right' or 'wrong' witnessing?

Langley: Yes, I think they can. Interpretation is conditioned by what we envisage the witness is implying. If an interpretation is different from what the witness actually intends it to mean I would say it is wrong. This does not mean that the client cannot become aware and work it out in therapy.

Jones: Would you say from this, that, in some cases, part of the role of the dramatherapist is to offer a reparative experience of witnessing to the client, by the therapist behaving as a 'good witness'?

Langley: I am not sure that clients connect somatic roles with embodiment work. They may, for example, find exertion affects breathing and other physical phenomena. I think it is in social roles that they can reach an unconscious transformation through embodiment. This may later be cognitively recognised; for some people, though, I doubt if cognition comes into it.

Jones: I very much like this identification of somatic roles and social roles in terms of reflection – so are you saying that the dramatherapy space can be an arena to explore and experiment with alternative ways of these aspects of being without the strictures of cognition?

Langley: I think this is linked with the first point that there does not *have* to be cognition. I think this is one of the advantages dramatherapy has over verbal therapies. Cognition may not come until there has been time for reflection – not even in the same session – or it may not become apparent to the client at all. Freudians see projection and identification as primarily defensive. I wonder if they can also be used in dramatherapy as a defence in a 'not me' situation. Time is limited within provision such as the National Health Service (NHS), and we often do not see clients long enough to overcome barriers. Is it possible to reinforce defences through drama?

Jones: Two things: I wonder about the role of clinical supervision here – do you think that supervision has a role to be the therapist's and client's audience, as it were, adding an additional reflective space? The other question is: why do you see a dramatherapist's misinterpreting as being such a problem for a client? You talk about the witnessing part of the dramatherapist in terms of audience, director and interpreter. . . . Often when I read interpretations made by some therapists in the literature I feel that they are made by someone who is not a good critic – they seem to offer a meaning that makes sense to the therapist, but not necessarily to the client, for example. There is, I think, naturally a need for therapists to feel that the work has impact and therapeutic efficacy and this can affect what they think they see. I sometimes feel that the therapist needs to be better trained in seeing the 'work' from different angles, developing a better capacity to be a critic drawing on different possible meanings. Do you see a part of the witnessing being allied to the role of theatre critic as well?

Langley: This is a very good point which I had not previously considered. I do agree with you both about the need for the training of dramatherapists and the possibility for the witness. This may take a long time to happen. I ask myself – does it have to be cognitively recognised to have maximum effect? Can it be negative for the therapist or group? I used to work in a unit for offenders with mental health problems and often wondered if re-enactment of crimes, although helpful to the protagonist would give ideas to other group members who were not so mentally aware.

Dialogue with Adam Blatner: 'Only through a mobilisation of viewpoints can people develop a more mature consciousness'

These issues of interpretation, the role of the dramatherapist and witnessing are developed in the following dialogue with Adam Blatner. It starts to look at ideas concerning the nature of narration, the ways in which clients see themselves and the way they experience the narratives of who they were, are and could be within dramatherapy. It looks at what Blatner describes as the different ways of experiencing oneself that the client can encounter in dramatherapy: a 'mobilisation of viewpoints'. Holloway has talked of the importance of particular aspects of this in dramatherapy: the interface between 'self, other and world at large . . . to simultaneously perform, and evaluate the reactions of others; to be actor and critic within the same corporeal and chronological space' (1996: 138). He sees dramatherapy's 'heart' as 'the invitation to become the active agents within our own dramas. . . . This is the aim of my dramatherapy sessions: to provide a process where people can move from a sense of being overwhelmed by external events to opening up new ways of seeing themselves as actors in their own lives' (1996: 139). Blatner parallels this when he defines drama as action, a thing done. He asserts that unlike the 'talking therapies', conflicts and problems can be approached through metaphorical representation. By enacting an unfamiliar role it is possible to experience new ways of being. Exploring a familiar role facilitates the 'discovery of a new perspective on life . . . and this act can change the client by offering new "narratives", new ways of seeing their roles and themselves' (2007: 55)

Connections to practice and research in this book

The discussion of issues Blatner refers to concerning the nature of witnessing, meta-role and change, can be found on pages 190–191 and 257. Other examples of clinical practice relating to narrative approaches to dramatherapy, the experiencing of different aspects of the self and of being witnessed by other group members or the dramatherapist and the nature of change can be found in the following:

- Chapter 4 Novy: The Narratives of Change project: dramatherapy and women in conflict with the law (pp. 69–82)
- Chapter 6 Chipman: Expanding the frame: self-portrait photography in dramatherapy with a young adult living with cancer (pp. 109–118)
- Chapter 10 Sajnani: Mind the gap: facilitating transformative witnessing amongst audiences (pp. 198–205).

Jones: When I originally wrote about witnessing I had in mind the beneficial effects of having an audience. In the new edition one of the therapists talks about this process bringing out other aspects of audience-related phenomena. I'd be interested to hear your response to Stirling Twist's comments about 'presence' and about the negative possibilities of witnessing:

> Being witnessed in unhelpful ways is tantamount to not being witnessed at all I think. If the story has never been told because of a lack of trust in the available audience, or has been told and not heard and reflected back with care, then there is no repair, but maybe there is more hurt. The listener isn't present. And when the listener isn't present the presence of the teller is impaired or even denied.
>
> (Stirling Twist cited in Jones 2007: 107)

Blatner: Yes, this reminds me of the way in psychodrama that a mistaken or intentionally distorted double or auxiliary response may stimulate the client to correct. That draws on an interesting and obvious dynamic – the 'you don't understand!' feeling. But there needs to be an associated sense that such protest will be received well and there will be support. In contexts where one is frequently misinterpreted and there is an obvious bias to any interpretation other than the official therapist's impressions – e.g. the experience of too many patients in psychiatric hospitals – one becomes demoralised and ceases trying to be understood.

Anyway, yes, having someone who listens, re-tell parts, even fragments, can be part of empathy, and as I've written about mutuality, having the freedom to correct someone's responses is also an important opening. Being ignored is one message, but having someone witness you and come to conclusions that don't fit your self-system; being told 'I know what you think' and it really doesn't fit, is even more crazy making. What if the analyst's (or psychiatric aide's or nurse's) 'interpretation' is half-true, but also half-untrue? This is a very common problem interpersonally – having significant others who hold seemingly un-correctable opinions about you. I told clients 'I won't come to any conclusions about you without your permission or agreement.' People often forget their power on others, that their withdrawal may seem to them 'inside' like just giving in to inhibitory tendencies; but that from others' view-points, their withdrawal may seem like a rejection of the others! Only through a mobilisation of viewpoints – there's a phrase – can people develop a more mature consciousness with a wider circle of caring.

Jones: I like that phrase – 'mobilisation of viewpoints' – so is part of what you are saying there that the content of the therapy may be less important than the process? That the dramatic form – for example:

- the capacity or experience of being able to shift viewpoints in a session
- allowing yourself to move from engulfed actor, to witness, to being a director looking at your life
- being able to move outside your own situation to play the role in someone else's drama.

. . . that these might be the key part of the dramatic process in the therapy for the client?

Blatner: Yes, in general – that shifting viewpoints – you say that well. How-ever, phrases like 'the key part' may be presumptuous. There are so many healing elements that I hesitate to say which ones will be 'key' for any given situation, nor do I think that we can know for sure; nor do I think that it is necessary to ascertain what is key! (I'm reminded of how we as older parents of now-teenagers to middle-adults get feedback of what these now articulate younger people remember of parenting – and it's often things we elders have for-gotten, or remembered rather differently! Ha ha!)

Jones: I'd be interested in your thoughts on the life–drama connection. In your discussion of meta-role you talk about the importance not only of the role play itself but the way the client changes their awareness of themselves and the world around them. I wanted to try to articulate the need for the client to be able to make con-nections between the world of the therapy room and the world outside. The temptation for some being the ability to make changes in their therapy work but not to be able to relate that back to their life outside. I guess I'm thinking there of the interconnection between the client's narratives, the narratives presented to them by society outside the group, the roles they create and take in psycho-drama or dramatherapy and their roles outside. What are your thoughts/responses to the notion of a 'life–drama connection' as a key process?

Blatner: Well, I don't expect this to happen automatically. This is con-sidered together with the client:

- So what are we learning here that is relevant to your life?
- What do we need to do to make it more relevant?

Box 3.6 **Excerpt: Adam Blatner: empowerment and meta-role**

Patients or clients are being viewed as needing more 'empowerment' and that includes their role in the process of therapy itself. In psychodrama, for example, I talk to the protagonist as if we are not only going to address and analyse the problem at hand, but equally important, the protagonist is going to learn the ways that we approached the situation so as to be able to implement these skills in addressing future challenges (2007: 9).

In neuroscience, Ramachandran (2004) describes the function in humans of the capacity for not just representation, but 'meta-representation.' In role talk, there are then the two levels: the role, and the broader range of when and how that role may be played. At first, there is little variability; this is what Moreno meant by 'role taking.' A child playing a fireman has a few stock phrases and general actions, based mainly on imitation. This is true also for an adult learning a new role. As the role is learned, one begins to become a bit more flexible and creative, at which point it might better be described as role playing. With more self-awareness, though, one advances to role creating, and more actively using meta-role functions. This might involve the person modifying his or her behaviour in a variety of ways by asking questions such as:

- Which role should be played here?
- How involved do I choose to be in this role?
- How explicitly conscious am I that I am playing this role, or balancing more than one role?
- How am I being perceived in this role? How effective am I in this role?

(Blatner 2007: 7–9)

The theme that Eric Berne (who developed Transactional Analysis in the early 1960s) brings up is making a contract: What is it you'd like to change? How would we know if it were indeed changing? Role training is part of my thinking of how we might use drama in this way: Let's set up a problem in your anticipated future – preferably near future – and explore how else you might respond? Rehearse it until you feel a bit more confident. When you return, we can sharpen up your responses even more. The spirit of spontaneity involves a re-engagement – the 're' is a re-minder of process. This all relates to what you said before about shifting from audience to actor to co-director to other roles:

- in the mirror technique: where a client reviews the scene from a distance
- in the double: allowing another to help you hear what you say, help you listen for what you wouldn't ordinarily admit, and what thoughts come to you but you tend to push away.

Many other psychodramatic techniques place the client in a slightly different frame or viewpoint and this is crucial to the nature of therapeutic change.

Dialogue with David Read Johnson: 'As the therapist and client play, the play is increasingly about what is real, while remaining play'

The dialogue concerns dramatherapy in relation to notions of a 'play space' and ideas about the benefits of the changes this arena can offer. Dintino and Read Johnson have summarised this in relation to a specific way of encountering the space in dramatherapy, as 'developmental transformations'. Here the 'condition of free play' and improvisation is seen as central: the therapist attempts to create and sustain a 'play space' within the session, being an 'imaginal form of interaction in which both clients and therapist understand that what goes on is pretend, and is more than real ... the inner worlds of the clients are revealed, as the therapist non judgementally responds and enters into them' (1997: 206). The following dialogue explores the nature of play, improvisation and the notion of transformation within dramatherapy.

Connections to practice and research in this book

Discusssion relating to issues Read Johnson talks about concerning the nature of play, transformation and the relationship between the play space and living can be found on pages 74 and 230. Other examples of clinical practice relating to playing, developmental transformations, the idea of the dramatherapist as player and the life–drama connection can be found in the following:

- Chapter 10 Sajnani: Mind the gap: facilitating transformative witnessing amongst audiences (pp. 198–205)
- Chapter 13 Vaughan: 'The river of my life – where things can break and things can mend' (pp. 249–256)
- Chapter 14 Madan: Saisir les étoiles (pp. 263–272).

Jones: In your Developmental Transformations (DvT) textbook, you say: the theory needs to be self-negating, in that it needs to act in such a way as to remove itself from the foreground of thought: [therapists] are able to place that theory into the play space as a play object, subject to transformation with everything else.

Do the therapist and the client play with theory together on some level (if everything is in the play space . . .)? If you say 'yes' – how does that happen?

Read Johnson: The fundamental principle is to be able to play with, that is, place into the play space, whatever is on the client's mind. So first this means that if a theoretical idea or concept arises within the therapist's mind, which is not placed into play, the therapist must have tools to allow the thought to form, rest in consciousness, and then pass on. That comes with training and mindfulness. If however, the client brings up, or perhaps senses in the therapist, a conceptual idea (e.g. 'is this my oedipal complex?', 'am I being inauthentic?', 'is this an archetype?', or 'am I unconsciously repeating a trauma schema?'), and these ideas do occasionally arise in clients, then the therapist and client should place these ideas into the play space and play with them (e.g. 'is this my trauma schema?' 'why yes, it appears to be so! And an awfully cute one, I might add.' 'I can't believe this; my uncle always told me I was cute before he abused me.' 'I know . . . (becoming uncle) and are we ready for our bath, sweetheart?'). Whether or not the concepts are clinically true or accurate is in some sense irrelevant to the play. They are not irrelevant to an understanding of the client, but in the embodied encounter of the therapy, their truth value is not relevant. One client asked me, after years, 'okay, so now I want your real inter-pretation.' 'My real interpretation? How can I give you that, you know this is developmental transformations and in our theory we don't give real interpretations.' 'I know, but I'm special, and I want you to give it to me.' 'Okay, here it is . . . (a real interpretation is given) . . . So now you have it.' '. . . I don't believe you, you just made that up!' 'No, really, I gave the real one.' 'I don't like it, whether it's real or not . . . maybe we'd be better off just playing with all this.' 'If you insist!'

Jones: Would you say, then, that the dramatherapy session *is* the play space for client and therapist? You have referred to 'the boundary between the play space and the real world': is there any part of the time and space in dramatherapy that is *not* within this place? Wondering about the relationship you talk about above regarding such a boundary between the client's 'play space' and the 'real world' – whether it is different from the idea of the 'life–drama connection' in the core processes where there's a relationship, but also a

---

Box 3.7 Excerpt: David Read Johnson: developmental transformations and the play space

Developmental Transformations (DvT) is a practice involving the continuous transformation of embodied encounters in the play space. As a practice, it may be applied in a variety of fields, including as a form of psychotherapy, education, acting training, spiritual practice, social change or recreation. It may also be practised without reference to one of these frames (2005: 1).

DvT takes place within the playspace and therefore all participants must enter the play space, including the therapist in psychotherapy. The playspace is a performative space and a dramatic space. The leader/ therapist's job is to engage the interest of the clients in entering the play space, and informing them through example of what the play space is. The primary element to successful practice is the leader's capacity to enter the play space rapidly and deeply, from the beginning of the session. Many times participants will engage in other forms of play that they believe are the play space, but are not, and the therapist must help them discover it. Other participants may know what the playspace is, but have such restricted playspaces that they can barely play. Again the first step is for the therapist to find a way for the client to enter (2005: 15).

(Read Johnson 2005)

---

differentiation between life outside and inside the drama-therapy space?

Read Johnson: Interesting question. In Developmental Transformations, the therapist's job is to engage the client in the play space. If the therapist and client discuss issues outside of the play space, that is fine, and often occurs, but that is not Developmental Transformations.

The implication of the 'life–drama connection (or differ-ence)' is based on the idea that in the drama, we are not playing with what is real. In Developmental Transform-ations, as the therapist and client play, the play is increas-ingly about what is real, while remaining play. Thus, one might have a conversation about an issue, a true issue, of the client, only in a 'play space' mode, that is, with parentheses, or a wink. It is the parentheses that makes all the difference, for it is acknowledgement that each of us are performing our lives, that we are constructing the ideas we hold of the truth, of reality, and this mutual understanding that each of us is constructing our reality, that is the play space, allowing for the tolerance of the other's ideas, for forgiveness of our own biased perspective, for the fact that each of us perceives the world from our own angle. In this way, DvT attempts to place 'reality' within the conditions of the 'play space', which transforms everything. I can have a conversation with you, Phil Jones, about how you feel about being a professor, and this conversation will have a certain quality. We can also have the same conversation, only I introduce it by saying: 'I would now like to ask "Phil the Professor" how he feels about being a professor.... Professor Phil, what do you think....?' This kind of conversation will have an entirely different quality, even if the words spoken are exactly the same.

Applying the conditions of the play space to one's real feelings and views is the same process as 'mindfulness,' as developing a strong 'observing ego,' as achieving an appreciation of 'diversity,' as reaching 'tolerance,' only a bit more fun than these serious sounding goals. In usual interactions, we signal to the other that they should not mess with our 'views' of reality. In the play space, we offer those same views, but signal that the other is free to play with them. It is quite freeing, actually.

Jones: I think the life–drama connection doesn't separate out the experience in the dramatherapy space from that in life outside. It proposes the idea of a connection as crucial – if the life–drama connection isn't there then the client and therapist might create a 'world apart' in the dramatherapy space where change, difference, development may occur but is not reflected or translated into the client's life outside. Now there may be a time where the client needs to create, deliberately or unconsciously, a 'world apart' in the dramatherapy space, but I think it important that therapist and client bear in mind that the relationship between the dramatherapy space and that outside the therapy needs attention. You talk about DvT having 'some relevance' to engaging with relationships in the same paragraph as saying: 'To be able to feel comfortable on the swaying boat in a rough sea, not only to walk on solid ground.' Would you suggest that drama has particular capacities to provide comfort . . .?

Read Johnson: Yes I do. But of course that begs the question of what is comfort. I think that Developmental Transformations in particular, improvisation in general and dramatic playing to some degree can be very helpful in soothing our turbulent souls. Paradoxically its helpful action is not through avoidance of turmoil or conflict, not through a calming salve or positive reassurance, not even through acts of kindness or protection, but by bringing forth the fears attached to the spirit world, the hidden depths, the transcendent desires, and giving form to the ephemeral – really a form of transubstantiation. Through this we gain perspective, tolerance and appreciation for our truly unique situation as human beings. Dramatherapy is a form of desensitisation, a way of understanding and a path for energetic release. The result is often one of greater inner peace, and greater capacity to sustain intimate relations with others.

Jones: In the description of dramatic projection I refer to Ensor's idea of the mask as a hard shell for soft creatures to hide behind and the paradox which Brook speaks of, that the 'mask is the expression of somebody unmasked' (Brook 1988: 219). That discusses mask, specifically, but I like that image very much for some of the work that can happen in dramatherapy: the idea of Ensor's shell has a different relationship to role than to masks for me. At times, I think, the role or persona can play a part in hiding, or providing a shape that the client can experiment 'growing into' – trying on, to see if it could be a possible shape they might want, need or could explore – or it can provide a necessary shield to hide behind or to protect them whilst growth happens. In my experience the client, at certain times, might need to be clear that this is 'not them' and that it is definitely a fictional creation. At others, though, I feel it can be important for the client to live with ambiguity; a lack of clarity about the lines of what is pretend or fictional identity, and what they see or own as themselves – to be unclear (to take some of your terms) and to be involved in possible duplicity, possible ambiguity in a way that doesn't even make clear if what they are doing is ambiguous – because that would, in itself, be too clear! What they are doing, in a sense, shouldn't be 'looked at' by themselves as client or by the therapist. To me that lack of responsibility and ownership, the absence of needing to 'read' what they are doing, or have done, can be a crucial part of how dramatic projection can be effective. I think this may be a different take on what theatre/play lets the audience/actors know, than your comment: 'Theatre, and play, must let the audience know what they are experiencing is not actual, or it cannot be theatre.' Do you agree that this is a different angle on the need for theatre to 'let the audience know what they are experiencing is not actual, or it cannot be theatre' or do you see the process I'm talking about in a different way?

Read Johnson: Well, much here. I am in agreement with all that you say about mask. The mask simultaneously reveals and hides. In the case of a mask made of cardboard or plastic, the client knows that it is a mask. In the case of our everyday social-role behaviours, many times we don't know that these are masks also. That is why we believe our behaviour and our thoughts are real, not theatre. DvT attempts to bring the client to an awareness that these states are masks also, or performances, which frees them to decide whether to keep them going or not. By subjecting the client's social-role behaviour to the conditions of the play space, and through repetition, masks that are no longer needed, that have burdened the client, become experienced as contingent, as chosen, and only then can be taken off. After all, few of our clients tolerate keeping the cardboard mask on for very long ... it is fun for a while but then it becomes restricting and they take them off. Try having your clients keep their masks on for an hour or longer! Our identities are masks that we have not taken off, that we feel we can't take off. DvT, by turning them into theatre, allows the client to 'let them go', especially those that have 'become encrusted' and are no longer necessary. In our sessions, when a client reaches this point and lets go of the habitual behaviour, what emerges from behind it is truly new, young, or as Ensor said, soft. This is our method of journeying to the source by the via negativa that Grotowski called for, of removal. It is a beautiful thing.

Jones: I found the *Being in Proximity* text lovely to read, and moving. I feel hesitant to ask about it, in a way, because it feels as if it should just 'be' there – so you may not want to respond to this one and that's fine. Can you say what you see as deep play here, and how it relates to the image of the intensification of flow? (See Box 3.8 p. 60)

Read Johnson: Form and formlessness, we ride in between these. Forms arise and are the banks of our river; our river is that stream of consciousness, that energetic presence that surges mysteriously through the substance of our bodies. As Buddhist understandings have taught us, it is through the letting go of forms, of embracing absence, that the turbulence of our minds/consciousness is diminished. Thus, as the banks of the river move further apart, the flow of the river slows down: being alone at the shore or at the edge of a meadow or on a mountaintop, the great expanse softens us and we often feel more at peace. The rush and tumble of our daily lives, the many activities, duties, emails and demands, and

---

Box 3.8 **Excerpt: David Read Johnson: being in proximity to the other**

. . . such encounters range in distance from those that allow plenty of room between us for manoeuvring, the encounter being about presentation of our surfaces to each other, to those more personal in which we come in contact with our proximal spaces, that is, the spheres of immediacy that surround us and that define our personal space, in which we interact with most acquaintances. Then, moving further inward, where our proximal spaces overlap with each other, we enter intimate spaces, and then even further . . . territory we know as deep play or presence.

. . . as the banks of the river narrow, the stream moves faster.

(Read Johnson 2005)

---

mostly the presence of other people, especially in proximity to us, brings these banks of the river close together, and our energetic presence rushes chaotically, becoming white rapids of excitement or burden.

Buddhist intentions are to achieve peace by moving the banks of the river apart, and thus one must move away from others, from activity, from doing, and through retreat, meditation and breathing, quiet the spirit. Developmental Transformations does not aspire to these heights. We are more interested in those moments when one is engaged, the river is flowing rapidly, one is in proximity to another and all possibilities of action are immediate and potential. What then? In our worst moments, this is the time we act out, become violent, say something we don't mean, become symptomatic, freak out. DvT training helps one not do these things. Deep Play is a state of being in which one is very much in close proximity to another person, the client or clients, very much filled with the imposing forms of our lives, and very much in the rapid rush of the moving stream of associations, but while maintaining one's equanimity. One can calm the breath and breathe deeply and evenly while meditating in a mountain retreat, that is Buddhism; or one can breathe deeply and evenly after throwing oneself out of an airplane and falling rapidly through space, that is Developmental Transformations. DvT is not needed if you are on the beach, on vacation, or at the ashram. DvT is needed if you are stuck in rush-hour traffic, are late for an important meeting, and your cellphone is dead. But that is really a metaphor. Deep Play in the clinical setting occurs between the therapist and client or clients who have been involved with each other for quite a while, and who in so many ways have come to love each other, and the intensity and energy of that intimacy would usually lead to some form of acting out, but in this case, does not. This not acting upon one's deeply held feelings and associations about being with another, and just letting the impulses move through one, is deep play.

Dialogue with Helen Payne: 'It is emotional intelligence which is being developed . . . since feelings are located first and foremost in the body'

The dialogue concerns dramatherapy in relation to movement and the body. The following dialogue explores the nature of the self and non-verbal aspects of dramatherapy, connecting with Read Johnson's ideas about the nature of the presence of the therapist and contemplation in relation to the therapeutic space and relationship. The dialogue also looks at embodiment, play and authentic movement in relation to dramatherapy.

Connections to practice and research in this book

Discussions drawing on the issues Payne talks about concerning embodiment and the non-verbal in dramatherapy can be found on pages 119 and 257–258. Other examples of clinical practice relating to the nature of the therapeutic relationship, presence and witnessing can be found in the following:

- Chapter 6 Chipman: Expanding the frame: self-portrait photography in dramatherapy with a young adult living with cancer (pp. 109–118)
- Chapter 5 Haste and McKenna: Clinical effectiveness of dramatherapy in the recovery from severe neuro-trauma (pp. 88–95)
- Chapter 11 Dokter: Embodying difference – to join or not to join the dance (pp. 210–220).

Jones: You say 'The body provides direct access to feelings, the unconscious and the imagination in the right hemisphere which are not mediated by words and logical thought found in the left hemisphere.' (Payne 2009: 9) I wondered about your thoughts about the relationship between meaning making through words and meaning making through bodily expression without words?

So, for example, in the group members' perceptions of change and impact you summarise a key part of this by saying:

'Participants stated that they had been enabled to understand how their emotions or life situations had an effect on their bodies and how symptoms were triggered, but also how these could be avoided or how they learned new strategies to cope with any new symptoms in a different way' (Payne 2009: 32) and the 'learning process' (Payne 2009: 33).

Payne: This is an important point you bring. In my understanding of the process at work in the case of these patients, it is emotional intelligence which is being developed and tapped. Since feelings are located first and foremost in the body it is the embodied felt sense that needs to be accessed. Following that verbal language can then be a bridge leading across to the left hemisphere whereby conceptual thought is brought to bear on the experience and learning in its broadest terms can be said to have taken place. This is embodied learning however not solely cognitive. A cognitive understanding (such as reading about the material) of how feelings about life-events can be a trigger for stress related conditions such as medically unexplained symptoms, anxiety and depression, cannot bring about change alone. This understanding has to be located first and foremost in the body resulting in sustained change unlike when reading self-help books or in a cognitive behavioural therapy approach, for example. The approach has to be flexibly implemented, i.e. able to be personalised in such a way as to be individually tailor made for that particular person's psycho-biosocial profile.

We term our approach 'learning through the bodymind' to emphasise the personal learning, as in personal development, aspect and to prevent stigmatising people who frequently say that by attending 'psychotherapy groups' they are made to feel they are 'mad' or 'mentally sick' and so on. They report they have often felt 'put down' by medics that the very real and debilitating bodily symptom they experience is 'all in the mind' and that they have a mental health illness.

When working in the arts therapies with people with learning difficulties, i.e. who may lack some functional cognitive capacities, it is also the emotional intelligence which is being worked with such as in the talking therapies as in Valerie Sinason's work.

Having the opportunity to create meaning from bodily symptoms by exploring their characteristics, context, onset circumstances – antecedents – has been found to relieve distress for some patients.

Jones: You talk about 'Moving and witnessing was introduced, depending on the participants' needs in the group setting.' (Payne 2009: 10) One of the group members in 'Body as Container and Expresser' talks about 'witness and mover' (Payne 2006: 164) and you talk about the 'inner witness' (Payne 2006: 166) Can you say something about what you understand by this term 'witnessing' – who witnesses who and the relationship between witnessing and embodiment?

Payne: Initially, it is normally the facilitator in the role of witness. The

---

Box 3.9 **Excerpt: Helen Payne: embodiment, authentic movement and witnessing**

Group themes, feelings and dynamics are embodied symbolically in the work. For example, themes such as resistance, support and trust can be put into movement with a partner, as can how we believe we are seen, how we feel we are seen and what is actually seen by others in relation to self and the symptom. This can be done through participants adopting either the role of witness and mover as in authentic movement and having time for transition and reflection. Often these roles can be creatively weaved in as a way of entering into mindfulness experiences whereby the present moment is honoured.

(Payne 2009: 12)

---

quality of this witnessing is crucial. It is not observing or watching, looking at or noticing even. It is regarding the other with compassion and love. The intention is always benign; to be a supportive presence. The inner witness is the part within each one of us who is aware of our actions in the world . . . could be seen as our inner critic or judge, and not always very benign! This aspect is placed in a role outside of the one who is in the role of mover who is moving – expressing through natural bodily movement or stillness – from deep within – doing, making an action or not. The intention of the witness here, whether it is as the facilitator or another participant in the group, is to be fully present to the mover, and to themselves (as in a microcosm of the relationship of the inner witness to the self) without expressing, but noticing the experience they have in the presence of that mover. This experience may fall into categories of interpretation: bodily sensations, feelings, thoughts, kinaesthetic perceptions (feeling a need to move as a response to the expression of the mover), imagery, stories and so on. Gradually the witness is experienced as supportive and nurturing and sometimes a unitive experience is felt when both witness and mover find, from the languaging following the experiences, that a mirroring has taken place whereby both embodied experiences match each other. The witness holds or contains the embodied responses she has had in the presence of the mover until after the mover has returned and chosen to speak about her experience in the movement to her witness. Both witness and mover have embodied their experiences, in the mover this is expressed and reflected upon later, in the witness it is contained and expressed only when it is met by the mover mentioning that movement in her story.

Jones: I'm interested in your introduction of the idea of contemplation into the act of therapy, for example when you talk about the 'contemplation of our internal world through movement of the body' (Payne 2009: 161). Can you say why you chose this term and what you see as the benefits for clients?

Payne: Contemplation is a form of prayer or meditation, a way of making contact with the Divine or a higher consciousness. To do with honing the soul perhaps; a vessel for making a relationship with something larger than our little 'i' beyond the everyday. It is content – free which is where the mover and witness begin with a feeling of emptiness. Not feeling the need to 'have to do' anything. Letting whatever emerges come through without control or editing from the ego. The term provides for another possibility, for something unknown to occur. The participants may receive the description of the approach which uses this term, along with that of meditation through movement, as a way to enhance their spiritual journey as well.

Part 2

Clinical practice and practitioner research

Ethics statement

All permissions for the use of any material have been gained from clients and settings following the ethical protocols of services, authorities or associations. This has included full consent and assent and details have been retained. All names of clients in this volume are pseudonyms and no locations of service settings are given.

4 The Narratives of Change project: dramatherapy and women in conflict with the law

Christine Novy

Box 4.1

Questions about practice

- How can narrative therapy relate to dramatherapy?
- Can dramatherapy redress the impact on women of gender blind treatment within justice systems?
- Can clients be consultants within the development of their own therapy?

Research perspective

- The use of vignettes in research
- Clients as co-researchers
- Qualitative group interviews

Client perspective sample

'I found that with this approach I made progress quicker. Because I've been in therapy when the person is sitting down and she listens and she listens, but after a while I get lost. Perhaps she thinks that talking about it will help us see things. But I found that you don't take this approach. You listen, but it's the objects that help us find the words. Each of us listens because we've all come here to understand.'

Introduction

The project described in this chapter was hosted by a community organisation in French-speaking Canada that assists women in conflict with the law[1]. As the title suggests, the project was designed for women in transition to give a shape and history to their progress. Methods revolved around creating and performing personal stories, and included creative expressive processes from dramatherapy as well as a number of ideas and practices from narrative therapy. Several ideas about stories and their use in therapy informed the project's methodology. Among these, an idea shared by dramatherapists and narrative therapists alike: that our lives and identities can be represented in different ways and from varying perspectives; that life stories are, indeed, creations and, as such, they can be created or constructed differently. This multi-storied perspective carried through the entire project. Its broad aim was to instill in the participants a sense of agency in the shaping of their lives (Epston and White 1992; White 1995).

The project was first piloted during the summer of 2005 over seven consecutive weeks. At that time the coordinator of the organisation contacted a number of clients who she thought might be interested. These were former clients of the organisation as well as women currently on probation, parole or receiving community supervision. Five francophone women, who ranged in age from 29 to 59 in age, took part. Two years later I invited these same women to participate in a second six week project. Three of the women accepted my invitation, and their narratives of change will be the focus of this chapter.

By way of introduction, I provide, below, a brief description of the first project, along with some more general information about women in conflict with the law and their treatment within the criminal justice system. My intention is to show how certain features of the methodology were shaped by considerations of context.

Contexts

The first project

When I explained dramatherapy to the original participants, I suggested that the different methods we would be working with were like lenses through which they might view their lives, and that each lens would offer a different point of view. I used the lens metaphor, in part, to convey the concept and

---

1   The organisation provides a variety of services at various stages of the detention process, both within prison and for women offenders on parole, suspended sentence or probation. These include community supervision, half-way housing and a 'stop shoplifting program' as an alternative measure for women accused of economic crimes.

practice of dramatic projection in dramatherapy: 'the process by which clients project aspects of themselves or their experience into theatrical or dramatic materials' (Jones 2007: 84). I also wanted to introduce the idea of discernment.

Narrative therapists, Freedman and Combs write:

> We are born into stories, and those stories shape our perceptions of what is possible. However, we don't usually think of the stories we are born into as stories. We think of them as 'reality'. Stories have the power to shape our experience of reality.
>
> (2002: 106)

The dramatic activities and media that we worked with during the first project were intended to loosen and open up that 'reality'. This involved what Jones describes as 'a play shift': taking 'reality' into the play space of our meetings and treating it in 'a way that encourages experimentation' (2007: 166). Projective methods from dramatherapy and 'a questioning approach' from narrative therapy made it possible for the participants to unravel the themes they had chosen to explore. Repositioned as audience to their lives they were now better placed to comment on and re-evaluate their experience.

Research shows that the majority of women in conflict with the law come from disadvantaged backgrounds, and that a high percentage of women serving a prison sentence have experienced physical or sexual violence (Canadian Association of Elizabeth Fry Societies 2000). Even so, mental health systems continue to emphasise bio-medical over social factors in women's lives, and there seems to be little understanding of the context in which many women are criminalised (Pollock 2008). One of the purposes of the project was to challenge the belief that the difficulties in the participants' lives were a reflection of their identities (White 2007). A cornerstone assumption in narrative therapy is that people are not their problems. In narrative conversations problems are externalised by changing adjectives that describe a person as problematic into nouns (Morgan 2000). This verbal technique, similar to the process of dramatic projection in dramatherapy, provides 'people with a place to stand which makes it possible for them to give expression to their experiences without being defined by these' (White 2004: 60–61). When a participant expressed feeling overwhelmed by thoughts of unworthiness, for example, I suggested she externalise these negative thoughts, using fabric and other objects in the room, as though they were an actual obstacle on her path. Then I asked: 'If this obstacle had a voice, what ideas would it talk you into about yourself?' 'You're stupid', she answered. Other participants answered my question with 'you don't deserve to be here', 'you won't accomplish anything'. As they spoke these words I asked if they heard echoes from their past and whether particular people or places came to mind. Tracing the thoughts in their head back to their childhood origins helped the participants to see that they were not truths, but one person's words. In this way, long-held beliefs about personal culpability were called into question (White 1995).

A question guiding our creative process was 'how do the changes in the participants' experience of themselves during their work with personal narratives affect the way they live their lives outside the project?' (Radmall 2001/2002). This question was largely inspired by an idea from narrative therapy: that the stories we, or others, tell about us have real effects on the way we live our lives. While some stories generate possibilities and inspire hope, others have limiting, unhelpful effects. As the example above illustrates, these more limiting narratives are often created by others: people in positions of authority who hold the power of definition (Morgan 2000). Another participant described her experience: 'Because I have a criminal record, the police don't take me seriously. I think in their eyes I am worthless. They see me as a liar, a thief, an addict.' During the project the participants were invited to step out of these and other limiting stories, into a play space where their own knowledge about their lives was privileged.

Evaluating the project

Forensic literature is largely focused on men and high security populations (Baker and McKay 2001). There are very few studies that centre specifically on women in conflict with the law. The Canadian Association of Elizabeth Fry Societies (2000) provides statistics that account for this gender-bias. The majority of offences for which women are charged are non-violent, economic or drug related. As such, women represent less than 5 per cent of all individuals serving sentences of two years or more. A number of studies draw attention to the gender-blind treatment of women in prisons and within the criminal justice system. Recommendations are made to include women's views, where possible, in the design and on-going development of services (Department of Health 2000; Department of Health 2002; Canadian Association of Elizabeth Fry Societies 2000). A World Health Organisation report on women and mental health (2000) is equally encouraging of qualitative research to help clarify the meaning women themselves give to their experiences.

Encouraged by these recommendations I invited participants in the first project to join with me in its evaluation. My intention was to use their suggestions to inform future provision of the project. The consultation process also strengthened the project's therapeutic objective: to privilege the participants' special knowledge about what suits them in their lives. As Epston and White explain, 'When persons are established as consultants to themselves, to others, and to the therapist, they experience themselves as more of an authority on their own lives, their problems and the solution to these problems' (1992: 17). In my planning for the second project I drew from the participants' feedback to pinpoint effective practices. Non-verbal dramatic languages, projective methods and a 'questioning approach', in particular, seemed to offer helpful building blocks for creating and sharing personal stories in new ways. In my description of the second project, below, I will discuss in more detail how each contributed to the process of change.

The second project

The second project also included a consultation process. This time, following Jones' vignette research methodology, I consulted the participants, more specifically, about their perception of the nature of change experienced by them within the therapy (Jones 2007). This group interview was audio-taped, transcribed and translated into English and, with the participants' consent, is excerpted in the following account.

I begin this account by introducing the participants and the theme that each chose to explore during the project. I then describe the process and progress of our work together over six meetings: what took place, the drama-therapy and narrative therapy processes and media used and the participants' responses to these. Description is interspersed with reflection and commentary: my own, as I reference some of the theories underpinning my practice, and the participants', which I have inserted into the text in quotation marks. A fuller account of the participants' reflections features in the 'Reflections on theory and method' section.

The participants

Initially I met with Louise, Carole and Solange individually to explain the second project and its research component. At these meetings they informed me of developments in their lives since the first project and we explored together what their focus might be this time.

During the first project Louise chose to explore the abuse she had experienced as a child. Finding a language to 'give form to what was haunting me' marked a turning point for Louise and in the months following she wrote a book about her life to help other abused women. In Louise's words: 'I've lived theft, rape, prison ... my usefulness is linked with my life story.' But her past still weighed heavily on her and she hoped, this time, to lift more of that weight from her shoulders. At the time of the project the term of her community supervision was drawing to a close.

Carole had wanted to understand why, in her words, she never felt happy. 'Negative thoughts and feelings', she estimated, took up 80 per cent of her life. During the first project she was able to trace these negative thoughts and feelings back to their childhood origins and begin to de-centre their influence in her life (Epston and White 1992). Since then, she told me, she was questioning her unhappiness rather than allowing it to overwhelm her. During our meeting Carole spoke about her shoplifting offence for the first time. She described it as a 'rebellion against my situation' and a catalyst that began her search for understanding. In this project she wanted to understand why she still felt angry.

Solange stayed in the organisation's half-way house following her release from prison for a drug trafficking conviction. Since then she had successfully turned her back on drugs and was pursuing a college education. Solange's daughter had been legally adopted by her own adoptive parents at a time when she was unable to care for her. Her goal was to continue to make positive changes in her life in order to create a stable home for her daughter. In the first project Solange had chosen to work on sexual abstinence and self-respect. At our meeting she described some of the choices she was making that demonstrated a growing self-respect. She said she wanted to use the second project to talk about her progress and to affirm her commitment to the choices she had made: to be faithful to herself and to God.

Description of the work

Week one: experience near

At our first meeting I laid out a selection of fabrics of various colours, textures and patterns and we talked together about how the participants might use these props to build a three-dimensional image of their theme. Carole said that she wanted to explore anger but that she couldn't think of any images. I asked how she might characterise the anger: Was it like a volcano? Or like fire? She said it was 'underground, like something bubbling beneath the surface.' The image seemed to provide Carole with a way into the activity and she expressed new confidence in her ability to convey her experience.

Traditionally, because of their professional position, the therapist's words and 'expert knowledge' are privileged. But the social constructionist world view informing narrative therapy suggests that meaning 'is always something to be negotiated' (Freedman and Combs 1996: 28). Throughout the project I paid close attention to the politics of story creation. This meant carefully considering whose knowledge, perspective and means of expression were privileged as stories, were made and made sense of. Narrative therapy's 'questioning approach' assisted me in the negotiation of meaning. Questions like, 'Is this a helpful image or not?' followed by an invitation to explain 'Why?' and 'Is this something you would like to explore further?' or 'Are you drawn to something else?' lead to an awareness of choice, both in the participants' experience and in their storytelling. In this instance, the 'questioning approach' ensured that Carole's ideas, not my own, were at the centre of our work together.

Once their three-dimensional images were complete, the participants shared their work. Carole had placed herself inside her sculpture. She had wrapped fabric around her shoulders and thighs and placed a white veil over her head. As she described her creation she shared her discouragement. She said that it was impossible for her to be under a veil and that she wanted to change her experience but did not feel she had permission to do so.

On the other side of the room, Louise had used some black fabrics and a chair to create an image of a person hanging. She said the image represented her despair over the circumstances of her daughter's life.

Beside Louise, Solange had spread out a patchwork of different fabrics to represent her life and identity. In one corner she had placed a folded square of red fabric representing feelings of anger about a recent conflict with a house guest. Solange explained her intention, not to allow herself to be taken over by this anger. She spoke confidently about her decision to turn the anger in to peace and said it was a pleasure to see herself reflected back.

In dramatherapy, non-verbal expression is viewed as a first step towards creating meaning (Andersen-Warren and Grainger 2000). The process of dramatic projection mediates, as Jones writes, between 'inwardly held feelings or life experiences' and 'outer expression in drama' (2007: 83). Participants in the first project spoke about 'the non-verbals' providing them with an 'emotional language' and a way 'to speak from inside'. Aside from its weight, texture, size and colour, fabric imposes a minimum of information. The participants arranged the fabric props to create their own product and imprint their own interpretation (Jones 1991). As they did so, they later explained, the words came easily. The fabric's colour, its weight and feel as they interacted with it, evoked sensations and associations, offering an 'emotional language' with which to both foreground and communicate their own perception of their experience. Language then made dialogue possible.

In my planning for the project I was reluctant to assign a particular focus for our work together. 'The idea of the "better story"' as Hoffman warns, immediately introduces hierarchy 'and puts the therapist in the position of editor-in-chief' (2002: 223). If the project was to be relevant to the participants' lives, rather than the other way around, its methodology needed to be flexible enough to encompass different interests. The customary shape of dramatherapy includes a warm-up, main activity and closure. In group work, the main activity can take various forms: 'one or more individuals dealing with an issue; a group as a whole working together with a specific theme or focus; or all members of a group working on their own material with each other in small groups, pairs or in the large group' (Jones 2007: 13). I chose the latter because it would allow the participants to focus on their individual interests. It also created a forum for them to witness each other's stories, to negotiate meanings together through conversation and to experience their lives connected around shared themes, values and commitments. As Solange summarised at the meeting's end, 'we learned together that our stories are all associated.'

In preparation for our next meeting my thoughts turned to story development. Small world storytelling with objects came to mind as an activity that might assist the participants to place their theme in its larger historical and social context. The activity involves using small objects to create 'a miniature representation of a much larger reality' (Jones 2007: 151). Because the objects are small and easy to move around the storyteller can interact with their story much like a theatre director directing a cast of actors. I decided to bring along two bags of small figurines: one that contained family dolls and furniture, the other animal and fantasy characters.

Week two: the plot thickens

Each of the participants arrived with fresh appraisals of what they wanted to explore in the project and so I suggested they build a story to illustrate their new understanding. I emptied out the two bags of figurines on to the table in the middle of our circle and invited the participants to choose what they would need. As they set about their task I offered some simple story grammar as a guide: Who is the protagonist/s? Where is your story taking place? When: in the past, present or future, or a combination? What happens?

There was a childhood theme in each of their stories. The toys' associations with childhood play seemed to make it easier for the participants to bring past events into the dramatic present. Louise used the small family dolls to tell the story of the abuse she experienced as a child. She said that when she saw the toys she felt like a child again and travelled back in time. Carole shared a similar experience of transport: 'When I had the figurines in my hand, my story became clear: I was a child, I wasn't happy. I didn't feel loved or understood.'

Solange had patterned several different scenes from her past, present and future. As she shared her small world she explained how each toy's unique characteristics contributed to her story. She first introduced her adoptive parents: a roving eyeball to represent her mother, 'because she watches over everything', and a green-monster finger puppet to represent her father 'because he is a mean judge.' Her 'vision of the future' revealed a dream to re-unite with her eleven year old daughter. The roving eyeball and green-monster finger puppet were presented as obstacles in her way. Once again Solange drew on the toys' symbolic potential to illustrate her response: a Tin Tin comic book detective figure to represent 'reflection leading to a plan of action' and a dolphin to represent her commitment to 'freedom of expression'. These skills and values, Solange clarified, would help her stand up to judgement.

Solange later explained that seeing her future represented in this way strengthened her resolve to begin the process: 'to prove that I am capable of looking after my daughter.' In all of their stories the smaller-than-life-size objects helped down-size the problem stories' influence in their lives, making room for more hopeful stories and inspiring new resolve to make real-life changes. Beside the scene from her childhood Louise assembled another scene that showed herself in the future speaking to an audience of children about the risks of drugs. While Carole ended her story with a statement of resolve to live life on her own terms.

Weeks three and four: in the role of expert

A lot had happened for each of the women since our last meeting: setbacks as well as promising new developments. Solange, in particular, had had a bad week, including disappointed expectations and acting in ways that went against her values. She was tearful as she spoke about how confused and tired she felt. Both Carole and Louise took turns to respond to her distress with acceptance and understanding: 'Why do you feel so guilty?', 'It's okay to slip back.', 'Making changes isn't easy.'

Narrative therapists Freedman and Combs write about the persistence of problematic stories: 'People have usually been living them for a long time. Often their local culture includes attitudes and practices that support the problem-saturated story. It is not at all unusual for an alternative story to fade between therapy conversations' (1996: 195). Among narrative therapists there is an understanding that these new, preferred stories require the support of a community if they are to survive. Increasingly I saw my role in terms of keeping the participants' alternative narratives about their progress present and alive in our work together and I noticed that they, as audience to each other's stories, increasingly took on that role for each other.

In the time remaining we planned for our next meeting when two staff members from the organisation would be visiting our group. In dramatherapy it is unusual for an audience to be called in to witness the work (Jones 2007). Narrative therapists, on the other hand, actively promote contexts in which accounts of progress can be acknowledged and supported. I welcomed this opportunity to strengthen the life–drama connection. At the same time I recognised the need for careful planning. I wanted to ensure that the witnessing experience was supportive and acknowledging for the participants. To structure the meeting I suggested a TV chat-show format in which everyone would play a role: the participants, as guest speakers, would share from their experience and understanding; the guests, as members of the audience, would respond to their testimonies; and, as chat-show host, I would facilitate the interviews. The participants liked this idea and each chose a theme for the interview. Louise decided to speak about turning her back on the past and choosing a better life. Carole would talk about the challenges of personal relationships and how to manage these and Solange decided that she would play herself five years in the future and speak as an expert on how to manage desires.

Between meetings I prepared a script of interview questions. My questions were constructed in 'a grammar of agency' and designed to position each participant as an expert on the process of change (Epston and White 1992: 18).

Questions like: What made it possible for you to turn your life around, in spite of what you were up against? Can you tell me more about how you did this? I also prepared some questions for the audience. Questions like: What were you most drawn to as you listened to Carole talk about her experience and why? What does this say about what Solange stands for in life? What difference will hearing Louise's testimony make to your work with women in conflict with the law? (White 1997). During the meeting itself, I interviewed each participant in turn. I then interviewed the audience members and the participants became an audience to their responses. The clearly differenti-ated roles of audience and performer heightened everyone's focus and concen-tration, creating a climate of attentive listening and acknowledgement (Jones 2007: 102).

Along with my interview questions, the fictional world of a TV chat show heightened the expert role, and seemed to make it easier for the participants to speak with confidence about their progress. The audience members also played an important part in the creation of perspective (Jones 2007: 104). The participants had an opportunity to listen to a retelling of their story through someone else's eyes. At the end of our meeting when we talked all together about the experience, Louise said she had a sense that 'my life is important', Solange spoke about how helpful it was to review the past and see her pro-gress more clearly and Carole spoke more confidently about her progress: 'I'm making good choices. I'm finding myself to be a good person.' It seemed that by making their narratives of change more available to others, they were now more available to the participants themselves.

Week five: narratives of change

The participants frequently used the French word *cheminement* to describe their progress, both in the project and in life more generally. *Chemin* means path; however, there is also a verb *cheminer*, which roughly translates as 'to advance progressively over time'. A 'going forward' is implicit in the word *cheminement* and it carries a sense of personal agency, as in *mon chemine-ment*, my progress.

Since this would be our last meeting with a play focus, I wanted to provide a creative way for the participants to see their progress over the course of the project and proposed that we collaborate on a map that showed their different *cheminements*. We taped three large pieces of paper together and drew a circle in the middle to represent the project, where all of their paths would meet and interconnect. The plan was for the participants to begin by mapping their *cheminement* before and leading up to their participation in the project, as well as their forward movement after the project.

I used a flip chart to demonstrate the activity in outline and offered some metaphors (crossroads, a stopping place etc.) that I hoped might shift their experience in to visual images. Solange and Carole chose markers and found a place on the map to begin, but Louise said she felt uncomfortable with the art materials and that all she could feel right now was depression. She was prepared to have a go nonetheless and see where the activity might lead her. Louise used a black marker to draw two parallel paths which reached halfway to the group circle. She explained to me that the two paths showed her choice not to go the way of depression, but that she was not sure how to link the path she had chosen to the circle. She had drawn a black hole on the path of depression and I asked if she could draw what was in the black hole. I also wondered what had contributed to her taking the alternative path and whether she could draw that. These questions seemed to make it possible for Louise to continue with her drawing. The two paths eventually joined and led to the group circle where she drew a picture of childhood play.

When the participants spoke about this exercise they confirmed that mapping their process in this way was encouraging. Carole described the map of *mon cheminement* as 'research in to my wellbeing. It was everything that we'd lived over the project. My "me" grew bigger.' I asked her what it was like to see her *cheminement* as a progression and she said she was proud: 'It gives me a lot of hope.' Solange explained that it was also helpful to witness each other's progress: 'It seems like Louise drew the whole project, from the beginning. Like the image (black hole) you drew first Louise, I remember you phoned me in despair that first week. It was her personal journey. It touched me because it was encouraging.'

Using narrative or the French equivalent, *cheminement*, as 'an organizing metaphor' (Freedman and Combs 1996; Bruner 1986) and, in this way, linking different experiences over time, conveyed movement and contributed to the notion of change (Epston and White 1992; Denborough 2004). To see that 'obstacles come my way' and 'things crop up', but 'I learned that life carries on' and 'I make some progress' and knowing 'that you won't be judged if you take some steps backwards' was encouraging for everyone.

Week six: co-researchers

At this final meeting Solange, Louise and Carole were interviewed all together about their experience during the project. I was curious to hear their evaluation of the methods that we worked with and, more specifically, their understanding of whether and how these were helpful. To begin the interview they were invited to choose a moment or moments that stood out in their experience of the project. I then asked each in turn to describe this moment and to reflect on its significance. The group interview was audio-recorded and later transcribed and translated into English. In the 'Reflection on theory and method' section that follows, I take the participants' thoughts, meanings and language as a starting point for my theoretical reflections on the methods used in the second project.

Reflection on theory and method

> Before I would always defer to others. I defined myself in relation to others. Now I have begun to define who I am myself. In short, I've taken a big step forward.
>
> (Carole)

> It didn't really impact my life outside, no, but it helped because it freed me. I would arrive home and I'd be less consumed by darkness. I had dark thoughts when we started. I don't have any now.
>
> (Louise)

> It was all the questions, the sharing that we did together, the openness, the respect for my faith, the welcome . . . all of this contributed to my self-respect. It's not everyone who understands what I am living and how I am living. The group's respect, the way we communicated amongst ourselves. We didn't judge anyone. This kind of experience really helps me.
>
> (Solange)

As these three testimonies show, each of the participants experienced transformation at some level of 'being, thinking and relating to their lives' (Jones 2007: 126) as a consequence of their participation in the project. In the following discussion I reflect on their thoughts about how 'finding words', 'seeing', 'playfulness', 'questions', 'the group itself', 'being mirrors for each other' and 'my role' contributed to their being able to separate from what was known and familiar and arrive at new conclusions about their life and identity (White 2004: 60).

Finding words

Carole remembered our first meeting and how, initially, she 'had no words' to describe her experience. 'Doing the sculpture', she explained, 'it all came out easily and I found words to explain what I was feeling.' I asked what made it easy. 'The objects', Carole answered, 'it's the objects that help us find the words.' She gave the example of using a veil to cover her face: 'my emotions were veiled.' The objects provided the participants with a language to express and represent their experience.

Seeing

The objects also made it possible for the participants to see their experience represented. Louise explained how creating and seeing the sculpture of a hanging person changed her ideas:

> After I put together the hanging man, oh, it was like someone had

stabbed me in the heart. Making it and seeing it really made me feel something. And then I said to myself 'my god' and I had goose bumps looking at it. I'm depressed but I mustn't let myself go that far.

Louise's account fits with Jones' description of dramatic projection: 'the process by which clients project aspects of themselves or their experience into theatrical or dramatic materials . . . and thereby externalize inner conflicts' (2007: 84). Jones goes on to explain how 'the dramatic expression enables change through the creation of perspective.' For both Louise and Carole, externalising the problem in this way diminished its influence in their lives. Carole explained that once she saw 'the things that make me suffer' she discovered that they 'are less powerful than I thought.' In Louise's case, the darkness was more persistent. As our last meeting illustrates, it was necessary for her to work with equal persistence to separate herself from its influence.

Playfulness

The women used words and phrases like 'openness', 'trust', 'I played', 'I lived things', 'when I come here I feel like a child, I open up' to describe their participation in the project. Despite the seriousness of the problems they had chosen to explore, there was often a mood of lightness and laughter during our meetings. In the fictional world of our play space the participants enjoyed a 'playful relationship with reality' (Jones 2007: 88). Nonetheless, I sometimes questioned whether our work was contributing to build a new, positive social context to the participants' lives. Louise frequently described the anxiety she felt living in her neighbourhood, where even a knock at the door could feel menacing. Poverty seemed to work against their efforts. The relationship between the participants' lives outside and our weekly creative process at times felt tenuous.

It wasn't until consulting the group about their experience that I learned the full extent of each participant's confidence in these 'playful approaches to serious problems' (Freeman, Epston and Lobovits 1997). Louise spoke about her 'trust in the fabrics and in the objects that we worked with.' She explained that without the opportunity to 'work with what was inside' she quickly would have lost interest in the project. Carole added:

I found that with this approach I made progress quicker. Because I've been in therapy when the person is sitting down and she listens and she listens, but after a while I get lost. Perhaps she thinks that talking about it will help us see things. But I found that you don't take this approach. You listen, but it's the objects that help us find the words. Each of us listens because we've all come here to understand.

Questions

Some of the activities themselves evoked memories of childhood play and, as such, provided the participants with an opportunity to bring new insight to their childhood experience. The small world storytelling activity was particularly significant for Louise: 'When I made the story I felt like crying. I felt that I was four years old and my body was crying.' In spite of the immediacy of her experience as she built her small world, Louise explained that she was able to tell the story with an adult's understanding: 'Now I know what was going on. Today I've made sense of it. When you are a child you can't say what you want to, but as an adult you can.'

The projective methods that we worked with during the project made it possible for the participants to step more fully into positions of authority in relation to their own lives and identities. During our second meeting the opportunity to create a miniature representation of a much larger reality repositioned each participant as the artistic director of their life story. From this new vantage point they each seized on the occasion to retell 'the history of the present' and, in doing so, to privilege their own understanding. Placing the problem in its historical context, for instance, unmasked the relations of power surrounding it. As Louise explained: 'When you use the toys you see that someone else was responsible and it shows that it didn't just start today. It started fifty years ago and I'm still affected.' 'The value in this exercise', Louise concluded, 'was to feel understood without being judged.'

Jones uses Brecht's term 'reader' to characterise an engagement in dramatherapy more oriented towards reflection and meaning making (2007: 95). In the two examples above, as Louise shared her small world and narrated the story of her childhood, she was better placed to comment on and re-evaluate her experience. In Jones' words, she 'became a reader rather than a victim of her experience' (2007: 111).

From this more distanced perspective it was easier for the participants to discern between stories. As Carole explains:

> When you can see it, it makes it possible for you to say 'your life is this way and you don't like it, so what life do you want?' Let's say one life, two lives. I find I keep falling into the first. But now I'm in the second life and I don't want the first life any more. I really don't. And now I know that I don't want it any more.

And Solange: 'To say: that's unhelpful, that's helpful, how do I want to live? If it's unhelpful, well next time I'll say no. I did it this way. I'll do it that way next time. In other words, I am beginning to choose which events make up my story, and which stories about my identity contribute to moving forward in my life.' Here the life–drama connection is very much in evidence.

The group

Solange lived through some difficult moments both inside and outside the group. When I asked what brought her to the group each week, she said it was her *cheminement* and, more specifically, the encouragement she felt at each meeting to continue on in spite of the setbacks. For Solange it was the group itself that was the most helpful. She thought their shared history, the absence of judgement and the encouraging way that the other participants acknowledged her progress all contributed to her self-respect. She explained that coming to the group was about taking care of herself.

Louise also talked about the group as a source of friendship. She described how the 'chance to get out of the house and meet people' worked against the darkness and explained that the new confidence she felt was 'a feeling of not being alone'. Later on, like Solange, Louise spoke about the group encouraging her *cheminement*: 'Like when Solange says "you're doing well Louise, don't give up", just hearing that pushes me forward . . .' All of the participants played a role in acknowledging each other's progress and keeping it alive. Throughout the project time spent in conversation, as the stories took shape, as well as in response to each story, was *as significant* for the participants as time spent independently and actively engaged in creating.

Mirrors for each other

Witnessing each other's progress was also experienced as encouraging. As Solange explained:

> We've all grown. Not all in the same way, but we all see now that we've grown. That's what's fun about a group. It's like the people in the group are a mirror for each other. Carole might say something and I see myself reflected in it.

There were a number of exchanges during the group interview that illustrated Solange's mirror metaphor. For example, Carole was the first to speak about her experience in the project and identified Solange's ability to stand by her own truth as a contributing factor to her own progress:

> To say 'I belong to a faith. I believe in God. And I know that there are a lot of people who do not believe, but I'm not going to start telling myself I shouldn't believe.' That helped me. Respecting her in that I made a discovery.

When it was her turn to speak Solange picked up on Carole's earlier comment:

Solange: I've learned because she has grown and I have grown too, through her.

Christine: How did this help you?

Solange: What she did helped me too: to accept myself and the choices that I make. To stand up for myself. Seeing her process to assert herself. Because I'm learning to assert myself too.

Their comments and stories lend credence to Morse and Morgan's findings that 'bringing women together poses a direct challenge to isolation and to women defining themselves as "flawed" and "different" and "alone"' (2003: 41).

My role

In my facilitation of the project I used collaborative ways of working to foster a culture of acknowledgement in which the participants felt they, and their ideas, were listened to and respected. I welcomed their questions and suggestions as we went along and, since French is my second language, I appreciated the rephrasing, clarifying and negotiation of meaning that followed when I introduced guidelines for the activities. The participants said that they had a lot of freedom to follow their own preference during our meetings. But also that the different processes and topics that I introduced encouraged them to think differently. Carole describes how this played out:

> Like when we did the drawing, I'll use that as an example. You took a piece of paper and drew some lines and some circles. And I hadn't thought about it in that way, not at all and so I said to myself 'She's telling us what to do! Because she's drawing lines and circles and I would never have thought of that.' Especially for me, being someone who respects other people's ideas. I said to myself 'no, she can't mean that everyone should draw lines and circles . . .' And it's true you brought in an idea but we ended up doing it in our own way. You were able to guide me, to make me think, but I ended up expressing what I wanted to express with other symbols and in other ways. When we don't feel like we have any good ideas and we have no words . . . but we always ended up taking what you brought; and often we'd say 'my god, what am I going to do?' but we ended up, like magic, giving a form to what we feel inside and by saying what we have to say.

Conclusion

In this chapter I set out to represent the voices, experiences and preferences of three women who have come into conflict with the law. During the project the participants were invited to create and share stories of identity in which their own knowledge about their lives was privileged. The participants were also involved in telling the story of how their stories were created. At our final meeting, they joined with me to reflect on the nature of change experienced by them and to evaluate the project's relevance to their lives. In the 'Reflection on theory and method' section I hope to have shown how their analysis of the methods that we worked with helped me as a practitioner to isolate the real effects of our work together. Indeed, the consultation process raised new questions for me about the role of our participants in the co-creation of dramatherapy theory and practice. Their commentary would seem to offer helpful guidelines for future work with women in conflict with the law, and others who are marginalised and misrepresented in our society. In summary, therefore, I shall outline some general implications for practice inspired by this collaborative enquiry:

- Dramatic props (fabrics, figurines and art materials etc.) provide a language with which to articulate experiences that cannot initially be expressed with words. For people whose knowledge has been disqualified they offer a means with which to convey their own perception of events and, thereby, experience themselves as more of an authority on their lives.
- Dramatic props can be used as storytelling media to represent experience and to give a visible shape and trajectory to people's lives. Using figurines, for example, events from the past, present and future can be placed side-by-side to create a storyline. A person who can see the story they are telling is better placed to comment on and re-evaluate their experience. It is easier, for example, to see their lives as moving forward and, from their 'now' location, to place past difficulties within a context of progress rather than regress (White 1995).
- By actively witnessing one another's progress, the group members, the dramatherapist and, on occasion, specially invited guests, work together to encourage perseverance and a new discernment of choices.

Acknowledgements

Special thanks to the three participants who took part in the project and who generously share their stories and reflections in this chapter. Thanks also to the two coordinators of the host organisation for their warm hospitality and on-going support.

5 Clinical effectiveness of dramatherapy in the recovery from severe neuro-trauma

Eileen Haste and Pat McKenna

Box 5.1

Questions about practice

- How can dramatherapy be of use to clients living with the effects of severe neuro-trauma?
- How can the social model of disability be relevant to dramatherapy?
- How can the approaches of neuropsychologists and dramatherapists be relevant to each other?

Research perspective

- Non-participant structured observation
- Semi-structured interviews
- Client-comparative ratings of dramatherapy in relation to other therapies

Client perspective sample

'Helped me work out things from being here after my illness – things from the past. Quite therapeutic – It helped me to see the pressure I was putting on myself before the illness – by shifting what objects stood for in the session – it showed me how I could shift things in life. . . . Whole way of working was very interesting, very clear. It helped me to gain insight into the past and has far reaching consequences for the future' (Greta).

This chapter describes a study undertaken in a neuro-rehabilitation hospital to investigate the clinical effectiveness of a short course of dramatherapy delivered individually to ten patients recovering from severe neuro-trauma. It was led by Dr Pat McKenna, the neuropsychologist at the hospital. Eileen Haste, working as a freelance dramatherapist, was employed to deliver the programme of therapy. In the following text we shall refer to ourselves by our first names.

Introduction

The majority of people in a neuro-rehabilitation unit share the legacy of severe trauma from a sudden, life-threatening event, which leaves devastating consequences affecting physical and/or cognitive status. The psychological effects of such trauma are aptly described by Duggan and Grainger as 'capable of shattering our equanimity to such a degree that we are cut completely adrift from our existential moorings and thrust into an ocean of fears and inadequacies, a turmoil of existential chaos' (1997: 64).

At the same time, the individual has to negotiate his/her new role as a patient and meet the expectations of family and staff (as well as their own) in adjusting to disability and in learning new skills. This process is an intensification of social relations, described by Duggan and Grainger as keeping:

> ... our balance among the conflicting demands and pressure of the social networks that sustain us, but also distort our judgement, circumscribe our awareness and most important of all, restrict our freedom to be ourselves. We are pulled this way and that in the present by others present.
>
> (Duggan and Grainger 1997: 105)

Contexts

The model of disability

The study explored the use of dramatherapy in mediating adjustment to neuro-trauma within the hospital setting. The rationale for this lies in the power that subjective power has to change the individual's relationship to actual or external reality. Johnston (1996: 205–210) in her model of disability described the failure within the health setting of current practice and measures of outcome to allow for this crucial stage in adjusting to physical disability. The medical model of care, which has characterised the health service for most of its existence, has viewed health mechanistically as a lack of physical infirmity. In rehabilitation terms, this criterion looks to objective physical measures such as mobility, physical strength and lack of physical disability to gauge recovery.

This traditional model of disability, which was embodied in the (1980) World Health Organisation model similarly assumes a simple causal link from 'physical impairment' to 'disability' to 'handicap' (Patrick and Erickson 1993).

Unlike the social model of disability, which argues that it is society's social and physical constructs that disable individuals, the medical model focuses on the physical and neglects to acknowledge the part our emotional life plays in our well-being and quality of life.

This simple linear relationship does not hold up in clinical experience. A 'good outcome' following rehabilitation often exists alongside social or emotional misery and distress. In examining and integrating psychological models of adjustment (emotional, behavioural and coping models), Johnston proposed that impairment also gives rise to mental representations which can affect coping behaviours and moderate relationship between impairment and disability. Johnston further found that mental representations could predict level of disability when coping behaviours (as taught by therapists) did not. To maximise the chances of a positive adjustment to disability rehabilitation, programmes need to address mental representations and subjective perception in patients.

In the early 1990s the health service developed a psychosocial concept of health to incorporate quality of life and which included a state of subjective well-being. This move was reflected in the World Health Organisation, WHOQOF Group 1994 which then defined quality of life as:

> An individual's perception of their position in life in the context of culture and value systems in which they live, and in relation to their goals, expectations, standards and concerns. It is a broad ranging concept incorporating and affected in a complex way by the person's health, psychological state, level of independence, social relationships and their relationship to salient features of the environment.
>
> (WHOQOF cited in Patrick and Erickson 1993: 27)

In practice, there still remains the problem of how to redress the balance and nurture psychosocial well-being within the healthcare setting. This study reflected one attempt to consider the beneficial effects of dramatherapy within the traditional medical model within a regional neuro-rehabilitation unit.

The neuro-rehabilitation unit

Patients within a neuro-rehabilitation unit have to adjust to physical disability and/or cognitive deficit affecting such things as perception, memory, problem solving and communication and to the position society's attitudes and lack of provision can place them in. All of these difficulties can cause a dramatic shift in self-identity.

Patients are expected to deal with their changing circumstance and complete a major part of their recovery within the institutional setting of the hospital wards and departments. The traditional therapies (physiotherapy, occupational therapy, speech therapy and neuropsychology) necessarily address the objective world and the fact of disability. These therapies are essentially performance oriented in nature, so reinforce the fact of loss and change. In contrast, a dramatherapy programme offers release to the individual from the immediate present and time to explore those parts of the subjective world untouched by the present loss. It offers opportunities to progress through a period of gentle play and rediscovery of self and the environment.

> By attending to fantasies and by indulging 'playful' thoughts, actions and feelings, individuals come in to contact with their own unique aspects which are not captured by what society or culture dictates concerning work and love. It is precisely in play, therefore, that we are able to reach deeper levels of individuality . . . Play allows individuals to be in contact with experiences that maintain a sense of old identity while at the same time helping them face the changes following brain injury. If patients are not helped to have symbolic experiences involving work, love and play (i.e. their individuality) after brain injury they remain fragmented and fail to develop a sense of direction or identity.
>
> (Prigitano 1989: 428–430)

Within the dramatherapy programme, it was Eileen's intention to address this aspect of a patient's recovery. This study represents an attempt to evaluate formally the effects of dramatherapy intervention on the recovery process following severe neuro-trauma.

Referral

Referral to the program was made by Pat, as the neuropsychologist. There were several constraints to be respected within the context of a health care setting, existing therapy timetables and the timescale available to carry out the research. In particular, care needed to be exercised in predicting the likely length of hospitalisation for each patient. Consequently, the selection criteria were broad to allow inclusion of any patient with a traumatic event to the central nervous system producing severe and sudden disability. Ten completed the course; six patients were recovering from a traumatic brain injury, one from a cerebral vascular accident, two from removal of a cerebral tumor and one recovering from Guillain Barrie syndrome, a disorder in which the body's immune system attacks part of the peripheral nervous system. Five clients were male and five female. Ages varied from sixteen to sixty-nine.

Patients were encouraged to attend the dramatherapy session, but made an individual choice as to whether to continue with the programme. The code of ethics outlined by the British Association for Dramatherapists (www.badth.org.uk) were carefully adhered to. The clients' interests were put first and all clients were made aware of the study, the process of the research and the nature in which feedback and observations were to be gathered and used and their consent was obtained. Care was taken to emphasise that this was not part of usual therapy, but an extra and experimental venture for patients who might be interested in taking part and that attendance was voluntary and patients could leave at any point. Indeed we were aware that for patients, being fully informed and involved as an equal partner in the venture can be experienced as empowering in the vulnerable life situation of being a patient. Thus all stages of the procedure were fully described, and consent could only be given after a period of a week when the patient had had time to consider.

Description of the work

The therapy began with an introductory session in which Eileen met with the patient in order for her to prepare an individual programme of activities based on the interests of the participant. The following week, therapy was commenced on a one-to-one basis with the participant meeting with Eileen and this occurred for one hour each week for five consecutive weeks. For the efficacy of gathering data for the study, feedback and observations of the programme were gathered in several ways. After each session the drama-therapist filled out two questionnaires. One, devised by the neuropsychologist, helped to gauge the responsiveness of the participant. The other, devised by the dramatherapist, aimed to judge the appropriateness of the material for the particular individual. In the fourth session, a video camera was positioned in a corner of the room to allow later observation by the neuropsychologist. Only the neuropsychologist had access to the film. Following this fourth session, the neuropsychologist also filled in these checklists after observing the session on video. Within a few days following the last session, the neuropsychologist carried out a semi-structured interview (with participants), which was tape-recorded . . . The central questions were how enjoyable or worthwhile the course had been to them and what relationship this had, if any, to the rest of their experience in the hospital. They were also asked to rate the importance of the two main therapies, physiotherapy and occupational therapy, as well as dramatherapy in their rehabilitation programme.

We considered it important for Pat to observe at least one session, for two reasons. First, it was important for a neuropsychologist to monitor the effect of any cognitive difficulty in engaging (e.g. visual neglect where the patient might have been attending to materials only on one side of space). Second, in such a subjective form of therapy, it was considered necessary for a second non-participant observer to view the interaction in order to carry out an assessment of its efficacy. However, this needed to be done unobtrusively. Thus, in the fourth session, a video camera was positioned in a corner of the room to allow Pat to also observe the session. Participants consented to this, and in relation to confidentiality, only Pat as part of her observation role would ever have access to the film. Following this fourth session, Pat also filled in the checklists, after observing the session on video. Within a few days following the last session, Pat carried out a semi-structured interview with participants which was tape-recorded in most cases (the facility was not available for the first two). The central questions were how enjoyable or worthwhile the course had been to them and what relationship this had, if any, to the rest of their experience in the hospital. The questions were open-ended and encouraged the expression of anything that the participant felt relevant or would just like to say. This method of feedback encourages freedom of expression, and incorporates room for the participant to say whatever they wish about any aspect of their experience they consider relevant to their situation. It allows for dialogue and clarification and divergence. This semi-structured questionnaire approach thus allows for individuality of personal experience and its efficacy had been shown in previous studies carried out by Pat. This methodology, which targets the expression of exactly what the participant wants to say, contrasts with the distortion possible, if not inevitable, in tick-box questionnaires where the outcome can only be within the preset parameters set by the tick boxes and questions.

They were also asked to rate the importance of the two main therapies, physiotherapy and occupational therapy, as well as dramatherapy in their rehabilitation programme (see Table 5.1).

Following the fourth session of the dramatherapy course, both Eileen and Pat had filled in the checklist measuring engagement of the participant in the session. There was good concordance and most participants scored close to, or at, ceiling indicating that they were able to both carry out the activities and interact appropriately with Eileen.

At the end of the entire series of interventions Eileen sought to define the results of the therapy from the practitioner's point of view, by outlining the ways in which she felt the therapy had been of benefit to the patients. This process also proved useful in the analysis of the qualitative data (see Qualitative analysis: the ways in which therapy was effective). She defined four distinct processes that she had perceived during the sessions. They were that clients were able to:

1   Take control of details in the environment that effect or can enhance their ability to be themselves, i.e. create a personalised space.
2   Enjoy or rediscover the nature of play, creativity and spontaneity.
3   Develop existing skills and discover new abilities and therefore experience the role of creator.
4   Gain insights into the nature of their psycho-emotional processes. This was achieved by translating their inner world into a concrete manifestation, which can then be observed from a new perspective.

The ratings of importance to them in relation to their recovery and well-being from all therapies from each participant are as seen in Table 5.1.

Table 5.1 Frequency ratings of importance of therapy to treatment

	1	*2*	*3*	*4*	*Total*
Physiotherapy	0	0	1	8	9
Occupational therapy	1	2	4	2	9
Dramatherapy	0	2	4	3	9

(4 =very important)

Content of dramatherapy intervention and individual experiences

Given that all the clients were convalescing from physical trauma, assessment showed that a focus on dramatic activities that related to objects, play and image-based work would be more relevant to the ways the clients could best engage in the medium. All clients were given the choice to determine the ambience of the room. They chose the lighting mood and music. In engaging clients in the dramatherapeutic processes Eileen found that using objects was the single most appropriate medium. Most patients were engaged in using objects in some way. There was a great range of objects available to use in this work. One bag contained random items, such as a hinge, model dinosaur, key, conker, mirror, button, candle. Another contained natural objects and another was a magpie's hoard of shiny bits; marbles and beads. All of these objects were small enough to fit on the palm of a hand. There was also a bag of scarves and fabrics. Eileen used these objects to initiate relaxation, play or self-reflection depending on which intervention was perceived as most appropriate. The use of objects was enhanced and complemented by the additional use of visual images, music, percussion instruments, sound recording equipment, making materials and maps. Eileen encouraged a sense of play by presenting objects to a participant. By choosing those that resonated with the participant Eileen then invited them to create a context for the objects, e.g. a character, a story or landscape. This then would be the stimulus for further exploration in which participants engaged in a free flow of ideas.

In some cases a similar activity took a more symbolic direction where objects were assigned meanings relating to the participant's emotional language. Objects were placed in patterns where the distances and relationships between them were perceived as metaphors of their own emotional processes. At other times objects and images were used as a sensory stimulus to assist participants in relaxation. Pebbles were used to help focus a participant on their senses, whilst visual images and sound effects would accompany them on an imaginative journey. Eileen found that in this setting the objects created windows for them to reconnect with their former selves and the world outside the institution. They also formed bridges to a client's imagination and ideas, making their inner world more tangible. As Chesner puts it: 'Objects are easier to work with than abstract ideas, and ideas can be made more accessible by "concretizing" them with the help of objects or props' (Chesner 1994: 64). Using materials to create miniature landscapes has long been a recognised technique in therapy. In this study Eileen found that working with objects opened up many avenues, enabling people who were physically limited to engage in a range of processes. Even though most of the work took place on a tabletop, the work was expansive and involved several dramatherapy core processes.

Dramatic projection and personification was witnessed in Greta and Ned's case (see case studies). In both cases they created constellations with objects that symbolised aspects of their inner landscape. By reflecting on the relationship of the objects to one another and by shifting them, they gained fresh perspectives on their emotional processes. As Jones states:

> The client can feel more powerful, more able to physically change the materials and life events or issues they represent. This in turn through analogy, makes the clients more able to feel empowered to make changes in terms of real events or issues.
>
> (Jones 1996: 142)

This was particularly true in this setting where engaging clients in physical activities would have had the opposite effect in dis-empowering clients. Play, recognised as another core process in dramatherapy (Jones 1996; 2007), was a significant part of sessions for Mike, for example (see case study).Whilst Greta and Ned naturally used the medium to relate to their inner landscape Eileen didn't invite a discussion on the interpretation of themes or images that clients created unless they did themselves. Given the length of the therapy programme, Eileen felt it inappropriate to initiate exploration on any other level than the participants chose for themselves.

The following descriptions provide background information on a sample of the participants and give a brief overview of their experience and attitude to the dramatherapy.

Case studies

Greta

Greta, aged 35, was a young artist who had severely impaired visuo-perceptual skills following a brain haemorrhage. For much of the time, Greta's rehabilitation programme reinforced the loss of basic levels of skills in which she had excelled before her illness. For her, dramatherapy sessions were comforting and comfortable and allowed her to experience the sheer enjoyment of her creative skills freely, the impairment being irrelevant. In this way, she could again experience continuity of self. She often expressed this, both in her use of the space and in her comments during sessions. Of equal importance to her was the space and medium it provided for her to work through problems she needed to solve, by using the materials as metaphor and objects of projection.

Greta, during one session, placed a few autumn leaves and white shells in a pattern on the table. It was a simple constellation. Greta explained that it represented a gentle figure with the nature of an angel who came to her during her time of convalescence. It was clear that the feeling of the angel's presence was very significant to her and her feeling of safety and well-being. In a later session, using objects more consciously to represent what she felt her strengths and vulnerabilities to be; Greta began placing the same leaves and shells around the core of this constellation. She realised that she had unknowingly created the angel again. She interpreted this by recognising that the angel was the mirror of her core being. This deeper understanding of the healing figure gave her further comfort and belief in herself. During another session, using a brushing percussion instrument, Greta recorded the sound of the angel's wings moving. In the following sessions she would spend part of the time in a meditative state, listening to the sound of the angel's wings moving. This came to be a deeply peaceful time for Greta. Another time Greta had created the image of a bird learning to fly. In the next session she reported that an occupational therapist had commented that Greta reminded her of a young bird also learning to fly. She recognised the echo. With this and the angel in mind Greta lifted her arms to feel the space in her armpits and experimented with the feeling of flight in her hands. Whilst dynamic physical work wasn't an option for any of the clients it was important not to underestimate the significance of the smallest of gestures.

Mike

Mike, aged 41, was recovering from the removal of a brain tumor, which affected mobility and coordination. New to the use of a wheelchair, he had also to contend with visual and auditory impairment as well as continuous pain and facial disfigurement. For him, the main benefits of dramatherapy consisted of restoring self-confidence and demonstrating his creative abilities, as well as showing him that he could adapt this facility in other ways than he had in the past, allowing him to express some hope in the future. Mike was naturally efficient and organised and found the inconsistencies in communication and changes in timetables, which occurred in the hospital routine, very difficult to tolerate and these increased his sense of helplessness. By reconnecting him to his abilities and giving him back some control, he found dramatherapy increased his self-esteem and redressed the balance. Mike used the objects to create landscapes which, when photographed, were used to illustrate a story he had previously written, about a journey to Saturn. With cloths, little figures, beads, strings and threads Mike took time to work the materials and find the right shapes. In creating this photo-story Mike was not only director for a while but was also able to escape into the world of his imagination.

Mike had been positive about the treatment and when he was readmitted seven months later agreed to be interviewed again. The following account is included as an entire sample of one interview and in the subsequent qualitative analysis we draw on the interviews as a whole. Here Mike makes some pertinent points:

Pat: So it's actually seven months on. Have you thought much about that dramatherapy you did since?

Mike: When I looked through my drawers at home which I keep for my cassette tapes and my photographs from drama group. . . . I remember then of the times I used to come up for those sessions. I sometimes think about the things I've done and what was involved and look at those lessons. When I had to make a layout of what was supposed to have been the landing space on the planet Jupiter with all rocks and bits of string and everything. I must admit it looked good. . . . I mean when I went to occupational therapy I was working to improve my condition because of my condition. And when I went to physiotherapy I was doing the same there, but when I went to dramatherapy it was nothing to do physically with my treatment. And well, being in this place I found it was as much a social thing as well. I didn't consider it as a treatment. It was as nice for me to think that I could get out of my system. I knew I could come up here and I wasn't depressed. I wasn't angry. In fact I used to get lost in my subject.

Pat: Do you think it provides a positive sense of your ability to adjust disability? Does it give you something to help you?

Mike: Yes. Well it . . . after the dramatherapy I realised that I could do something as an activity at home. And keep my mind on it. And to escape. I've never done it before. Since I've been ill I really haven't had the patience to do anything. Even at physiotherapy I couldn't keep my concentration very long. I've been told that. I was miles away. I used to get involved for so long, but I wouldn't be interested then.

Pat: When you were doing physio in Rookwood?

Mike: I did have a lot of hurt, as far as I'm concerned . . . is grief. Because I think I lost my life then. Basically I did at the end of the day, that's my livelihood gone. Dramatherapy helped me, made me believe that I could do things which don't actually connect me with being disabled or my disability. I can escape out of it. . . . Well when I used to come to dramatherapy I used to escape being misunderstood and come in and doing my stuff, listening to music and talking in general I realised then I'm not just a patient. I'm a human being as well. I'm being understood on that level. Because it may have been a therapy, but I wasn't being a patient here I wasn't being treated as such. So I behaved as such. So I didn't feel so helpless any more really or misunderstood. So when I went back to the ward I wasn't a patient. I was a normal human being that wasn't very well.

Pat: Did it change your ability to assert your needs while you were in hospital or to negotiate decision making processes in your treatment? Did it give you confidence, I suppose?

Mike: Yes it did. Yes in the same way as being misunderstood before. It's hard to explain it, but knowing that I'd been very ill and very restricted. I couldn't move, I couldn't move the wheelchair at all. I was very dependent. But like I said before knowing that when I came here afterwards I realised I wasn't just patient after patient. I was a comparatively normal person who has just ... maybe begin to rationalise things that had gone wrong as far as my treatment. My appointments, my let downs had been concerned and if I hadn't come to dramatherapy I think I would have still been the same. I would have still felt put upon. I would have still been the patient. The underdog. But now as far as treatment is concerned. I'm not saying now, but after the dramatherapy I didn't actually call the shots, but I had a voice in making those decisions. And because I had more confidence in myself I was able to do that. I was able to do that more confidently.

Ned

Ned, aged 30, had suffered a third head injury which left neither obvious physical deficit nor primary problems with language, perception or memory and he was above average in intelligence. Ned's overriding cognitive deficit was of the 'executive syndrome' which had never been recognised before, even though it was suspected that it had first been acquired in his earlier head injuries. For most of the time, Ned was dogged by a sense of being disjointed in life and being led by others and he described a part of him that felt helpless, worthless and confused; a feeling that he hadn't 'quite got the grip of what's happening' all the time. In dramatherapy, he was able to experience a continuity of self that pre-dated his head injuries, when he was happy playing alone for hours in the countryside and on the beach. The contribution that dramatherapy provided was to allow him to clarify what way of life suited his needs and personality.

During one session he created a collage of two very different objects. One represented him as a materialist who worked for money to pay for a good car and a good time. The other was a person who cherished the outdoors and could spend hours watching colours change. Ned took a stone in the shape of a heart and instinctively placed it in the centre of those objects which symbolised the nature-loving side of his personality. He explained that he realised that that was where his true self felt acknowledged. This simple gesture had the potential of nurturing the germination of a decision and allowed him to plan a blueprint for work and living which also became part of his community programme. Ned did go on to research the possibility of training in dry-stone walling. Some five months after discharge, his social worker rang to request a list of dramatherapists in their local area.

Reflection on theory and method

Qualitative analysis: the ways in which the therapy was effective

The transcripts of the interviews with the participants were studied at length individually and comparisons across transcripts made. The individual ways in which the therapy was perceived to be beneficial to participants were grouped into core categories where they echoed themes of other participants. From this the following four categories emerged which showed remarkable congruence with those which Eileen had produced independently (see previous section).Thus these categories emerged through a process of initially noting common themes, successively refined by re-reading each transcript, and considering the strength, commonality and variations across them.

Creating a personalised space: contrast to traditional therapies

All the ways in which the participants described the therapy as being effective, lay in its contrast to traditional therapeutic interventions. This reflects the first process described by Eileen as the opportunity for participants to take control of details in the environment that effect or can enhance one's ability to be oneself, i.e. create a personalised space. Six of the nine participants who were able to feedback at interview gave clear accounts of this process, part of which reflected a balance between freedom and structure woven into activities, tailored to suit the individual's creative needs and personal style, which also empowered the individual and made them feel in control of the procedure. Greta described this as follows:

> Eileen had the sensitivity to find my creative way . . . came from my inner space, which was painting . . . That approach, that Eileen developed concentrated on what you enjoyed.

Mike and Graham expressed this as being able to listen to their music as and when they wanted and Mel described this most directly in the following way:

> She was quite easy to go along without any structure, but she'd also have been content to keep it in control and not go wandering off . . . She didn't make any demand of you.

Rebecca described the sensation of empowerment thus:

... it was really peculiar ... normally with the therapist, you think 'they're the therapist, I'm the patient'. When I was with Eileen it was like she was my friend. The only difference was that I was in a wheelchair. So that helped me see really 'what difference does it make?'

All of the participants had been in hospital at least several weeks and many for months and some were acutely aware of the ways in which they were vulnerable to becoming institutionalised. Participants listed the opportunity to leave the ward as a benefit in itself. As an antidote to institutionalisation, the therapy was much valued:

> You get pushed and pulled around a lot in an institution. Clothes, untidy, little things, being woken up too early. Riled me a lot – insensitivity. Got me away from the ward.
>
> (Greta)

> ... its time out from being a patient ... you just felt it was a change from sitting on the ward, the horrible magnolia walls. ... It gets you out of that rut of routine ... The nurses control the environment, they control when the lights go on and off, when the TV goes on and off ... the routine of a hospital decrees when you eat ... you can become over-whelmed in a sense of the routine.
>
> (Mel)

Creating an environment within the dramatherapy session in which participants felt able to make decisions about the direction of their own experience was integral to creating a positive foundation on which to develop further work, but more importantly, was integral to them feeling empowered and therefore positive about themselves.

Indeed the significance of this aspect of the therapy is illustrated in how often it is commented on by participants.

Escapism and enjoyment

'It was an hour I could almost forget about my condition ... I was using my imagination, I was forgetting'. Mike here describes what happened when he was allowed to rediscover play, creativity and spontaneity.

This sense of escapism from the ward and their current situation was the most commonly reported benefit, clearly described by eight of the participants. Their awareness of sheer pleasure during the sessions demonstrated for them that subjective experience need not be dependent on, nor reflect, actuality and that pleasure could be accessed on a regular basis even in stressful or distressing life circumstances. Sharon's consistent and positive response to whether she enjoyed dramatherapy was always to say 'yes'. Given that she was not able to give any more elaborate responses beyond the monosyllabic, this sparse but persistent response could reasonably be taken at face value.

Mel experienced escapism most acutely:

> I actually forgot I was sat in the [wheel] chair and almost at one point went to stand up and go . . . It's more than an hour away from the ward. It's an hour in a different . . . doing something that you want to do . . . its something that you could totally enjoy and not really know at the time how much effect it's having on you until you, like I said, until you get back. And then you realise 'here we are again'.

Awakening creative potential and improving self worth and confidence

Seven of the group actually produced creative works e.g. poems and paint-ings, five of whom described a consequent process of feeling empowered which contrasted with their previous feelings of dependency, worthlessness and sometimes hopelessness. While the previous level of engagement led to a positive state of mind this level of engagement provided concrete evidence of an ability to make a positive contribution, and be of use and worth in sometimes novel and experimental ways. Thus, it became apparent that a negative and unproductive future does not inevitably follow the fact of dis-ability. Mike particularly benefited from discovering his creative talent and described how this cascaded to enrich his self image:

> . . . and it was nice to express what I thought – never done that . . . not since I was in school . . . Though I can't do those things again [referring to impaired coordination preventing playing on a keyboard] this reminded me that I was still fine in my head, I can still be creative. . . . The chance of being even a little bit creative – because I can't play music anymore, make anything, basically can't do anything, and therefore can't express myself, it is reassuring that haven't really lost it up there. . . . I don't know why but – like exercise and when I leave the premises I'm still exercising, feel more confident. Therapy apart from body and mechanics is important. Brain still needs something.

Mel, who described becoming estranged from creative activities in the normal course of her very busy life as a working mother, was delighted with the opportunity to re-explore the experience and consequent empowerment:

> And it was nice to be able to do something that looked lovely and was nice to do and was very textural, which helped a lack of sensation in my hands. . . . As we get older we just get so involved with going out to work, earning money, doing housework. [On creativity] I can still do it, it's okay to do it. You always think 'Oh art . . . I'm not going to be very good at that'. But the positive thing is there's always something creative in

everybody. Whether it's, not exactly draw or paint, but just use objects to make a picture, or make a story or poems or something like that. I really enjoyed doing pictures. It wasn't something that you had to do. I liked using the fabric. It was nice to be able to do that. To take that away . . . that you are still able to do something worthwhile in the community.

Rebecca was delighted to discover she could still write poetry and had been skeptical at first. By examining poems she had written as a teenager (five years ago and three years before her accident) she first identified similar feelings between now and then. She was surprised at the ability she had demonstrated and did not feel that she still had the creative ability and had no conscious intention to attempt a poem. After using word maps in earlier sessions, Rebecca produced a poem spontaneously and effortlessly in the fourth, videoed session. Rebecca's head injury had affected the motor control of her vocal apparatus and she was very difficult to understand, so that conversation was slow and Rebecca often had to repeat herself and even spell out words before they could be understood. Through poetry, Rebecca could have a potent voice. John's case, perhaps most clearly, embodies the act of creation, empowerment and usefulness for the community in producing a piece of work clearly specified to be made available and used by others, as a gift outlasting his mortality.

The opportunity to experience themselves as empowered played a significant role in rebuilding a positive self-identity for the patients. Participants were able to reassess their recently adjusted identity and recognise that they were in fact potent individuals.

Psychotherapeutic process

Three of the group, Greta, Ned and Rebecca, were able to both engage in the creative aspect of the therapy and direct it towards examining personal issues. Mel saw this potential, but did not wish to use it in this way. She also pointed out that the limited number of sessions could curtail this aspect of the therapy. For Mel, the other three aspects were what she needed at that time and she was able to clearly articulate this:

> It's too short a time to have a counselling relationship as such, but like I said she's very easy to talk to and very understanding. You could use it in that sense if you wanted to, but I didn't use it in that sense.

Greta, whose artistic nature needed no time for re-acquaintance with the creative process, almost immediately focused the sessions on salient issues in her life:

> Helped me work out things from being here after my illness – things from the past. Quite therapeutic – It helped me to see the pressure I was

putting on myself before the illness – by shifting what objects stood for in the session – it showed me how I could shift things in life. . . . Whole way of working was very interesting, very clear. It helped me to gain insight into the past and has far reaching consequences for the future.

Ned took a little longer to discover this potential of the therapy but was able to clarify certain areas of confusion in his life:

It made me sort my thoughts out a little bit. It made me realise that there's two definite sides to my character . . . There was a small stone in the shape of a heart which I ended up putting in the countryside which made me realise that's where I really wanted to be. It made me kind of realise things about myself which I suppose I'd always known, but I hadn't really though about. I think it helped me realise aspects of my character. I think it actually helped me know what I wanted which is half the battle. Because to be honest with you I've had no idea for a long time what I wanted to do. Basically I've just gone from the one job to the next job and then I've got frustrated because it hasn't really been what I really wanted to do, but it was just because it was paying the bills and so I was doing it.

For these patients, who chose to use the therapy in this way, it proved to be an effective medium for them to gain clarity about their internal processes. However, the majority of these participants did not use it in this way. Furthermore, one person was used to self-examination as part of their creative life style. We consider this to be significant. At such a time patients are physically and emotionally vulnerable. This study suggests that when people are newly traumatised with such a depth of change and loss, and having to navigate a new environment away from their own home and routine, their current psychological need is for reaffirmation, empowerment and hope. It was felt that any self-examination should be client led and embedded within a positive framework.

Within the pleasures of the process of empowerment, benefits experienced by the group reflected deeper engagement with the process. This included a sense of escapism and enjoyment, the awakening of creative potential and improvement in self confidence as well as a means of gaining insight into one's inner world. These reflected the same processes described by Eileen in terms of rediscovering the nature of play, creativity and spontaneity, experiencing the role of creator and gaining insight.

Status as therapy

Finally, with the exception of John, each participant was asked whether they thought dramatherapy was a luxury or an essential element in their treatment. Only three people (Joanne, Graham and Sharon) described it as a luxury or irrelevant to their treatment and progress. Joanne described it as 'nice but not essential', Graham thought of physiotherapy as the only relevant treatment for his needs, Sharon tended to give monosyllabic answers or to say 'don't know', but rated all therapies as equally important and gave no real indication of having valued dramatherapy. Maurice described it as being 'not a luxury, could be an essential part of treatment', but this appeared not so much a conclusion from his personal experience (given he had not really engaged in the process) as the semi-automatic response of the cultured professional. The remaining participants thought it was an essential element in treatment. Their responses were as follows:

> Not only a good complement but stands alone, more beneficial than OT at Rookwood.
>
> (Greta)

> I think it's not [only] a complementary element but a necessary element.
>
> (Mike)

> For me, yeah. For people certainly with my character, it gave me the space and the time.
>
> (Ned)

> I think people will really benefit from it. Because it is time out in more senses than just time away from the ward, it's time out from being a patient. It's time out doing something creative. Doing something that you want to do. Listening, just quiet. I think it will get people, especially people who've been here for a long time; it gets you out of that rut of routine. It makes you think a bit more.
>   It should [be an essential part of treatment] . . . because it makes you feel better about yourself.
>
> (Rebecca)

For those patients who found they are able to engage with the medium of dramatherapy, the study indicates that it is potentially of significant benefit. Whilst there are many ways in which participants chose and were able to engage in the material, the feedback suggests that whatever the nature of their experience, they felt the benefits acutely.

The effects of dramatherapy

Qualitative data from this small group of participants provide some evidence that dramatherapy can be an effective method of intervention for some individuals in their rehabilitation following neuro-trauma. In describing, in depth, the effects of dramatherapy on a few carefully studied participants it was possible to gain some insight into the psychological mechanisms of adjusting to neuro-trauma. In the analysis of the feedback, a clear symmetry between the ways in which the participants benefited and those defined by the dramatherapist emerged, increasing the validity of these conclusions. These were; to redress the balance of power within the hospital setting so that patients were allowed to experience control over their environment, to experience fun as an antidote to the negative circumstances of their illness, to be empowered by their own creativity and to examine their own psychological processes in a gentle supportive therapeutic framework.

The results show that an individual's perception of impairment influences how disability is experienced and mediates coping behaviours. For instance, Mike and Rebecca both fed back that the course acted as a spur to aid them alter their perceptions of the nature of their impairment. Mike recognised he still had power to be creative and effective in his life and felt more detached and less of a victim to the vagaries of bureaucratic timetabling and organization; a view he was still expressing seven months later. Rebecca gained a perception of herself as no different from others, apart from being wheelchair dependent.

Notwithstanding these positive reports on the therapy, not all the participants benefited to the same extent nor in a homogeneous manner. Within the research framework of this project, the amount of dramatherapy these patients received had to be uniform and delineated by the constraints of the research protocol. The dramatherapist had originally envisaged ten treatments as being a reasonable exposure to the medium, particularly as most adults express a lack of confidence and some wariness of involvement in the creative arts. This wariness was increased by the term 'dramatherapy' which was misleading for both the participants and staff who could often not override the belief that it was to do with acting. This occurred even with the full, written description of therapy at the introductory stage. In this series, Greta, the artist, initially 'thought of drama as not pleasing' to her. Ned described 'having reservations' and 'not being really sure what it involved'. The fear of having to perform also occurred for artistic endeavour as expressed by Mel:

> First of all, I thought 'I'm not going to be any good at this art stuff and whatever' . . . initially I've always felt that I'm not very good at arty things. I thought 'will I be able to do this?'

Most of the patients were thus taken on at a very vulnerable and disrupted time in their lives. It is of note that with such little exposure and in so short a time the participants were able to respond so well. The constraints posed by certain cognitive deficits and by pre-morbid personality traits also needs consideration in appraising the therapy at an individual level. These interactions were not systematically explored in this small sample nor were they the focus of this study, which sought to assess the benefits of the therapy.

The question of boundaries of application is an important one in targeting the subset of patients who will maximally benefit. Setting these boundaries is not easy. Though it would appear reasonable to assume that compromised insight might impair ability to benefit from the therapy this was not necessarily the case. Some participants, who had impairments of the executive system which did compromise their ability to integrate and monitor their intellectual and psychosocial behaviour at the higher and subtler levels of functioning, benefited particularly well. Others, with more pronounced difficulties in ability to monitor their thinking processes had greatly restricted or dubious benefit. Pre-morbid personality factors also appeared to influence motivation within the therapy, but how far previous experience or lack of it in creative activities can influence outcome needs to be determined.

Similarly, the amount of exposure to the therapy needs to be explored. Overall, the participants rated the importance of dramatherapy as equivalent to occupational therapy but not as important as physiotherapy. Yet their exposure to these therapies was not equal. In contrast, each participant would have received almost daily physiotherapy and occupational therapy; often for some weeks before the dramatherapy commenced and for very many weeks after. They received only five single sessions of dramatherapy spread over some weeks (usually five, sometimes four). The parameters of exposure needed to achieve maximum creative, psychotherapeutic and long-term benefit, also need to be mapped, so the timescale of sessions can be tailored to suit the needs of individuals.

This project demonstrated how addressing the inner, subjective world of a small group of patients and allowing them to experience their own creativity could give them access and insight into their own strengths and intrinsic worth. This process appeared to boost successful coping within the hospital setting. How well this extends to the community, which is arguably more important, is a further avenue needing exploration. It is within the setting of the community that coping mechanisms are really tested for long-term adjustment to disability. Psychological coping is so intimate a part of physical coping that any physiotherapy gains made in hospital can easily be lost if psychological coping is inadequate. Hospital life does not prepare patients for the attitudes of society to disability and the effect these attitudes have on disabled people. Fitzgerald describes how science, bureaucracy and organised religion have played an important role 'in shaping the construction of disability as the broken, incomplete and imperfect self, as the case requiring management, and as the object of pity or charity' (Fitzgerald 1997: 407–413).

The move by health service in the early 1990s to revisit a psychosocial concept of health has been reflected in several government initiatives in recent years. Specifically in relations to neurological conditions the government launched the National Service Framework (NSF) for Long-term Neurological Conditions (Department of Heath 2008). This framework was designed to transform the way health and social care services support people living with long-term neurological conditions. Central to the framework are aims to assist people in independent living, care planned around the needs and choices of the individual and joint working across all agencies and disciplines involved. It sets out markers of good practice that describe the services the NHS and Social Services need to provide and aims to reduce differences in the treatment, care and support people receive now, because of where they live or because of their cultural background.

Whilst these intentions may not specifically outline the social model of care, where it is recognised that barriers, prejudice and exclusion by society (purposely or inadvertently) are the ultimate factors defining who is disabled and who is not, the Framework's intention to deliver person centred care is at least aspiring to it.

The White Paper published in 2006 which outlines the NSF entitled *Our health, our care, our say: a new direction for community services* (Department of Health 2006) and government best practice guidance entitled *Now I feel tall: What a patient-led NHS feels like* (Department of Health 2005) also intimate a clear move in this direction. The Disability Discrimination Act (Office of Public Sector Information 1995) defines disability using the medical model – disabled people are defined as people with certain conditions, or certain limitations on their ability to carry out 'normal day-to-day activities. But the requirement of employers and service providers to make 'reasonable adjustments' to their policies, practices or physical aspects of their premises follows the social model. In 2006, amendments to the act called for local authorities and others to actively promote disability equality. However a survey conducted by the Social Neuropsychology Research Group at the University of Exeter (2008) commissioned by Headway, the brain injury association, exploring how people feel about their brain injuries revealed that the NSF has as yet had little impact. Indeed it showed that people with brain injuries experience disturbing levels of isolation, discrimination and prejudice. Furthermore, it revealed that discrimination is coming from social prejudice and also in the form of a lack of requisite care and attention from health, social care and other statutory agencies. In fact 60 per cent felt they had been discriminated against by one or more statutory service.

Conclusion

Within this context dramatherapy, alongside the other arts therapies, can play a significant role in celebrating the individual and in placing his/her emotional experience central to their recovery. Whilst there is arts therapy provision in the neuro-rehabilitation service in the NHS, private and voluntary sector this is usually represented by art therapists (Weston 2004). Indeed Art Therapy in Neurology, a group set up to promote an understanding of the particular issues associated with working with clients who have neurological problems was granted Special Interest Group status by British Association of Art Therapists (BAAT, www.art-therapy-in-neurology.co.uk)

in October 2002, the need for which indicates a growing awareness of the value of an arts therapy presence in these services. In the USA art therapy has been established for longer in neuro-rehabilitation treatment units. 'Neurological art therapy' is recognised as a speciality within the profession indeed the neuro art therapy certificate allows practitioners to train in the use of art to enhance cognitive functioning. However, there remains little evidence of dramatherapists working in these settings. The results of this study support the case for further incorporation and development of this therapy in the acute rehabilitation setting and exploration into how it might impact on longer-term coping and adaptation. In particular it illustrates that a personalised space within the rehabilitation setting, play as a form of therapy and the use of dramatherapy to examine intra-personal psychological processes, can be important for patients' well-being, empowerment and self-esteem and can enhance the success of their recovery.

6 Expanding the frame: self-portrait photography in dramatherapy with a young adult living with cancer

Lindsay Chipman

Box 6.1

Questions about practice

- How can self-portrait photography be useful to clients undergoing cancer treatment?
- What forms of social exclusion affect people with cancer?
- What role can embodiment and witnessing play in dramatherapy?

Research perspective

- Case study
- Taxonomy of roles as assessment
- The core processes as evaluation

Client perspective sample

'Being (or, striving to be) "self-sufficient" can have its downsides. Especially when time is not on your side . . . constantly ticking, not stopping to allow one to stop think and then react with composure – or better yet, see the consequences of her decisions . . . so she can make the *perfect* choices "this time around". *no* margin for error . . . tick tick tick – make up your mind, move along . . . – *no* margin for error . . . tick tick tick' (Gaïa).

Introduction

Photography has had a long history as an adjunct to verbal therapies, but very few references exist to its use in dramatherapy. This chapter will examine the use of self-portrait photography in the context of dramatherapy clinical practice, working with a young woman diagnosed with Stage II breast cancer.

The client was seen on an ongoing weekly basis over a one-and-a-half-year period in private practice, having been referred by a non-profit organisation working within a major Canadian hospital. Clinically, the individual approach centred on processes of role play, embodiment, self-portrait photography and witnessing. Similar to the methodology called *Photo-Theatre of the Self* as developed by British photographer Jo Spence (Martin 2001; Spence 1988; Spence 1995; Spence and Martin 1988) this process addressed issues of identity, powerlessness and changing social relationships. Since Spence's auto-photography process was done outside of any formal counselling context, this case example will illustrate how self-portrait photography can be applied to key dramatherapy theories in a formal counselling context (Chipman 2009). Also addressed will be relevant ethical, legal and clinical issues that may arise when using photography in a therapeutic context. Clinical issues such as shifts in self-identity, interpersonal conflicts, living with serious illness,and management of depression and anxiety will be explored.

Case study: Gaïa

Contexts

Reason for referral, cultural background, family and diagnostic history

For the purposes of this case study, the client will be referred to as Gaïa, and is a 32-year-old young woman diagnosed with Stage II breast cancer. Gaïa is from a Haitian background, born in the United States to her birth family, but raised by a French Canadian adoptive family beginning in early childhood. Her diagnosis was given at the end of December and her treatment began with an axillary node dissection, which was performed during the following January to remove a lump in her breast. Gaïa also underwent fertility preservation, consisting of in vitro maturation and vitrification of ovules, costing upwards of 2,000 Canadian dollars. Cancer treatments often cause infertility, a gamble Gaïa was unwilling to take despite financial constraints. Gaïa began chemotherapy in March during which she had a regimen of prescription medications, self-administered injections and blood transfusions. She terminated chemotherapy in August and began radiation treatments at that time. She had a total of 25 radiation treatments that occurred once a day, completing this portion of her treatment in October. The end of December of the same year marked the end of her treatment with a PET/CT scan to assess the treatment results. She was given her results in January, which indicated that she was in remission.

This referral came from a non-profit organisation within a hospital in a major Canadian city with a mandate to provide free psychosocial, practical and humanitarian support for cancer patients and their families, and is committed to the offering of compassionate care and understanding to enrich the lives of cancer patients during their treatment process. I had met Gaïa in a Creative Arts Therapies (CAT) support group that I co-facilitated with a social worker from the above-mentioned non-profit organisation within the hospital. Gaïa's first session occurred only a couple days after her initial diagnosis and prior to any treatment interventions. Gaïa's own personal interest in self-portrait photography and self-initiated artistic practices influenced her request for individual support outside of the hospital. As my expertise had been in the use of self-portrait photography in dramatherapy and Gaïa had already been involved in auto-documentary projects, the fit of approach was extremely relevant. The case study portion of this chapter will focus solely on the therapeutic interventions of the individual dramatherapy within private practice.

Relation to other disciplines of education, psychology, and/or medicine

Because of the special medical and psychological needs of young adults with cancer, a multidisciplinary clinic was created for young adults with cancer at the referring hospital. This larger team consists of specialised medical and mental health professionals sensitive to the unique treatment, research and support aspects of young adults and cancer. Several free supportive psychosocial programs are available to young adults with cancer at this hospital, many of which incorporate action in their interventions. Public lectures are made available to patients, families, friends and the community at large in order to provide relevant and accurate information about the multi-faceted effects and treatments of various types of cancer. This forum also allows for patients to educate medical, mental and support staff about patient experience. Gaïa actively participated in many of these free services and used them in concurrence with one another to achieve a sense of overall community support. She used psychosocial and educational hospital services, individual dramatherapy in private practice and personal artistic projects in conjunction, desiring a holistic approach to her healing and health.

Relationship between clients' needs and experience of therapy

Young adults living with cancer face particular challenges specific to their developmental life-stages and various cancer diagnoses. Young adult patients living with cancer are presented with unique developmental tasks and psychological and relational stressors. According to Thomas, O'Brien, Senner, Treadgold and Young (2006) the specific developmental tasks of individuals aged 18–25 and 26–30 are:

- developing physical and sexual maturity
- acquiring skills for adult roles
- increasing autonomy
- furthering education

- realigning and developing social relationships with members of both genders
- developing social skills through peer oriented interaction
- developing self-image
- life planning
- pursuit of career.

Cancer can interrupt or disrupt many of these processes, lending adversity to many young adults diagnosed with cancer.

Gaïa had been involved in a long-term relationship and the pursuit of a career prior to diagnosis. Once faced with the life-altering series of treatments, both of these aspects of her life were challenged. Prior to Gaïa's diagnosis, she had started a part-time employment as a receptionist. She was diagnosed with cancer one week after having begun her new job. Gaïa was eligible for 12 weeks unemployment insurance as of January 2007, but because of a six week processing delay for disability insurance, she only received this money in May 2007, leaving her struggling financially for several months. During this delay, she also applied for welfare (social assistance), which was also only granted in May of 2007. Because Gaïa was from a single-income household after the dissolution of her long-term relationship with her live-in boyfriend shortly after diagnosis, having cancer became not only a physical struggle, but also a financial one. At the age of 32, leaving her family home several years prior to her illness, Gaïa had been enjoying her independence and sense of autonomy. With cancer, she was forced to rely more on others, this being especially difficult when needing financial and emotional support from her parents.

The concept of loss when faced with life-threatening illness is one that impacts multiple aspects of an individual's functioning. According to Sourkes, loss can be 'conceptualised along three intersecting axes: loss of control, loss of identity and loss of relationships' (1982: 31). Similarly, Miedema, Hamilton and Easley (2007) identify issues relating to loss of control and transformation of identity in their grounded-theory research based on interviews with young adults diagnosed with cancer. Gaïa spoke consistently about her overwhelming need for control. She described feeling the need to structure and organise everything from the physical, such as appointments and treatments, to emotional expression, like the amount of time allowed for crying. Several aspects of her experience of living with cancer created the sense of a loss of control over body, self-identity, and personal relationships. This was a huge source of anxiety, sadness, and personal chaos for Gaïa, as she had to seek a way to conceptualise, organise, and externalise these multiple losses. Not only did she need to mourn what was in the past, she needed to find a way to conceptualise her present and continually transforming sense of self. Reaching out to her parents for emotional and financial support caused a shift in the parent–child dynamic within the family. Because of the assumed independence of being a young adult, it was difficult for Gaïa to shift to a position of greater dependence on her friends and family. Consequently, some relationships grew stronger and others dissolved. Sourkes (1982) and Miedema *et al.* (2007) reflect on how living with a life-threatening illness can impart a sense of isolation, where patients feel their lived experience makes them 'different' from their peers. Gaïa felt limited physically due to the effects of her cancer treatments, emotionally because of her lived experience and socially since she became financially restricted. All of these factors contributed to potential moments of social exclusion, isolation, and loneliness. The gravitation towards an action-based approach to therapy is not at all surprising for this population. Once again, both Sourkes and Miedema *et al.* underscore the importance of action in effective coping skills when dealing with life-threatening illness.

Description of the work

The first sessions

The first four sessions focused on gathering information regarding personal history, family history, relationship history, past psychological interventions, previous mental health issues, current medical condition and psychological functioning, present stressors, creative coping skills, support systems and therapeutic goals. Prior to any photographic work within the dramatherapy sessions, both client and therapist signed consent for photographing, video-taping, and audio-taping during therapy form. Other forms such as informed consent and fee/cancellation policy were also agreed upon prior to commencement. Since working with self-portrait photographs in therapy presents both legal and ethical concerns in terms of confidentiality, copyright, record keeping, informed consent and professional liability proper research and establishment of procedures for private practice were in place *prior* to interventions. As emphasised by Weiser (1986) it is important for those interested in this type of methodology to engage in the necessary research, protecting both themselves and their clients when using photographic representation in a therapy context.

Therapeutic goals included the creative expression of Gaïa's changing self-identity, the management of the emotional aspect of living with cancer, stress reduction and continuance of personal relationships. Therapeutic goals that specifically pertained to the dramatherapeutic approach were the externalisation of personal conflicts, the transformation of self-identity through role exploration and the development of self-awareness through embodiment. Witnessing was a core process throughout all therapeutic objectives and was the perceived route to change. All therapeutic goals were set by both therapist and client, addressing the expansion of her creativity and spontaneity when dealing with adversity and unexpected change. Since Gaïa's diagnosis, she identified multiple financial, emotional and relational stressors, which meant she had to re-evaluate her lifestyle and how the elements contributed to her illness and ultimate recovery. This re-evaluation of her lifestyle also called into question aspects of identity. Wanting to be an active participant in her treatment and recovery, Gaïa sought ways to visually represent, narrate and record her experiences. At the time of her entry into individual therapy, Gaïa had been working with a local professional photographer on a documentary project about her living with cancer. Photography had always been a medium of interest to Gaïa; it also became an obstacle for her to overcome while having cancer, especially in terms of redefining her body image and concept of beauty. Because of several factors such as age, interests and intensity of approach, there existed a very strong therapeutic alliance. This positive alliance would also become apparent in Gaïa's frequently expressed wish for a personal friendship. She was constantly aware of restrictions in terms of contact outside of the therapeutic context, but Gaïa would continue to fantasise about social situations where we could enjoy each other's friendship. It was clear to Gaïa and myself that our 'real relationship' was healthy, that we both were able to have reasonable and appropriate wishes and interactions with one another (Weiner 1998: 198). Just as important as our 'real relationship' was the respect of the boundaries of our relationship and our 'working alliance', which was clearly reflected in Gaïa's acknowledgement and respect of the limitations of our relationship outside the therapeutic context (1998: 200).

Landy's (1993) taxonomy of roles is a standard method of assessment I use in my private practice. Having based much of my methodology on the Photo Theatre of the Self work by Spence (1995) and role theory, my emphasis on the aspect of roles in identity formation was paramount. These roles would serve as the basis for later work using self-portrait photography in dramatherapy. I would also use this assessment throughout the therapeutic process in order to evaluate progress and change. In session three, Landy's role assessment highlighted several key roles, which contributed to Gaïa's stress around self-identity. There existed difficulty with 'living with ambivalence' between contradictory roles of seeing self as 'beauty/hero' and not being the 'sick person' (Landy 1993). She had intertwined her own perceptions with those of others, becoming confused when trying to identify personal versus socially held beliefs (1993). The role of 'mother' was also identified as significant, but at this time in the process little focus was placed on her relationship with this role, but later in the process, the 'mother' role became central to the work, as this role symbolised multiple experiences of loss.

Developing work

Frequent cancellations and rescheduling occurred during this time, as Gaïa was in the crux of her chemotherapy treatments, often becoming ill, exhausted and physically overwhelmed. In the following sessions, my intention was to situate the roles from her assessment within the body, developing her mind/body awareness and exploring the physical sensations associated with her sense of self. Use of *mirroring techniques* simultaneously drew awareness to her body and its relationship to me as therapist (Emunah 1994: 150–154). Many issues regarding body image arose, especially around physical limitations due to side effects from cancer treatments, these occurring often in comparison to me. I often felt as though I was the mirror of what she had physically lost (flexibility, ease of movement, hair, slim, etc.) and when this was reflected to her, she had a 'flash' of how she wanted to construct her image of the 'sick person' in the upcoming session.

Session 8 marked the first photographic session, where Gaïa was assigned homework of finding costumes, props and music. Self-portrait photography sessions were structured with me in the role of therapist/photographer and Gaïa in the role of sitter/client. Prior to the Gaïa arriving, I would prepare and design a mini-lighting studio in the therapy space with backdrop, tungsten lighting, and digital camera equipment. Initially there would be a warm-up to music chosen by Gaïa. This music would always be associated with the role being explored in the photographs. Gaïa would dance and sing to the music while changing into costume and setting up props. I would act as witness to this process, awaiting her to step onto the backdrop. Once Gaïa was ready, she would begin posing for photographs. I would reflect to her what I was seeing and she would give me feedback regarding how she was feeling in the role and in her body. Based on this feedback, I would make framing and artistic choices, aimed at re-creating the emotional state she was describing. Once photographs were taken, she would de-role by a similar process to her warm-up, whereby she would dance and sing while removing costume, putting away props and setting the room back up as an office. As therapist, I would participate in the de-rolement, transitioning back from the role of photographer to that of therapist. This occurred through mirroring of her dancing, often having us create a dance around the clean-up.

Every self-portrait photography session would then be followed by a session devoted entirely to the witnessing of images. No alteration of the digital images was done prior to sharing them with Gaïa, as it was important that the client be the director of the photographs. Gaïa gave titling and verbal feedback as she viewed images. Most of the time she would sit, quietly ensconced in the visual display. As Weiser emphasises, significant time should be devoted to the viewing and processing of images, as this seemingly quotidian activity often becomes emotionally charged (1986, 1999). This session coincided with a decline in health and the day after her 32nd birthday. Several of the images made her feel uncomfortable, having had to surrender some degree of control to me as photographer to interpret her experience. Some of the pictures had her confront aspects of her health that she had not yet accepted, such as weight gain and alopecia. Ultimately, she began to redefine her sense of being 'beauty' and how to live with the contradictory nature of this role and 'sick person' (see Figure 6.1). She quickly saw the 'beauty' in the pictures when what she initially saw was the 'sick person', ultimately indicative of the adaptation of her role system.

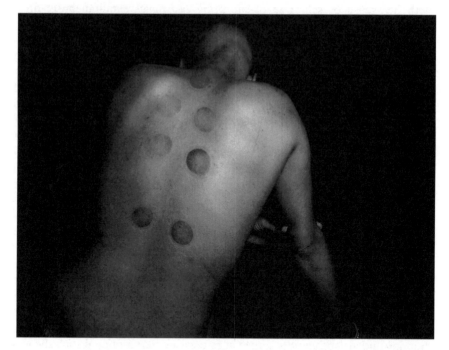

Figure 6.1 Self-portrait of Gaïa in the role of 'sick person' (2007) Lindsay Chipman.

The sessions that followed marked a decline in Gaïa's health and sub-sequently in her attendance. Four sessions in a row were cancelled, culminating in her fearing that I would interpret her absence as a dismissal. This period in therapy marked the emergence of themes of abandonment, mostly a projection stemming from Gaïa's tumultuous childhood, rejection by her birth mother and having been left by her boyfriend. Traditionally Gaïa functioned as an independent person, never relying on others, preferring to be her own support. Asking me for help became an obstacle, bringing in to question Gaïa's own fears of abandonment. She openly questioned whether she was a burden to me and whether or not I would grow tired of her, eventually forced to leave. Further photographs were delayed at this point as issues of abandonment and social exclusion became paramount. The above themes related primarily to the role of mother, especially in how she wanted to define herself in the future. Along with this exploration came sadness and apprehension when confronted with the possibility of being infertile. Struggle existed when thinking and acting on and engaging in romantic relationships, having been disappointed in the past when her boyfriend left at her diagnosis. Health-related constraints forced her to remain at home, often feeling too ill to attend weekly sessions.

There was a gap of two months where Gaïa cancelled several appointments and ceased to call to make new appointments. Leaving her the space to decide how she wanted to cope with her ongoing treatments, I did not call her to schedule sessions. The New Year and her notice of remission marked her return to individual dramatherapy and a new phase in her process with cancer. Gaïa re-appeared as if she had never lost contact, and was very distraught with her current life situation. She was in remission and felt unsure of her self-identity and future direction. Cancer had been her life's purpose and now that it was gone, she was mourning the structure and purpose it brought to her life. She was paralysed by fear, rarely leaving her home and recoiling from social situations. She experienced sleeping and eating disturbances, as well as symptoms of panic, anxiety and depression. Gaïa described feeling anxious, fearful, lost and as having a negative body image. I returned to the role assessment used at the beginning of the therapeutic process and found that the roles with which she felt conflicted were synonymous with the feelings she described: 'lost one', 'coward', 'worrier', 'mother', 'wife', and 'beauty'. Even though mother and beauty in the past had positive associations, they were now infused with panic, fear, sadness and anxiety. Many of these roles pertained to future direction and the apprehension that they would go unrealised.

After the role assessment and in the following session, Gaïa was alive with energy, which was a significant shift from the previous session where she was meek, anxious and quiet. Gaïa spent the week brainstorming ways to represent the place in which she now found herself, seeking that creative externalisation of her internally held state. She arrived at session 15 ready for another photo shoot. Again keeping with the previous structure of the self-portrait photography sessions, Gaïa began her warm-up and process of enrolment with me as witness. Relying less on the formal lighting studio, Gaïa moved about the room freely, creating an embodied narrative of the story she wished to tell (see Figures 2, 3, 4). In the session that followed, prior to viewing any photographs, Gaïa came with a list of words that kept reoccurring for her throughout the week while reflecting on the self-portraits. She listed to me all that had been running through her head 'fear, success, failure, expectations, normalcy, decisions, choices, obstacles, limits (who set them and what they are), capacity, finances, conventionalism, procrastination, sense of/meaning of my procrastination and self-sabotage'. Once again she was quietly engaged when viewing photographs and processed her emotional responses to them by titling images as they flashed on the computer screen. Many of her initial responses to images were in terms of body image but as she deepened her witnessing, she began to create the narrative of the woman in the pictures. A couple days later Gaïa sent me an email of the story of those images:

> She lived in a relatively simple world . . . or so she thought. How could it be? She went through something difficult with her head held high, inhaling faith and exhaling fear. Yet, when she finally ended up seeing the light 'at the end of the tunnel' she found herself LOST!!! Blinded by the light

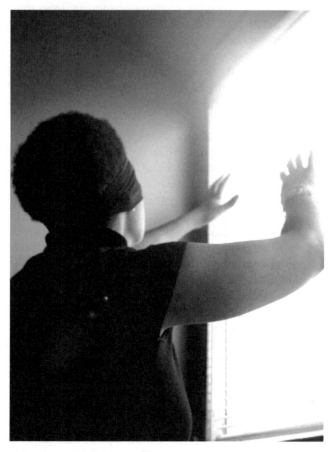

Figure 6.2 Self-portrait of Gaïa in the role of 'lost' (2008) Lindsay Chipman.

... or is it blindsighted? Caught by surprise ... unaware that this light would lead to so many questions, so many choices, so much insecurity. So much pressure from others (expectations/inquiries/desire to help) as well as self-imposed ... desire to please, to have answers, 'whip' back into shape ... to lead a 'NORMAL' life. Well equipped with fool-proof, multipurpose tools – her personal strengths (humor, determination, self-assessment), her support system's strengths (love, understanding, availability) – but not knowing what to do with them or maybe simply not how to use them to her advantage. Being (or, striving to be) 'self-sufficient' can have its downsides. Especially when time is not on your side ... constantly ticking, not stopping to allow one to stop think and then react with composure – or better yet, see the consequences of her decisions ... so she can make the PERFECT choices 'this time around'. NO margin for error ... tick tick tick – make up your mind, move along ... – NO margin for error ... tick tick tick – make those choices, come

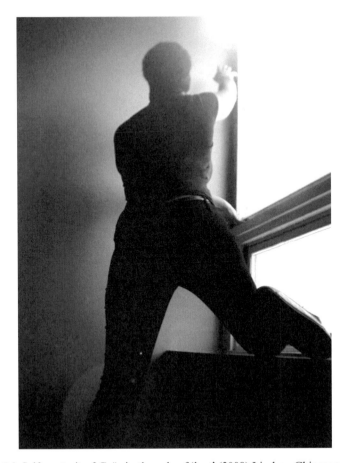

Figure 6.3 Self-portrait of Gaïa in the role of 'lost' (2008) Lindsay Chipman.

on now . . . – No margin for error . . . tick tick tick – so, what's new? Well I'm reaching for perfection . . . not allowed to make 'mistakes' 'this time around' – NO margin for error . . . tick tick tick. Truth is, I know I should just DO THE BEST I CAN . . . that's enough FOR EVERYONE . . . mistake = trying = making a valiant effort = OK = experience to learn from . . . but I feel like my back is against the wall . . . like I'm trapped . . . at the very edge of the ledge . . . what is my next step and where will it lead me???

The following session marked a huge change in Gaïa's behavior, motivation, and emotional outlook. She would come in motivated, excited about life, moving forward in the everyday when in past weeks she was unable to even think about day-to-day tasks. She applied for several jobs and began to feel hopeful about the future with little anxiety about making 'mistakes' or

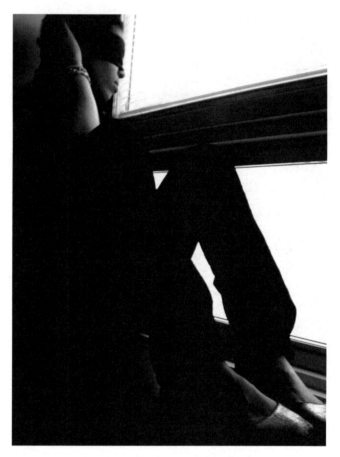

Figure 6.4 Self-portrait of Gaïa in the role of 'lost' (2008) Lindsay Chipman.

doing life 'perfectly this time around'. She described the previous series of photographs as helping her:

> Unscramble the thoughts in my head. It made me realize/accept/own the angst that I felt towards the 'what now' phase I felt stuck in. I realized I found myself using the expression 'this time around' a lot as if I were starting over instead of continuing. That may be what brought on the pressure I was putting on myself. I felt like I needed to start over and MAKE SURE I do things right, no, PERFECTLY . . . Coming to that realization and voicing it made me realise I was putting WAY MORE pressure on myself than I needed to. Mistakes, challenges are all part of life they build what we call experience . . . I am also very grateful as I realized that, BEFORE making the same mistake of letting stress and fear consume me . . . AGAIN!!! Cancer has made me a better person, not in the sense that I wasn't a good person before. It's more like I am a

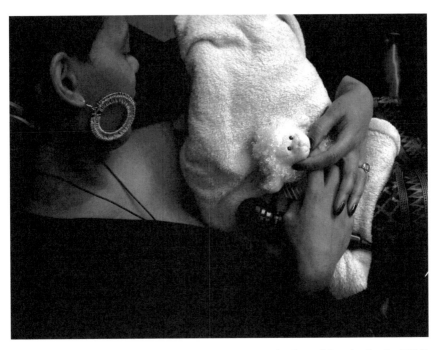

Figure 6.5 Self-portrait of Gaïa exploring future projection of 'mother' role (2008) Lindsay Chipman.

better person towards myself. I have decided to make decisions according to what makes ME happy and treat MYSELF in the same kind, caring, compassionate way as I have always treated others.

Despite Gaïa's improvement she continued to have anxiety regarding her future and said to me that 'I need to stop reaching for the impossible and I need to be reaching for acceptance'. The following sessions focused on exploring a 'future projection' self-portrait (see Figure 6.5). I felt that it was important for Gaïa to witness what the future 'could' look like, to serve as a landmark on her journey towards her goals. Before we were able to start these self-portraits, Gaïa had her anniversary of her first day in chemotherapy and exhibited phantom symptoms of being in active treatment. She cancelled due to feeling nauseous, exhausted and unable to leave her house. Session 20 was the photo shoot of the 'future projection' image. Gaïa showed up late but was full of energy, self-confidence, joy, and spontaneity, quite contrary to her emotional state when discussing her future. She was playful while embodying the 'mother' role, giving herself complete permission to fully experience the things she aspired to.

Gaïa used props and costume to personify qualities and roles she wishes for herself in the future; her earrings the symbol of her creative self, the microphone as her artistic self, her dress as her femininity and sense of being a woman, a stuffed animal and baby to represent her hope for children and to be a mother, an engagement ring to signify marriage and partnership and finally her 'Care Bear' socks to detail the quality of being caring for self and others. At the end of the session she talked excitedly about new job opportunities and overall hope for the future. She agreed that her anxiety had decreased and that significant changes had occurred over the past couple sessions. Gaïa was quick to say she didn't want to forget her process with cancer and her personal obstacles, as these were now an integral aspect of her self-identity. Gaïa showed signs of growth, change and greater awareness of self and others throughout the process. She also gained coping skills for communicating her story to others and developing a greater sense of self. Despite these improvements, Gaïa continues to struggle with anxiety regarding reoccurrence of her cancer and her future directions. Her individual dramatherapy process is ongoing and continues to be an essential part in her overall maintenance of health, both physically and mentally.

Reflection on theory and method

The potential of photography in therapy

For several years psychotherapists have used photographs as tools in the therapeutic relationship (Cosden and Reynolds 1982). Cosden and Reynolds exemplify the therapeutic value of photography in therapy and as a healing practice of its own: 'if a picture is worth a thousand words, the procedures involved in taking that picture also have great value' (1982: 19). There are several key assumptions that illustrate photography's potential as a tool in therapy and that have been discussed in the current literature. The general belief that photographs represent 'truths' can be used therapeutically; Weiser addresses the potential for photographs to provide 'factual emotional information', so that a client may gain awareness for future therapeutic interventions (2004: 24). Photographs also possess the unique ability to provide information about the physical self through the creation of self-portrait images (Chipman 2009). Self-portrait images allow the client to view parts of themselves that they are usually incapable of observing and can hold more information than what is visually represented (Weiser 2004). The historical components of photographs also contribute to its efficacy in therapy. Weiser contends that 'photographs always contain stories' and that they can serve as jumping off points for discussion in counseling (2004: 23). Photography as a tool has been widely used by consumers around the world. The familiarity of photography within our social traditions makes it 'user-friendly' and easy to propose as a therapeutic intervention (2004: 32). Photography in our everyday lives is not always perceived as an art making activity, relieving clients from the stress that artistic interventions may impose on them to create 'good art' (2004). For the trained psychotherapist, counselor, or any other mental health professional, the use of photographic tools is facilitated by the evolution of automatic, disposable and digital forms of cameras (Chipman 2009). If self-portrait photography is so user-friendly and approachable as a methodology, how can we, as dramatherapists, use this medium to its fullest potential and with the clearest of intentions?

Jones' nine core processes in relation to self-portrait photography in therapy

There exist exceptional similarities between the fields of therapy that use self-portrait photography and the theoretical underpinnings found within dramatherapy. Jones' *nine core processes* define how dramatherapy is effective and therapeutic by breaking down into nine core elements that account for the therapeutic potential of drama and healing (Jones 1996: 99). Similarly, these processes have informed my assessment, evaluation, and interpretation of clients' material when using self-portrait photography in my dramatherapy practice. If we look at the *nine core processes* of Jones as a way to evaluate change in Gaïa's self-identity, social relationships, and overall sense of health, we can clearly outline how and why self-portrait photography can work within a dramatic framework and orientation. Self-portrait photographs permit dialogue between client and photograph, allowing relationships and roles to emerge and be explored. Jones describes the function of dramatic projection in dramatherapy as communication between the dramatic material and client. Gaïa was able to project her internally held sense of self and relationship with others, into the embodied image, only later to have a dialogue with the finished image. At the root of this process is the idea that the client projects their internal world into the photograph, enabling them to examine their value system, belief structure and cognitive constructs (Weiser 1999). When Gaïa viewed images of herself, she saw what she wanted to see, a projection of her internally held image. There is also a projection into the embodiment of a client, where one poses for the camera they project their internally held image of the self into a body posture for the camera to capture. This is clearly illustrated in the image created by Gaïa used to represent the role of 'sick person', where she used body posture as a way to signify her belief about this role. Not only did Gaïa project her own internally held belief about the self, she also projected her internally held social belief about how others view illness. Dialogue during the witnessing of images centred on how others perceived her as the 'sick person' and her judgement of them for doing so.

The core process of *therapeutic performance* can clearly be seen in the process by which Gaïa enrolled prior to photographs (Jones 1996: 102). Also the use of props, costume, lighting and scenework is reminiscent of those used in theatrical performances to highlight, symbolise, and elicit emotion and mood in the audience. The overall self-portrait process involved performing, directing and creating of an image similar to the devices used in dramatherapy to externalise a client's internally held situation into the creative container. Similar to Landy's role method, Gaïa went through a process of enrolment, enactment, de-rolement, and reflection (1993). Within this we could observe her movement along the distancing continuum. In Jones' terms we could also see how Gaïa used the processes of *empathy* and *distancing* as related to the roles of audience/witness and engagement within the dramatic material (1996: 104; 2007: 95). When using self-portrait photography, the client is asked to embody various roles, emotions and scenarios in front of the camera, later to disengage from the creation of the image to witness the final product. In the act of witnessing the self-portraits, Gaïa was able to distance herself from the enactment of the photograph, moving towards confronting her 'self' in the portrait. During the enactment and photographic portion of the process, Gaïa was able to explore emotional affect and resonance within the creative process. She was encouraged to address the emotional effects of engaging in the self-portrait process, later to connect these feelings to everyday life. Through the creation of photographic images, Gaïa essentially externalised aspects of her inner world, only to dialogue with these to create new meaning.

The concepts of *impersonation* and *personification* from Jones (1996: 107) are both apparent in the techniques of self-portrait photography, especially when looking at the series of images where Gaïa embodied a 'future projection'. Objects were used to represent aspects, desired qualities and future aspirations for the self. As in Jones' core process, Gaïa had used 'objects to represent material' where there was also an engagement with the imaginary (1996: 108). Gaïa's natural creativity and spontaneity were heightened through the playfulness of the medium of self-portrait photography, allowing her to challenge reality and to reconstruct this through exploration and creative mediums. This addresses Jones' notion of *playing* (1996: 115; 2007: 88), allowing clients to express themselves through metaphor and symbol. In the image of Gaïa as the future projection of 'mother', the pictures are very much about the playfulness of this role and the ability of a mother to play with their child. Gaïa was absorbed in this play, able to fully engage in the play space and treat the plastic doll as a real child. When looking at the pictures a session later, Gaïa was astounded by the 'realness' of her laughter and playfulness caught in the still image, creating dual feelings of hope and longing. *Embodiment*, also from Jones' core processes, was constantly addressed throughout sessions, and served as a therapeutic objective when outlining goals (1996: 112; 2007: 112). Because Gaïa's cancer treatments had a large impact on her body, there was always an emphasis placed on her potential of body, of exploring different identities where the self may be transformed, and examining the various influences on the body. The simple act of embodying roles and emotional states for pictures would flood Gaïa with memories, traumas, and 'mind/body' connections in relation to her living with illness.

It becomes apparent when working with self-portrait photography the integral and constant use of Jones' core process of *witnessing* (1996: 109; 2007: 101). Much of what we seek to change about ourselves in rooted in a lack of self-awareness, of not truly being able to see ourselves. Witnessing in self-portrait photography is a process that is paramount in therapeutic change where there is a development of objective self-awareness. One of the most powerful experiences can be found not in the enactment but in the witnessing of self-portrait photographs, especially when the photographer is not under our control. The unique ability of photography to provide a client with the opportunity to witness the self from multiple standpoints is exceptional. Due to the distinctive ability of photography to create an instant concrete image of a person, clients can be instantly confronted with the image of self. Witnessing the self is facilitated by photography in the fact that it allows one to witness not only the actual image of self, but also the metaphorical and symbolic representations of self. The powerful process of looking at the self worked towards Gaïa's greater self-awareness, self-reflection and self-observation tools. Not only was Gaïa able to see what she believed to be her self, she was also able to see beyond that, to the future, to her aspirations, and to different uncovered aspects of self. Because living with cancer can become all-consuming with the involvement necessary for survival, the photographs also became the witness of what she had lived. They serve as memory or narrative, as proof that she struggled, lived, and survived.

Transformation in dramatherapy has been emphasised as one of the unique abilities of this healing modality to take everyday conflicts and to reframe them in dramatic action (Jones 2007: 119). Because self-portrait photography allows for a constant re-framing of reality and self, it allows for the client to take everyday conflicts and depict them through dramatic action. The ability of dramatherapy to transform the client's identity through creative exploration as cited by Jones is mirrored in photography's ability to capture that transformation in a tangible form. We already have evidence that self-portrait photography techniques possess the ability to transform reality through projection, metaphor and symbol. Through the process of self-portrait photography, self-perception may also be transformed. Objects have been photographed to represent aspects of self, consequently transforming concrete objects into something else. Since we believe that photographs represent truths, being able to witness the self in a snapshot doing something not previously believed to be attainable, incites real-life transformation through the witnessing of this rehearsal in front of a camera lens. Gaïa was able to transcend the fiction of her self-portraits, to take this image and put it into action in the everyday. She was able to transform her personal chaos into a photo-narrative, ultimately permitting her to continue her story and move beyond her obstacles. In both traditional approaches in dramatherapy and self-portrait photography, the client is asked to reflect on how they felt in the moment and how this relates to overall interpersonal functioning. Weiser talks about the idea of 'resonance' (1999: 121) and deeply identifying with an image as being integral to the therapeutic process, paralleling Jones' core process of *life–drama connection* (1996: 117).

Self-portrait photography's use of role theory

Jones addresses role theory in terms of its origins in theatre and psychology and how it has been applied in the context of dramatherapy methodology (1996). Jones describes the function of role in dramatherapy as:

> . . . describing a fictional identity or persona which someone can assume, and is also a concept used to understand the different aspects of a client's identity in their life as a whole. Both therapist and client can take on fictional roles during the dramatherapy session.
>
> (Jones 1996: 197)

This function of role can be undertaken in several ways in the therapy session through the enactment of a fictional identity of a past, present, or future self, or of an aspect of self (Jones 2007: 193). Emotional and cognitive elements of role are integrated through both enacting roles and witnessing roles, consequently shifting the relationship between the enacted/witnessed roles and those taken in everyday life. Both Gaïa and I were role players within the session, from the concrete roles of sitter/photographer, client/photographer, to more personal roles such as sick person/healthy person. Some of these roles were explicit in nature where Gaïa and I discussed and reflected upon how we enacted, interacted, and de-roled; some being more implicit such as those where I was clearly seen as other, seeing as I had no history of living with cancer and often stood for the socially held perceptions of the larger community. Within all dramatherapy role methods there is a universal process of '1) role play, 2) de-roling, and 3) assimilation' (Jones 1996: 208). In the self-portrait photography process that I use in my private practice, clients mirror this same core movement in and out of role.

Role theory has permitted the analysis and discussion of role in dramatherapy in terms of self and identity, relationship between role and personality, and theatre and life (Jones 2007: 203–204). The functions of therapeutic use of self-portraiture can include seeking and identifying self structure, making visible inner self, encouraging self-awareness and exploring self through fantasy (Spence 1988: 185). When reflecting upon her therapeutic use of self-portraiture, Spence sees that these images can 'enable us to have a better dialogue with ourselves' (Spence and Martin 1988: 3). Ultimately this demonstrates how self-portrait photography can be used to support interpersonal communication between inner structures of identity. Similar to the *photo-theatre of self* methodology of Spence and Martin, collaboration, play and self-portrait photographic practices, Gaïa was able to re-frame and re-integrate aspects of self and other into her everyday functioning. Gaïa experienced a shift in perception that speaks to the potential change that occurs through enactment and the communication of internal structures through external representation of Jones' definition of the therapeutic value in role theory (1996; 2007).

Reflections on the experience of clients

As Gaïa and I had always worked photographically, it became only natural to review the process and our relationship in the same fashion. After having been asked to reflect upon her therapeutic journey, the moments that stood out for her, and how our relationship worked within the process, Gaïa came to session 20 with a photograph she wished to create. Figure 6.6 represents the metaphorical and symbolic composite of all I asked Gaïa to reflect upon. This was the first time Gaïa chose to include me in her picture, illustrating how she viewed our relationship as integral in her growth and change.

As described by Gaïa, this photograph was a metaphor for our relationship and how this process had helped her. The metaphor centered on me giving her the tools (keys) and support (hand reaching out) to figure out her issues (lock in Gaïa's hand). She also described the position of her hand as open and ready to receive, which was generally her style in therapy. After this picture was taken, Gaïa commented on how she had changed, not just from having

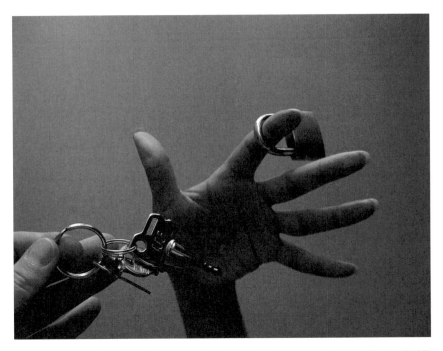

Figure 6.6 Portrait of the therapeutic relationship as perceived by Gaïa (2008) Lindsay Chipman.

cancer but also through the therapeutic process. She reflected on her relationship with the 'unknowns' of life such as her illness, having moved from a place of 'fear' to a place of 'trust'.

Conclusion

There exist similar processes between dramatherapy and self-portrait photography in terms of Jones' *nine core processes* (1996, 2007). At the root of both is a foundation built upon comparable principles, ultimately permitting self-portrait photographic techniques to be analysed in terms of their relevancy to elements found within dramatherapy (Chipman 2009). Despite difference in modality of communication, of theatre and photography both, nonetheless, fulfill aspects of the theatrical, audience and actor witnessing, story, role, and transformation (Chipman 2009). Hopefully this chapter will serve to inspire dramatherapists' intentional integration of self-portrait photography into their clinical practices. Since self-portrait photography is not part of dramatherapy training and since dramatherpaists do not necessarily have an awareness of the legal and ethical implications of such a medium; this section is a vital part of photography in dramatherapy, and definitely requires serious reflection and research *prior* to engaging in any self-portrait photographic techniques. More training and research is necessary regarding the employment of photography in dramatherapy, giving clinicians clear guidelines and confidence when using these techniques therapeutically (Chipman 2009).

Hopefully this case study will help inspire dramatherapists to explore the potential use of photography in clinical practice, providing greater awareness of its function within key dramatherapy processes. If anything is to be learned, it is that self-portrait photography is a very powerful technique with the potential for serious counter-therapeutic, ethical and legal, ramifications for both client and therapist (Weiser 1986). There exists a very seductive quality about self-portrait photography in therapy, facilitating its appropriation by other professions in mental health. Despite the cautions, it would be of great benefit to incorporate this powerful approach into dramatherapy training and theory. As I have previously stated, 'A picture is worth a thousand words, creating a plethora of narratives, with which clients may begin to re-story and re-frame their self-identity and their overall journey in life' (Chipman 2009: 72).

Specific Ethics Statement

Prior to publication, release forms were signed by the client giving consent to publish information gleaned from interviews and photographs for the purpose of peer reviewed journals and books, and to be used for conference/ lecture presentations. A detailed list of photographs was released for print with written consent from the client, to be specifically reproduced in the above chapter. All names, locations, and identifying information has been changed or omitted to protect the confidentiality of the client. The clinical practice and written content of this chapter is in line with the ethical standards of practice as outlined by the Canadian Counselling Association (CCA), the National Association of Drama Therapy (NADT), and the Art Therapy Association of Quebec (AATQ).

7 Dramatherapy with adolescents living with HIV: story making, drama and body mapping

Kirsten Meyer

Box 7.1

Questions about practice

- What does it mean to be a teenager in search of independence and to be living with HIV but having nowhere to speak about it?
- How does a society's political and cultural attitudes relate to the dramatherapy space?
- What issues arise in multi-agency work?

Research perspective

- Evidence gathering within a dramatherapy pilot context
- Use of written and verbal evaluation formats

Client perspective sample

How did drama help you?

- 'To have trust in the group and know how everyone is living with HIV-AIDS.'
- 'To keep secrets with other people and share feelings.'
- 'Being a gangster doesn't help.'
- 'It helped me open up, because some of the things we did had a lot to do with my experiences, like putting my personal feelings on the body map.'

(Group evaluation)

Introduction

What does it mean to be a teenager in search of independence and to be living with HIV but having nowhere to speak about it? What does it mean for the future of our country if we do not create spaces everywhere for our youth to be talking about it?

My country, South Africa, is but a teenager. We became a democracy 14 years ago and with it came freedom, excitement, hope and responsibility. And like a teenager we are faced with the same hopes and excitement, but also with feelings of loss, alienation and confusion. It is as if my country is aching to speak but does not know how. In a country with a history of unspeakable atrocities, human rights abuses, injustices, secrets, violence and imposed voicelessness, we have emerged into the twenty-first century with another kind of voicelessness: HIV. This is a secret that feels unspeakable for many, as having HIV is perceived as shameful, as if having the virus were confirmation of having done something really bad or sinful. When the weight of this secret becomes unbearable it seems difficult to find appropriate places to voice it.

And so, like a teenager, we are indeed struggling to find our identity and our voice.

Having emerged out of hundreds of years of imposed voicelessness, and finally finding a democratic voice, we find ourselves silenced yet again.

Contexts

When, on 11 February 1990, Nelson Mandela was released from prison after 28 years of imprisonment, he 'set into motion a wave of change that was to sweep over South Africa and give hope to millions of blacks who suffered under oppression' (Barbarin and Richter 2001: 1). His release signalled the beginning of significant political change and hope. Children born at this time 'symbolised the beginning of an era in which the nation would cherish its children irrespective of language, culture, or skin colour' (2001: 1). With the political changes that gave birth to a new democracy, our so called 'rainbow nation' was faced (and still is) with many complex social problems. Poverty, violence, lack of adequate medical care for all and an increase in HIV infection became the shadow of the hope of the 'New South Africa'. Never before was there a more important time to consider South Africa's children and what their future might hold. These children, born in 1994, are now adolescents and we are forced to ask if indeed we have failed them.

Like the political system, the health system has also seen significant changes; however, policy has been slow to transform into actual relief and access to all those in need. Most significantly, more government grants have been made available to those with disability, single-parent families and child-headed households. South Africa does not have a national health care system. The majority of South Africans seek medical care from major government clinics when in need. For those who can afford private medical health care and insurance the landscape is somewhat different. For most of the population, seeking health care means standing in long queues or visits to clinics in rural areas, sometimes a few hours' walk away. Steinberg, in researching the success of an antiretroviral project in the rural area of Lusikisiki in South Africa, highlights the challenges of access to health care in villages like this:

> A person who falls ill with AIDS in a poor African village is more likely to be attended to by a single nurse. She is treating dozens of cases every day, trying desperately to manage her workload. If one of her patients should fall ill with TB or pneumonia, will the drugs he needs find their way to the nurses' shelves? And if he requires intensive care, is there a hospital close by, one not so swamped by the epidemic's casualties that it has a bed for him to lie in and the spirit and the means to care for him?
>
> (Steinberg 2008: 83)

Possibly one of the most controversial legacies of the African National Congress (ANC) government is that it remained silent around HIV for far too long. Steinberg indicates the relationship between political power, denial and its impact on the response to HIV and the lives and deaths of people in South Africa:

> A new democracy is an era of resurging life. Sex is the most life giving of activities. That a new nation's citizens are dying from sex seems to be an attack on both the ordinary people's and a nation's generative capacities, an insult too ghastly to stomach. AIDS has given rise to accusation. Nowhere is this more evident that in the politics of South Africa's president, Thabo Mbeki, who questioned with bitterness whether the dying was caused by a sexually transmitted virus after all, and who asked caustically whether antiretroviral drugs were for the benefit of Africans or pharmaceutical companies.
>
> (Steinberg 2008: 6)

With this initial denial much of the work done in the HIV and AIDS context has been by non-government organisations, doctors who independently set up programmes, HIV activists and various health care workers. Beginning to move out of denial, but with some scepticism, in 2000 the Minister of Health released the 2000–2005 National Strategic Plan. This brought with it some achievements but not enough. (NSP 2007) During these five years there was no evidence to show that there had been a significant change in the prevalence of HIV. Realising what the devastating impact to the South African society. In 2003 the Government approved the National Operational Plan for Comprehensive HIV and AIDS Care, Management, and Treatment (CCMT). This meant that antiretroviral treatment became available at government hospitals and clinics. The roll out and implementation of the plan proved more difficult than expected (Steinberg 2008).

So within this broad context, what are the challenges facing our children and young people infected and affected by HIV? Steinberg frames the challenge in the following way: 'An epidemic that kills young adults in droves spawns difficult politics. How does a society absorb the death of its young? Whom does it blame?' (2008: 6).

According to the Department of Health (NSP 2007) South Africa has approximately seven million people in a population of 46 million who are HIV positive. Two million of these are said to be children and adolescents. However, South African social scientists are still struggling to accurately estimate the extent of the impact on children in the country (Higson-Smith *et al.* 2006). Gender also plays a role with women and girls being the most disproportionately affected: 55 per cent of HIV infected people (NSP 2007). In general much has been done since 1994 to address, at a policy level, the needs of children and young people in South Africa (Barbarin and Richter 2001). As with other HIV policies put into place, those concerning the policies around children have also not proven easy to implement.

The 65th clause of the United Nations General Assembly resolution on HIV and Aids stated that by 2005 member states will:

> Develop and . . . implement national policies and strategies to build and strengthen governmental, family and community capacities to provide a supportive environment for orphans and girls and boys infected and affected by HIV/Aids, including by providing appropriate counselling and psychosocial support, ensuring their enrolment in school and access to shelter, good nutrition and health and social services on an equal basis with other children; and protect orphans and vulnerable children from all forms of abuse, violence, exploitation, discrimination, trafficking and loss of inheritance.
>
> (United Nations 2001: 29)

In 2005, and in line with the international agreement, the South African government prepared the National Action Plan for Orphans and other Children made Vulnerable by HIV and Aids (South African National Department of Social Development 2005). This action plan calls for the implementation and evaluation of psychosocial models/programmes that offer care and support to vulnerable children, that can be 'scaled up to reach a much larger population group' (Higson-Smith *et al.* 2006: 4). Children and adolescents in South Africa infected or affected by HIV and Aids face many and varied challenges. Richter (2004 in Higson-Smith *et al.* 2006) provides a summary of eight ways in which HIV/Aids will impact upon children:

1   Poverty: with death and disability many families will become poorer as

they will lose the capacity to earn. As parents die, so children will lose their homes and access to family assets.

2   Dislocation: as families migrate and seek work, or return to their original communities to die, so will children be dislocated.
3   Family structure: many families will experience changes to their original structure. As parents of children die, many children will experience a change in the role of their caregivers. Many children will have grand-parents as their primary caregivers, who may be less able to respond to their needs. In some cases older siblings (mainly girls) may head up households.
4   Added responsibilities: many children will be forced to take on more adult responsibilities inside the home and outside.
5   School attendance: there is a strong likelihood that children will leave school early, thus impacting on the general level of education.
6   Neglect: many children will be less cared for and as a result become more vulnerable to abuse, illness and malnutrition.
7   HIV: with less adult care, many children will become more vulnerable to HIV infection through abuse and early sexual experiences.
8   Loss and bereavement: the impact of multiple deaths and losses will affect the emotional and psychosocial well-being of many children.

In this chapter I wish to demonstrate, by focusing on a dramatherapy group run with ten HIV positive teenagers, how the stigma of living with HIV can result in the unbearable weight of holding a secret, which has emotional and psychosocial consequences. Recent research has focused on the psycho-social needs of children made vulnerable by HIV/AIDS (Richter 2004) but what about our teenagers and their specific developmental needs? How do they begin to negotiate the independence that they are in search of whilst holding this 'secret'? How do we as a nation, who collectively hold this secret, face up to the reality of how living with HIV affects the needs of adolescents, our future generation? As Steinberg says 'when the history of this great epidemic is written, will it be said that an untold number of people died, not because the plague was unstoppable, but because they were mortally ashamed? Will it be said that several successive generations of southern Africans were decimated by a sense of disgrace?' (Steinberg 2008: 2).

How do we as a nation begin to find a voice to speak about this 'shame'? We need far reaching and diverse interventions. Dramatherapy may be one such intervention: however, working in the context outlined previously provides the dramatherapist with various challenges:

- as a new and developing profession there are, as yet, no public health system arts therapy posts
- major socio-economic and political challenges
- stigma and shame that surround HIV

- the psychosocial challenges for people living with HIV demands multi-disciplinary teamwork
- lack of funding
- lack of governmental organisational support and structure
- direct dramatherapy interventions are considered too expensive and not wide reaching enough
- arts therapy skills shortage, and African language barriers.

How then can dramatherapy be one way of providing a safe space for the expression of shame and fear using peer group interaction? Through the use of processes like role play, embodiment and body mapping, I will show how the group was able to express and explore feelings around being adolescents and living with HIV. While the dramatherapy space helped the group find a voice within the sessions, this voice was fragile and was silenced in the group time and again. The more important question is; did it necessarily help the adolescents find a voice outside the group?

Despite the therapeutic effects evident in the sessions, this chapter raises further questions: finding a voice within a dramatherapy session does not necessarily mean finding a voice in society, especially when that voice is deeply buried. What happens when that newly found voice is silenced? What does it mean when a nation cannot speak and is traumatised? Is it helpful then to provide a space that is in conflict with the social context? Or is that our challenge as therapists? Should we be working with teenagers in isolation? What about their caregivers and wider community? What about the stage of adolescence, do they not need space to do the work of adolescence? What does it mean to be living with HIV and negotiating this important life-stage? We are indeed left with more questions than answers when it comes to seeking appropriate psychosocial interventions to meet the needs of our children and adolescents. Furthermore, dramatherapy has its roots within Western European and North American cultures; if there is no connection with South African cultures how appropriate is this form of intervention?

I have been running dramatherapy groups over the past five years with HIV positive children and adolescents, in collaboration with an HIV focused NGO at a hospital in South Africa. Interestingly, despite the perceived success of the groups, the ongoing momentum needed to sustain a programme like this has been lacking. There is a continual high turnover of staff within the NGO, whose working conditions are very demanding. Up until recently, the majority of HIV work being done in SA has been by NGOs. Like many HIV programmes, there is a strong emphasis on getting the statistics right each month. Funders want to see impact on numbers and they want roll out. As a result, many projects are quite thin and lack depth, thought and ongoing monitoring and evaluation. All of this is to the detriment of qualitative psychosocial programmes. At times working in this field feels quite isolating. NGOs and individuals in the field can be quite territorial around their work, with not a lot of resource and skills sharing happening. If ever there was a time to break down barriers and territories then it is now. These kinds of difficulties that I experience are common to multi- or inter-agency work as expressed by Walker, 'some key barriers to multi-agency co-operation: differing functions of agencies which clash and compete; differing values and ideologies of agencies; and conflicting social policy and legislation' (2008: 222).

Atkinson, Doherty and Kinder (2005), in researching the barriers to multi-agency cooperation, found that funding and resources were the major challenge. They identified three main areas of concern:

1. conflicts within or between agencies
2. a general lack of funding
3. concerns about sustainability.

Their evidence suggests two perceptions regarding multi-agency work: the first being that budgetary constraints often force NGOs into assuming a minimalist role. The other perception is that multi-agency work is more effective for the sharing of resources and reducing repetition of work carried out. However, they go on to point out that when roles and responsibilities become blurred this can create further conflict when there is failure to move beyond existing roles. For example, 'participants reported that it required a degree of reflection, or even a capacity for self-criticism on the part of individuals and, at the same time, questioned their sense of identity, gained through following existing practice or procedure' (Atkinson, Doherty and Kinder 2005: 12).

In addition to the above challenges, much research and attention is focused around providing medication for only those children living with HIV ('medicalising the crisis'): 'a narrow approach, focused only on this group of children runs the risk of overlooking the health and psychosocial needs of very large numbers of vulnerable children living in communities affected by AIDS' (Richter 2006: 14).

So while their psychosocial needs may be recognised, little is being done to meet these needs. Even so, concerns around adherence to medication are building. Non-adherence to antiretroviral treatment (ART) results in drug resistance and an increase in infection. Teenagers have been shown to be particularly prone to non-adherence, especially if there has been a lack of disclosure (Brown and Lourie 2000) as well as social stigma. This in itself is an alarm bell. To what extent can non-adherence be said to be the result of psychosocial difficulties or even rebelliousness? And if teenagers are not given support in dealing with these issues what could this mean for future generations?

Description of the work

With the above contexts in mind I will describe and reflect on a second pilot dramatherapy group for teenagers on antiretroviral treatment (ART) that I ran in 2007. The group was set up firstly to provide the opportunity for psychosocial support to explore feelings around living with HIV, and, secondly to provide an opportunity for an HIV counsellor/facilitator to co-facilitate with the intention of possibly running similar focused groups with teenagers under my supervision as part of a sustainable ongoing project and skills transfer.

The overall treatment aims of the group were:

* To provide the adolescents with a safe space for the expression of feelings.
* To provide a learning space for HIV counsellor/facilitators to possibly run similar groups in the future.
* To provide recommendations regarding future possible facilitation of ongoing groups.

And the expected outcomes were as follows:

* Evidence to support the use of creative arts therapy as a useful intervention with teenagers living with a chronic illness.
* Evidence to support the need for psychosocial support groups for teenagers living with HIV.
* Evidence to support recommendations regarding a replicable model of intervention.
* Teenagers' increased adherence to medication.
* Developing and strengthening the teenagers' capacity to express their feelings, deal with difference, cope with loss and find sources of help and support.
* Investigating whether or not lay facilitators are able to use art and drama activities in a group setting to provide opportunities for teenagers to deal with issues associated with having a chronic illness, as expressed particularly in their having to take medication routinely.

Because of the limited number of sessions (12) and the use of a facilitator with limited skills and experience in working with teenagers, the co-facilitator was not expected to make interpretations, but rather to facilitate the teens' engagement with the activities as members of a group and through engagement with the themes of the sessions, to provide an opportunity for growth. There were additional benefits to working with a co-facilitator: while all the teenagers could speak English, it was not their first language and so working with a co-facilitator who could speak a number of African languages was absolutely necessary. The co-facilitator was male and this proved to be important in the group as none of the teenagers had 'present' father figures in their lives. Working with my co-facilitator was invaluable and I could not have done without him.

This dramatherapy group comprised ten teenagers and ran for a period of 12 sessions meeting weekly for an hour and a half. A number of people were involved setting up the group. These included a dramatherapist, HIV counsellors, facilitators, the programme co-coordinator, a psychologist, a social worker and the consulting paediatrician. All these people are involved with working with the teenagers at the clinic, either directly or indirectly through caregivers. This group met weekly for supervision and feedback on how the group was running. In consultation with this group we drew up the following overall aims and objectives:

- To provide an opportunity for teenagers to deal with issues associated with being teenagers and having a chronic illness.
- To encourage teenagers to develop and strengthen their capacity to express their feelings.
- To encourage teenagers to find and build a support network.
- To explore personal stories, experiences, challenges, hopes and dreams through art and drama.
- To learn to listen to one another.
- To evaluate whether this model of group can be replicated and run by HIV counsellors and facilitators.

Early stages

Recruitment to the group involved both word of mouth and direct referrals from the consulting paediatrician. She identified and referred specific teenagers to the group who were in need of psychosocial support relating to their HIV status. All potential group members were given an explanation of the nature of the groups and, where relevant, to their caregivers. Pre-group interviews were then held with all referred teens and caregivers to determine their suitability for the groups. Not all those interviewed were selected for the groups for various reasons.

Group selection criteria included:

- age
- gender
- awareness of HIV status
- suitability for group work
- suitability for art and drama
- individual teenager's developmental needs.

Group make-up

A closed group, composed of ten members (three male and seven female) ranging from 12 to 16 years of age was formed. Nine members were of various African ethnicities (Zulu, Xhosa and Sotho) and one was non-African. All members spoke English as either their second or fourth and fifth language. They had all been disclosed to about their HIV status (advertently or inadvertently). The majority of the group had lived with HIV since birth (MTCT – mother-to-child transmission) and one teen had contracted HIV through sexual abuse. All had experienced frequent hospitalisations and all were receiving antiretroviral medication.

Eight out of the ten group members had lost their mothers and one cannot begin to estimate the various other earlier bereavements and traumas that may have been present even if not disclosed. Six of the group members were being cared for by grandmothers, two lived in a children's home and two lived with their mothers. Fathers, as is often the case in South Africa, seemed to be completely absent, either through death, abandonment or divorce. None of the group members had contact with their biological fathers. Given that this was a short-term intervention, the consulting team decided that we focus sessions on various themes, but that the approaches be psychodynamic.

Sessions are focused around the following themes:

- introductions and orientation: who we are and why we are here
- my story . . . who am I and where do I come from?
- where do I find my support?
- being a teenager: changes and identity
- being a teenager: my emotions, my body and sexuality
- being a teenager: belonging and not belonging
- living with HIV: feelings
- living with HIV: medication
- living with HIV: talking about it
- my future and hopes: where do I find my support?
- reflection and preparing to close
- closure.

The group was designed to use methods such as body mapping, body sculptures, role play and image-making techniques. Each week we would begin seated on cushions with an opening ritual, followed by a deeper exploratory drama process. The body maps were used weekly as a form of reflection, onto which the participants could express their feelings and experiences from the session. We ended on our circle of cushions with a closing ritual.

While general group aims were formulated before the group began, in the first session the group was asked to say what they would like from the sessions.

What I want from the group:

- work with teenagers: learn about them and what they think
- to feel connected
- know more about different people

- learn more about being accepted
- to feel accepted and not be discriminated against
- learn how to deal with my status
- to be encouraged/motivated to drink my meds right
- not to be judged
- feel equal
- to learn.

The group's expectations for me were an affirmation of the need for groups like this to be run on an ongoing basis. Their need for a space free of judgement highlights the nature of the social stigma they live with and the burden of the secret they are forced to hold as a result. They also highlight the need for peer groups at this stage of life.

Development of active techniques

With only 12 sessions and a number of issues and subject matter to address, I began by trying to fill the sessions with too many active techniques. The techniques I used followed a developmental pattern: play, concrete, symbolic and dramatic play. While edging towards the beginning of symbolic play most of the techniques remained quite concrete. My understanding of this is linked to the nature of HIV in our society. Working with HIV and the social stigma attached to it feels as if we, as a nation, are still in a very concrete stage. We have only begun to acknowledge its existence and much is still repressed. In a sense, at a national level, we still have to awaken the body (the unconscious).

Play

We began each session with introductory and interactive games. The group generally enjoyed these and the opportunity to play. In keeping with my earlier arguments around a more concrete approach to the sessions, the group preferred structured games to the more spontaneous and imaginative ones.

Body maps

Body maps are created by clients and are life-sized, mixed media self-portraits. They have been used in activities concerning HIV to help express and explore people's experiences of their body: for example in IBIS' work with people with HIV and Aids (Kinghorn and Long 2006). I did not introduce body mapping as a structured directive technique, but rather as a creative and free space to play. I did not guide the group in how to create the body maps, other than in the beginning in drawing the outline of each of their bodies. We used the maps as a reflective tool; at the end of each session we would go to the body map room (adjacent to the therapy room) and spend 15 minutes putting feelings into maps. The group enjoyed doing body mapping and liked time to work on their own and chat causally amongst themselves. In the circle with me issues concerning language remained. While I can speak basic Isizulu I cannot speak it fluently, hence. I sometimes work with a translator. In this case I had a first language Zulu speaking co-facilitator who helped with translation. But I realise some things get lost in translation. Also we have 11 official languages in SA, so in any one group there will be a number of different languages spoken. In the framework we stress that any language can be used. So, when body mapping it felt like the group was free of this internal restraint and chatted and interacted far more easily than when sitting in a circle.

Journey maps

Based on workshops and research carried out by the Centre for Social Science Research at the University of Cape Town (2004) I adapted the use of 'journey maps' for the group. I wanted to use the journey maps as a way to help the teenagers identify feelings and express them in a concrete manner. There were a range of difficulties experienced by the group subsequent to being disclosed to. Some of these included not being able to speak about something that was directly affecting them. This same thing, from which the majority of their mothers had died from, presented in other forms through the body; for example, sore stomachs and anxiety. My therapeutic intention was to help the group begin to integrate what had happened to them by concretely creating a journey map onto which they could identify feelings and actual experiences, this way making the experience more real and bringing it to the fore. Journey maps also took an embodied form through the creation of a *walked journey* of adolescence. This embodiment of the transitioning of time was a powerful experience for the group.

Body sculpts

I like to work with body sculpts as a way into exploring issues. In my opinion, the most significant session happened through the use of body sculpts. (See session 8. It was in this session that I became aware of a shift towards more symbolic thinking in the group.

Role play

In a previous group run with a similar client group (Jones 2007) role play seemed very effective, specifically with this age group and the silence around HIV. Role play seemed to enable the teens to find a voice in the dramatherapy that they had not been able to access before. However, in this group it was not the same. There was much fear around role play, which I think speaks to the level of the repression: 'If I am to act it and embody it then will I be doing something bad; if I act it will I become it?' All had been told and threatened to not tell anyone. One mother gave her child antiretrovirals in the cupboard, for fear of anyone seeing.

Cameras

We also introduced disposable cameras as part of helping the teens to identify external support structures/people in their lives, as a way of building resilience. Each participant was given a camera to take home for the week and photograph themselves in as many different contexts as they liked. The photographs were then developed and the subjects formed part of one session through body sculptures. Here the participants were able to show each other their lives outside of the group. Some teens then decided they wanted to incorporate some of the photographs into their body maps.

Question box

In the first session we introduced a question box into the group. It had a place and there were always paper and pens. Any questions regarding HIV that the teenagers might have had were written on the paper anonymously and placed in the box. These were engaged with as part of the work.

These are the questions that found their way into the box:

- How do people get HIV?
- Why do people get it?
- How do people feel about it?
- If you have HIV I want to know how long you will live for.
- What do people eat when they have HIV?
- Why do you have to take pills when you have HIV?
- Why can't HIV be cured?
- Do white people have it?
- When will I have to stop taking meds?
- Why do we have blood taken every time we come to the clinic?
- Are antiretrovirals helpful to us? What do they do?
- After a person gets full blown AIDS is it possible to tell when he or she is going to die?
- Is it possible to have babies if you have HIV but are on antiretrovirals?
- How can you tell your friend that you are HIV positive?
- If you don't drink your medicine in the right way what will happen?
- When you are in love with someone and you want them to know

about the sexual abuse but you don't know how much that person loves you.

- I feel like helping *them* to be like us people.

The life of the group: themes and processes

Fragility

A therapeutic frame was clearly formulated with contract, time, space and group aims; however, this was a fragile group. This fragility manifested in illness, irregular attendance, ambivalence about the group, connection followed by disconnection with one another; speaking and silence; disruption and interruption. My understanding of this fragility is linked to the same feelings that possibly underlie forgetting to take medication, i.e. fear, denial and shame. Most of the group members had never been part of a group like this before, and much of their lives represented 'brokenness': family, school and community. Being in a group like this was very new for most of them. Twelve sessions was far too short to move beyond the brokenness. With the erratic attendance and some participants consistently arriving late, the group had a 'stop start' feel to it. Could this group be trusted? Would I as therapist leave them? Would I be there weekly? Who was this white woman from the outside?

In and out

Despite the fragility and the 'stop start' nature of the group, there were definite moments of cohesiveness and these happened sporadically. In session 7 only five members of the group were present and we explored feelings around having been disclosed to. I invited each person to create a journey map from the time they were disclosed to up to the present day. It was a quiet but meaningful session with various disclosures made between group members. The group seemed surprised at how many similar experiences existed between them. After the session they spent time talking with each other while they had juice and biscuits, and then left the clinic as a group. Previously they would eat in silence and then leave quietly one by one. My co-facilitator struggled through the session, saying to me afterwards 'the pain is too much' and yet I felt a real closeness beginning in the group and I wondered if we were moving into a new phase. Session 8, in my view, proved to be the most significant session of all. The session was powerful and was probably the only session that I can honestly say I saw the dramatherapy working therapeutically. There seemed to be a shift in the group; in their mood, in their level of reflection at the end of the session and in their interactions outside the space. For example, after the session I noticed the group members talking freely amongst themselves and leaving the clinic in a group. Previously they were quiet and left one-by-one. I came away at the end feeling we had found an 'in', only to arrive for session 9 and realise we were 'out' again. Only four group members arrived and they were back to being quiet and watching and silent. Had they shared too much? Could this group be trusted?

Stigma and shame: don't look at me

I have mentioned the stigma and shame that comes with HIV. The fear of being looked at and talked about was often spoken about in the group. My sense was that this was not only about outside the group but I wondered how much was present in the group as well. We know that adolescence is a time of self-absorption and self-consciousness. This was a highly self-conscious group. Despite the initial enthusiasm at the thought of 'doing drama' when opportunities arose (after much warm-up and ready making) for role play, the group became very shy. As I have mentioned the group seemed to be far more comfortable working individually on their body maps.

I wish I was still 12: growing up and coping

In session 5 I aimed to work with the transition into adolescence. I was aware at the start of the session that I wouldn't be there in the following session.

   This was the session in which the paediatrician was going to facilitate a question and answer session. As a group we built a teenager bridge from age 12 to age 18 created out of a variety of scarves. The group created their bridge quietly without much consultation with each other. Then they walked it following my invitations to take up an appropriate place. I guided them by asking the following questions:

1   Where are you now?

   a)   I feel angry and sad and confused, I don't know what to do.
   b)   I am about to turn the corner.
   c)   I feel like I am not a child but still in between.
   d)   I am here: I still want to play but I have to wash dishes.

2   Where do you want to be?

   a)   This is my 17; I want to feel more adult and able to cope.
   b)   I want to be able to choose and make decisions about which way to go.
   c)   I want to be 12 again and have no responsibilities.
   d)   I want to be able to make choices

During reflection the group commented on the burden of becoming teenagers and how they longed to just be 12 again with 'no worries'. We spoke about transitions and what it feels like to have to let go of parts of oneself or stages of life, e.g. childhood. I remember feeling quite moved at the end of the session as I know only too well that for many in the group a 'childhood' had not been possible due to circumstances.

When we met as a group again in session 7, we continued with the theme of journey, but this time the journey of disclosure. There were only five in the group this day and there was a very intimate and vulnerable feeling in the group. Each teenager visually mapped their individual journey from the moment of disclosure to present day. When asked to share aspects of their images with the group, some connections were made between them; for example, that four out of five had lost their mothers. My co-facilitator was very edgy during this session and found it difficult to be still. His mobile phone also went off during the session. At the end he said that this 'stuff is difficult with children'. He usually runs support groups for adults and finds talking about issues easier with them than with the youth.

I am normal

Session 8: finally it felt like the group was settling; more risks seem to be attempted and the group is more relaxed. As the group arrives Mpho says 'Hi Kirsten', it was the first time he had used my name. It felt like we had begun to talk and that the secret was broken. We opened the session speaking about what it means to live with HIV, what our fears are and what keeps us from talking. The group agreed that the worst thing was not being able to tell their friends and feeling looked at and laughed at when they go to hospital or when they return. One of the older girls, Lerato, said:

Lerato:	When I come back from the hospital I worry that people are looking at me and that they know where I have come from.
Therapist:	What gets you home?
Lerato:	I remember a trick a doctor taught me to tell myself 'I am normal'.

And so I felt this was an opportunity to invite the group into a drama/body sculptures. Lerato was assertive and willing and drama experienced, she volunteered to be the protagonist. I told the group that we were going to create a character who is HIV positive. I asked for a name. The non-African group member, Tracy, shouted out the English name Bianca (feeling quite marginalised and determined to have someone she can identify with). The group decided Bianca was 14 and lived in a suburb in a major South African township with her granny. Her parents had split but were not deceased. They decided she has known about her status for four years and that she has been going to an ARV clinic for ten years. So I invited Lerato, as Bianca, to sit on a chair. The rest of the group sat in a semi-circle facing her. I asked who could be next to her. They said the doctor and her granny. There were a number of volunteers who wanted to be the doctor but no one wanted to be the granny. My co-facilitator finally agreed to be the granny.

Bianca sat on a chair and next to her were the doctor, and her gogo (Isizulu for granny).

Therapist: Tell me about Bianca.
Lerato: She is a very emotional person.
Therapist: What does she feel?
Lerato: Sad, scared, confused and happy.

I invited the witnesses to take a coloured scarf to represent Bianca's feelings and to stand near her. Zandile took a green scarf to represent sad and said 'I am sad because people laugh at me.' Tracy took a red scarf to represent scared and said 'I am scared because I don't know what to say/how to answer people.'

Mpho took a multicoloured scarf to show confused and said 'I am confused because I am not sure how I am feeling.' Thulani chose a blue scarf to show happy and said 'I am happy because I know my status.'

The group was dead silent. Bongi who was left witnessing said 'Yo!' (a slang expression of shock).

My co-facilitator said 'Yo' quietly under his breath, and looked at me.

I held the silence and Bianca smiled.

Therapist: So what does Bianca need?

I gave her an open basket to receive scarves as symbolic representations of what she needed.

The group gave her:

- strength
- hope
- confidence
- trust
- normal feeling
- bravery
- support.

They put the scarves into the basket and we formed a circle around her.

Therapist: As her friends what do we want to say to her?
All: 'We still care for you' (all in unison).

There was not much time to reflect at the end of the session, but it felt appropriate. The drama had held the feelings.

How do I talk? Do NOT talk.

Session 9: in this session most of the group was absent. Gone was the feeling from the previous week: they decided they wanted to finish their body maps and work individually, not as group. I notice that the group is very tired today: are they depressed? I wondered about having worked the previous week quite symbolically. This week they seemed to revert back to the concrete and the superficial; their defences were back. Was the reality of the stigma and the outside world too much? I also had to acknowledge the reality that this group was ending too. I wondered out loud that before we go to our body maps, would we like to do a bit of drama? The group said 'OK'. I asked for volunteers, two girls got up. They decided they were two friends at school during break. A had noticed that B had been going to the clinic and wanted to find out if everything was alright. The role play began and ended in a few minutes. It felt superficial as the girl who had HIV in the role play could not and would not talk in role. When asked by her 'best friend' as to why she was always going to the clinic, she answered 'there is stress in my family.'

In reflection afterwards the girl who played the best friend spoke of her frustration at not being told the truth and thus not being able to help her friend. The girl who played the HIV friend reflected that even if her best friend disclosed that she was HIV, she would still not disclose her status to her. She would merely tell her friend to go to hospital to get medicine. Given an opportunity to speak, it still did not feel safe. The secret is deep and it is hidden and it will not out. The message is: *do not talk to anybody not even your best friend; you must be quiet.* Even if you would like to talk, you dare not. There is no other alternative.

Overall group themes

Some of the emerging themes during the sessions were:

- fear of stigmatisation and rejection if one discloses to other people
- understanding how one is infected with HIV
- understanding why medication is necessary
- forgetting to take medication and the underlying feelings
- the importance of not feeling alone
- the importance of being accepted and not judged
- the need to talk about one's status openly.

Participant evaluations of the dramatherapy

In the closing sessions participants were asked to evaluate whether their expectations had been met or not. They were also asked to fill out a short structured evaluation form based on a review of the aims. I have collated verbal and written feedback for general evaluation.

Evaluation of general group aims

1. To provide opportunity for teenagers to deal with issues associated with having a chronic illness and being teenagers.

- 'Before I started coming to the group I felt scared. Now when I come to the clinic I feel normal.'
- 'I wish we could learn about being teenagers like this at school.'

What was the most helpful thing about this group? Has anything changed because of it?

- Taking the medication.
- It helped me by knowing that I am normal just like everybody.
- I have changed by eating healthy foods.
- The thing that changed is my pills and now I am taking my pills properly.
- Taking ARV.
- Being able to share feelings with people who understand me and people who are in my position.

How did drama help you?

- To have trust in the group and know how everyone is living with HIV/AIDS.

2. To encourage teenagers to develop and strengthen their capacity to express their feelings.
   What did you like about the group?

- Knowing about each and everyone's feelings and status.
- Learning how to respect.
- To share feelings.
- Being treated equally and sharing our feelings.
- Not to be judged.

What was the most helpful thing about this group? Has anything changed because of it?

- Support and respect. I really appreciate what the group bought to me.
- To talk to other people.
- Being able to share feelings with people who understand me and people who are in my position.

How did drama help you?

- To keep secrets with other people and share feelings.

3. To encourage teenagers to find and build a support network.
   What did you like about the group?

- Being treated equally and sharing our feelings.
- Not to be judged.
- Being appreciated, 'cause I learned how to be special and that is something I lost when my mom left, so I liked everything about the group.

What was the most helpful thing about this group? Has anything changed because of it?

- Support and respect. I really appreciate what the group bought to me.
- To talk to other people.
- It helped me by knowing that I am normal just like everybody.
- Being able to share feelings with people who understand me and people who are in my position.

How did drama help you?

- To have trust in the group and know how everyone is living with HIV/AIDS

4. To explore personal stories, experiences, challenges, hopes and dreams through art and drama.
   What did you like about the group?

- Being appreciated, 'cause I learned how to be special and that is something I lost when my mom left, so I liked everything about the group.

How did drama help you?

- To have trust in the group and know how everyone is living with HIV/AIDS.
- To keep secrets with other people and share feelings.
- Being a gangster doesn't help.
- Listening.
- It helped me open up, because some of the things we did had a lot to do with my experiences, like putting my personal feelings on the body map. Thank you!

5. To learn to listen to each other.

6. To evaluate whether this model of group can be replicated and run by HIV South Africa facilitators.

7. What did you *not* like about the group?

- Nothing really, everything was good. The support I received was helpful for me and I will not like it if I have to leave the group.
- To celebrate.
- Being upset in the sessions.
- Children getting cross.
- Nothing, everything was fantastic and awesome.

Recommendations

Evidence from the above feedback suggests the aims on a concrete level were mostly achieved, for example, an increase in adherence to medication. At a group level having the space to feel accepted and not judged was the most valuable aspect of the group experience, as well as having the opportunity to share and express feelings and know that one was not alone. On a psychological and emotional level there did seem to be improvement in many participants' self esteem. With regards to the teens' relationship to HIV, themselves and their bodies, more work needs to be done. The secret resides deep and in the body and in society and I hadn't realised just how deep it was.

Reflection on theory and method

In this section I will reflect on the processes across groups I have run with adolescent HIV positive teenagers. According to Richter *et al.* (2006) most children affected by HIV do not need specialised psychological services. In labelling children living with HIV as orphaned and vulnerable, are we not unnecessarily pathologising them? How then can dramatherapy offer interventions specifically for teenagers that are about re-connecting with the social world and the self?

I will now briefly consider dramatherapy as an effective intervention in supporting adolescents diagnosed and living with HIV. It seems that dramatherapy is one choice of treatment for adolescents given that the internal chaos and emotionality experienced in adolescence demands external expression and acknowledgement. The interplay between expression and containment can help the adolescent gain control over her emotions. Adolescents need a safe space in which to explore real life with safety and distance. Drama allows the expression of pain and also engages 'the adolescent's strengths, idealism and healthful inner resources' (Emunah 1994: 103) In the case study discussed in this chapter, it does seem that dramatherapy provided a space for the 'unspeakable' (HIV) to be explored and externalised in a safe and distant way. However, the question remains as to how effective the intervention was, given the wider contextual complexities discussed.

Taboo

Death, sex and HIV are three of the biggest taboos in South Africa. Parents and caregivers find it very difficult to talk openly about these issues amongst themselves never mind with their children/teenagers: all these taboos are interconnected. You can't run a group on HIV without dealing with sex, death and loss at some level. Caregivers are afraid to talk and don't know how. They too need support. In previous groups (Jones 2007) we realised early on that you can't run group for children without groups for their caregivers.

In a study done on the psychosocial needs of children in the context of HIV/AIDS, Richter *et al.* (2006) found that you can't work with children in isolation. Children are best supported through strengthening caregivers' and households' commitments to the well-being of children. I would say the same applies to teenagers. Caregivers find teenagers difficult enough and struggle to find ways of communicating with them; coupled with HIV it makes the task even more difficult. Imagine having to look after a grand-child of your child who died of HIV. You may have already existing unresolved anger towards your child, firstly for contracting HIV and then for leaving you with an HIV positive grandchild. The situation is complex, as you haven't even been able to mourn the death of your child. And if you feel disappointment and prejudice towards your child for having contracted HIV, there is a good chance you may project these feelings onto the grand-child who is struggling to make sense of the same issues as well as the difficult life stage of adolescence. This group of teenagers was struggling with all these difficulties and, had we created a space for their caregivers to process some of their own difficulties, this would possibly have helped them in their development.

The peer group

The stigmatisation of HIV does not allow disclosure amongst the 'normal' peer group (at school or at home), so a psychosocial support group of adolescents living with HIV provides a space for the 'unspeakable' (HIV). It also allows for the normalisation of feelings and knowing that one is not alone. In terms of psychosocial support, the peer group aids in bringing teens out of isolation. The dramatherapy group I ran did seem to offer teenagers this very important space. Those teens who attended most sessions benefited and grew. As one teen commented at the end of the group: 'Before I started coming to the group I felt scared. Now when I come to the clinic I feel normal.'

Within the peer group there were slight developmental disparities in the group that affected the dynamics. However this was not necessarily negative; for example, the older teens could offer support and share experiences that were helpful to the younger less experienced group members. In the closing session the oldest participant commented: 'When I first came to the group I was surprised how much younger they were than the group I was in before. It was like I was with a bunch of learners.'

This was a positive comment in that she was expressing that she felt helpful and valued in that she could 'teach' the others. What the peer group also allows is a space to witness others.

Witnessing

In session 8 (see 'I am normal' p. 141) witnessing was powerful; while only one person got to be Bianca, all group members could identify with her. Witnessing is a powerful act that can enable transformation (Jones 1996, 2007). This has been evident in earlier groups too (Meyer cited in Jones 2007) in which witnessing another group member as a character speak the unspeakable about being HIV positive, enabled her to say to the group in closing 'I have something to tell you; I am HIV' (2007: 99).

In the group discussed in this chapter, Bianca took on the role others were afraid to embody. By creating a character other group members were able to project their fears and feelings into the character and then felt able to respond to this persona by speaking to her or about her as witnesses.

Distancing

One would assume with adolescents that the therapeutic method of distancing (Jones 1996, 2007) is appropriate, to prevent an overwhelming flood of emotions. The body maps provided this, as well as the image making activities.

Usually one works with the assumption that adolescents as a group need more distance with roles. In earlier work (Jones 2007) I observed that my group of adolescents needed less distance (given the distance South African society gives to HIV and the stigma attached to it); they needed an opportunity to feel their emotions and be less distanced. However, in the group I discuss in this chapter, it was not the same. Possibly what the journey and body map work provided was an opportunity to be outside of their bodies (given that illness/HIV resides in the body) and to project into the image material about their lives and situations that could give them space to 'see' what was happening to them – a process of externalising their inner conflict. This enabled them to reflect and find a language to share experiences that verbally seemed difficult for them.

Embodiment

Apart from two group members this was not a 'drama ready' group. I have spoken about the South African societal repression of HIV resulting in shame and stigma, in previous sections of this chapter. My hope was that dramatherapy, through direct physical work with the body, would enable a bodily awakening: creating an area to express and explore issues that could not easily be spoken about. The intention was that this would then enable the group to express their suppressed feelings and experiences to each other. This would, I hoped, eventually enable them to work with issues concerning their lives and HIV and help them to arrive at a new understanding of HIV. This was not to be. As a group, we seemed to be moving towards openness, but were not there yet. The group was very afraid to work with their bodies in the sessions. This area of their lives and identity needed more time to develop trusting relationships with me and each other, to develop group cohesion. These issues were reflected in other aspects of our expressive work. Role play, for example, became threatening: they were not ready. In the previous section on distancing it was discussed how the 'journey' and 'body maps' provided another kind of embodiment: through image making, rather than direct physical expression. Given the social messages that people living with HIV are given about their bodies, the map work enabled the group to look at their bodies from a safe enough distance. In hindsight this felt an important part of the process that was necessary before the group could physically embody roles. This relationship with the body emerged as a pertinent theme in the work and in the South African context as a whole. This theme was not fully explored in the group but is relevant for any further work that may be done. In Jones, identity is described as being rooted in the body, and if clients can experience physical change this may lead to positive identity change: 'The self is often seen to be realised by and through the body' (1996: 151) The challenge is to understand the bodies of these teenagers in relation to themselves and to a society that discriminates against HIV.

In the case of these teenagers, physical body work was frightening. It was as if their bodies had become stigmatised and they were cut off at an emotional level from them. My sense was that we needed to find ways to rediscover the body and connect with it, slowly and safely, before they could actually physically embody roles.

Not just about HIV

In this context a group that is psychodynamic in nature and focused around HIV, cannot only be about HIV. It will be about loss, bereavement, isolation, shame, illness, medication, sexuality, trust etc. and also building resilience and hope.

So many threads come together. Throughout the life of the group I came to recognise the importance of helping teens identify their strengths and capacity for hope in order to build resilience. Working in this context, as a therapist, one faces many challenges. In earlier work with children who had not been disclosed to I was left holding the secret and in a way colluding with the shame and the fear. This was a great burden to bear. I found myself feeling afraid to mention HIV when it felt like I should be finding ways of speaking about it. In this group with teens there was no secret, all had been disclosed to about their status but I also spoke easily about HIV saying it a lot as if in normal conversation. This was a much more comfortable way of working and seemed to enable to group to find their voice around it too.

In session 8 when Thulani said 'I am happy because I know my status', this represented something new and different for group, namely: I have HIV and I am happy I know it.

Conclusion

In summary, dramatherapy with HIV positive teenagers allows for: expression, containment and acknowledgement.

It seems that dramatherapy is one affective choice of treatment for adolescents who are HIV positive, given that the internal chaos and emotionality experienced in adolescence demand external expression and acknowledgement. The interplay between expression and containment can help the adolescent gain control over her emotions. Adolescents need a safe space in which to explore real-life with safety and distance. Drama allows the expression of pain and also engages 'the adolescent's strengths, idealism and healthful inner resources' (Emunah 1994: 103).

A peer group allows one to share experiences, move out of isolation and build supportive relationships. However:

- groups cannot happen in isolation, they need to be connected to the greater society e.g. schools, policy, homes and caregivers.
- caregivers need support too in finding ways of dealing with and communicating with teenagers.
- more research is needed on the psychosocial needs of teenagers living with HIV.
- working cross culturally demands understanding and sensitivity.

We face enormous challenges as our youth (adolescents) are in crisis. Over the years, South African youth have been victims of political and socioeconomic and cultural crises. They have been subjected to poverty, violence, inadequate schooling, loss of parents and now HIV.

We all face many challenges if we are to emerge intact. Our adolescents, living with HIV, are faced with critical challenges. Some of these are:

- stigmatisation and discrimination
- the relationship of the (ill or stigmatised) body to the self and society
- isolation and alienation
- peer groups difficult to find at school and home
- disclosure
- loss of parental caregivers
- developmental work of adolescence negatively impacted upon
- negotiating sexual relationships

- living with a chronic illness
- facing possible death.

We cannot hold the silence anymore. We need to speak and we need to help our teenagers speak. If we don't start somewhere where will we end? How many more lives and years will it take? Will we have any teenagers left, or will we have another generation of children born to these teens who have to hold the secret in silence? And so the shadow will remain. And when the shadow does not find expression . . .

8 Dramatherapy and victim empathy: a workshop approach in a forensic setting

Emma Ramsden and Mario Guarnieri

Box 8.1

Questions about practice

- How does victim empathy dramatherapy relate to the work of a high-secure NHS hospital setting?
- What impact can role work have?
- What issues arise concerning directive and non-directive approaches?

Research perspective

- Case study
- Group evaluation
- Focus group

Client perspective sample

- 'I wish I'd done this years ago.'
- 'I think everyone should be made to do this.'
- 'I didn't think I would but I really liked doing all the drama stuff.'
- 'I found it hard but feel I got something from it.'
- 'I've never done anything like this before it's so powerful.'
- 'It's not what I expected; I thought I was going to be made to be a tree.'

Group evaluation:

> There's something in dramatherapy that I've seen helps connect with the reality of the situation in a much more powerful way than talking about it does ... there's something about scenarios ... actually you're in the room and you're feeling it, you're feeling what

> it would be like being in that situation. You're there and there's
> no hiding away that this is what that person did, and this is what it
> can make people feel like . . . I think that's very powerful.
>
> Hospital staff focus group

Introduction

This chapter concerns an aspect of our practice as dramatherapists in a high
secure NHS in-patient psychiatric hospital in the United Kingdom,[1] where
we work with male patients who have offended and been sectioned under the
Mental Health Act (1983 – with amendments 2007). The Act 'permits the
transfer or diversion of mentally disordered offenders from the criminal justice
system to hospital at each stage of the legal process' (Davison 2004: S19).
In this chapter we focus on the use of a series of dramatherapy workshops
as an intervention within this population exploring the concept of 'victim
empathy'. We describe the working context and its process, provide reflections
from patients and colleagues from other professions and comment on implications for future practice. Our colleagues' reflections derive from a focus
group, which was facilitated with Phil Jones. The focus group setting enables
a group of people to discuss and explore a theme or topic together, often
within a defined open questions structure (Bryman 2001).

Victim empathy work within various forensic populations has been
developed over time by practitioners with multidisciplinary training, and
combines a range of theoretical perspectives. Forensic populations are those
where offenders, inmates and patients have become involved with the legal
system as a result of their offending behaviour. People who offend are referred
to often as either 'offenders', 'perpetrators' or both. In this chapter we use
the terms interchangeably to refer to the same meaning; that of a person
who has committed an illegal act against another person, people or object.
Practitioners such as drama specialists, psychologists, social workers, youth
offending caseworkers and therapists have applied their skills and knowledge
to work with offenders in order to explore the concept of victim empathy for
the individual. As we see in the following quotation, empathy is an essential
part of connecting with our sense of humanity:

> Empathy is what enables us to recognize another person's pain, even in
> the midst of tragedy, because pain cannot be evil. Empathy deepens our

---

1 For the writing of this chapter, we have obtained consent from patients who have undergone
this work and held a focus group discussion with colleagues we have collaborated with. In
order to protect patient anonymity the facts and events cited in case examples that appear
in the text have been altered to produce a representation of the patient's journey. However the
colleague quotations we include to highlight the process, are taken as verbatim from the focus
group transcription.

humanity. Its absence, whether at a collective level or in interpersonal relationship, signals the separation of human beings from one another and is an assault on the essence of what it is to be human. When perpetrators apologize and experience the pain or remorse, showing contrition, they are acting as human beings.

(Gobodo-Madikezela 2002: 7)

These connections of both thinking and feeling are used in the approach referred to in this chapter – the 'intensive victim empathy dramatherapy workshop' – which focuses on working with patients undergoing treatment for their violent offending histories. It is unique in the field of dramatherapy, certainly in high-secure services, and possibly in other forensic settings.

Contexts

This intensive victim empathy dramatherapy workshop structure explores the patient's capacity to identify with, understand and relate to the point of view of their victim(s) whether primary; the direct victim(s) of the offence, or secondary; those connected to the victim such as family, friends and colleagues, or bystanders (as witnesses to the offence). The main aim of this work is to provide a forum for the patient to connect with their offending behaviour, feeling remorse and a need for some form of reparation for themselves as the perpetrators, and their victim(s). Feelings, as highlighted in the following definition of empathy, play a vital role in our human experience '. . . to be able to feel remorse, one must be capable of empathic identification with . . . a specific person one values' (Thomas 1999: 131).

There are many factors and causes surrounding any individual case of offending. In dramatherapy we include aspects of the whole person, yet place emphasis on working psychologically with the offender, exploring the impact of their experiences. The majority of the patients who find their way to high-secure services and with whom we work have experienced damaging, destructive, toxic and dangerous attachments with parents, primary caregivers and other significant adults. Many patients have experienced terror in their early lives, with parents and caregivers themselves in need of care, leading to their inadequate or absent offering of basic, healthy care (see Maslow in Gross 2005: 119; Latta 2005: 226–251). As we see in the quotation that follows, a distorted attachment can lead to emotional deprivation:

. . . if the individual has not had the opportunity to simply be, his future does not auger well in terms of the emotional quality of his life. The likelihood is that this individual will feel empty . . . the infant who does not have the experience of a good-enough mother is prevented from developing and discovering the capacity to be.

(Abram 2007: 76–77)

In all cases, patients have experienced feeling out of control with life at the time of their offending. Their offences are so often expressions of deep-rooted anger, where feelings of remorse, empathy and forgiveness are impossible concepts at the time and often for a long time after the offence. Not until the individual, now incarcerated, begins to feel connected to a sense of community – receiving the safety of food, shelter and warmth – can he start the long and involved journey of learning to understand himself.

Positive affective engagement is a further aim of the work that we undertake. Our hope is to engender a sense of group feeling, mutual support and collaboration, whilst also acknowledging the individual nature of each of the patients, their offending history and commonalities between group members. As Barnes *et al.* suggest, feelings develop via increased communication between group members as their distress is understood outside of themselves: 'The therapeutic task is to translate the symptom into an understandable communication, so the subject is no longer isolated and withdrawn and there is increasingly free and open communication within the group' (Barnes, Ernst and Hyde 1999: 109).

Imagining being in someone else's shoes is described as one of the '. . . hallmarks of empathy . . .' (Cox 1992: xvi). It is an experiencing part of oneself that is inserted in order to gain the experience of the other, without losing one's own sense of reality (Hinshelwood 1991). This is the normal aspect of projective identification. Projective identification is a communication, projecting a part or aspect of oneself into someone else, in order to identify with and be identified by the other, with the aim of meeting one's needs. The pathological, or disordered mental functioning aspect of projective identification, is when the boundaries between the self and the object are destroyed by the loss of reality, a psychotic structure, which splits off parts of the mind, of evacuating unwanted feelings (ibid 1991).

In the intensive victim empathy dramatherapy workshop we engage with many drama and dramatherapy methods, developed, adapted and created over not only the past decade as dramatherapists, but also from our previous experiences of working with drama, film and theatre. For example, the Forum and Image Theatre of Boal (1979), improvisation work of Spolin (1998), acting out work of Cossa *et al.* (1996), empathy work by drama specialist Hewish (1992). Dramatic spontaneity and the nine core processes of dramatherapy, as developed and recorded by Jones (1996: 99–125) are central concepts that inform our methods of working. In the intensive victim empathy dramatherapy workshop focus is placed on the core process of the 'life–drama connection', where 'The notion of the life–drama connection acknowledges the therapeutic potentials of bringing life into contact with drama within a framework of intentional personal change.' (Jones 1996: 118). As one focus group participant commented, dramatherapy, in their understanding, '. . . helps connect with the reality of the situation in a much more powerful way than talking about it does, and because we spend time talking about empathy, but there's something about scenarios, actually you're in the room and you're feeling it, you're feeling what it would be like being in that situation. You're there and there's no hiding away that this is what that person did, and this is what it can make people feel like.'

The patient population, with whom this work takes place, is referred to as 'forensic psychiatry'. Forensic, meaning legal, '. . . is that part of psychiatry which deals with patients and problems at the interface of the legal and psychiatric systems' (Gunn 2004: S1). The three high-secure psychiatric hospitals that cover England and Wales in the UK are part of the National Health Service (NHS) rather than the prison system (HMP). '. . . prisons are not suitable places to treat people with serious mental disorders . . . we admit those who need in patient treatment to psychiatric units' (Davison 2004: S19). The term high security relates to risk, perceived and actual, both legal and psychiatric and of harm being enacted by the individual offender towards self and other.

> The nature of the task of the high secure hospitals may be regarded as uniquely challenging. It concerns the confinement of individuals within a social context at once both sceptical about and unrealistic in their expectations of professional abilities to protect the public from harm . . . Their [patients'] psychopathologies are such as to render the establishment of therapeutic alliances difficult and painful within the context of little hope of future change.
>
> (Deacon 2004: 93)

An intensive admissions assessment is undertaken during which time a mental health diagnosis[2] will be attributed to each patient, outlining something of their psychological damage. Throughout their stay in the hospital, each patient is offered medical and psychological treatment from his clinical team. The clinical team includes the assigned Consultant Psychiatrist, Primary Nurse, Lead Forensic Psychologist and Lead Social Worker. Together the clinical team discuss with the patient possible treatment options, both medication and otherwise. Individual and group therapy is offered from arts therapists, psychotherapists, psychologists, specialist nurse therapists, speech and language therapists and occupational therapists. Referrals for treatment are made via discussion in clinical team meetings attended by multidisciplinary professionals.

The intensive victim empathy dramatherapy workshop takes place on the hospital's specialist group therapy unit, where a range of treatment modalities are offered from a wide source of therapeutic frameworks. These include psychodynamic, psychoeducational and cognitive-behavioural. Some groups are closed and time limited while others are ongoing slow open groups.

---

2 See diagnostic manuals the DSM IV or ICD 10 for full details of medical diagnosis of mental disorders

Patients referred undergo a series of pre-group assessments to gauge their suitability for a specific group treatment.

Description of the work

The intensive victim empathy dramatherapy workshop is incorporated into two of the groups on the unit, the 'violent offenders group' and the 'sexual offenders group', the focus for this chapter is on the former. The group runs for between 14–18 months and is a closed group which means that the membership is agreed at the start of the intervention, and therefore no further members join during its life. The group often consists of between six to ten patients and has a facilitation team of four practitioners. It is aimed at patients with both a long history as well as a single act of violence. The overarching aims of the violent offenders group are to explore the issues around, and related to, the patients' experience and impact of these actions, from the perspective of victim and perpetrator, then looking towards risk reduction and preventing recidivism, by focusing on both the mental health needs and their criminogenic factors; i.e. the factors that potentially give rise to criminal behaviour.

The group operates with a four-phase structure:

1 Months 1–2: focus on group building, motivation, positive and negative effects of personal change.
2 Months 3–12: focus on the antecedents of violent behaviour and the experiences and perceptions of the victim/perpetrator dynamic.
3 Months 13–15: place emphasis on victim empathy focusing on perspective taking.
4 Months 16–18: explore relapse prevention, identifying areas of potential risk and strategising to prevent future violence.

A key aspect of the work is the organic evolution of the group's process by its members, using the phase structure as a guiding framework. Over time, and at their own pace, patients relate their experiences of violence, both as victims and as perpetrators. When discussing the impact of the overall violent offenders programme during the focus group session with our colleagues, the following quotations are noted: 'When [the patients] relay what they have done in the [therapy] group, the [intensive victim empathy dramatherapy] workshop is always the thing that sticks out in their minds.' 'The victim empathy workshop takes it to another level.' (Focus group participants) These quotations support the feedback received from patients during the closing session of the workshop and are consistent with feedback in previous workshops over the years. It seems that working in an experiential way with the lived experience of violence, enables the patients to enter into previously unconscious aspects of their psyche. Connections are made in the life–drama enactments and experiential sharing with others. Often we are given feedback by patients which indicates they are thankful in some way for being 'pushed' into looking deeper within. That working physically has enabled this looking to occur.

The intensive victim empathy dramatherapy workshop

We are both dramatherapists and facilitate the intensive victim empathy dramatherapy workshop supported by the group's regular facilitators – this always consists of nurse therapists and psychologists and can include other professions. In the particular series of workshops discussed in this chapter the group's facilitators consisted of a nurse therapist, two psychologists and a music therapist. There are two workshop sessions per day, for between three and five consecutive days. During the life of the workshop, patients will be invited to experience working and being together in a number of creative ways, using a variety of dramatherapeutic methods (for example, projective techniques with objects and each other, role play, reality-based enactments based around real offences). The patients in the workshop will be invited to explore being together using physical contact in exercises which require physical care and support working in pairs, small groups and the whole group. They will also be invited to engage in individual 'work segments', which are tailor made dramatic work tasks that focuses specifically on aspects of the individual's criminogenic history. Also to participate in group 'work segments' which explore the victim empathy concept and emergent feelings where '. . . destructive and vulnerable aspects of the self . . .' can be '. . . seen and explored creatively by the group, supporting each other and allowing themselves to enter into the safe and trusting environment which is enabled for them by the facilitators' (Guarnieri and Ramsden in Jones 2007: 109).

Patients explore something of their own traumas which are witnessed by other group members, themselves in turn identifying with their own personal experiences through the vicarious nature of witnessing (Cox 1992: 15). Sahhar, writing about the necessity for change, suggests that: 'Forensic clients are usually physically endangering . . . and their histories . . . provide compelling examples of how dangerous life was when they were young and vulnerable. This doesn't exonerate them of their acts, but it enables us to share their perspective – and that is an essential starting point for change' (Sahhar 2008: 6). The identification is multi-layered through dramatic enactment (patient–patient, perpetrator–victim, victim–perpetrator). Enactments are almost always moving and evocative of much grief, unexpressed anger, loss and despair of their own victimhood and their own violent actions. Professionals who work with forensic populations, ourselves included, believe it essential to explore the roles of victim and perpetrator symbiotically. We hold this belief because, as we have found, with this particular patient population, there can be an overidentification with the role of victim which can be used as a defence against acknowledging the perpetrator part of the self.

The workshop runs loosely on this following structure; seated verbal check-in; physical warm-up engaging in pair and whole group work; tasks and drama games; individual work segments with one dramatherapist facilitating and one involved, where applicable; role work group exercises connecting to the themes experienced in individual work segments; seated reflection with a focus on checking-in and closure.

Whilst any group works on a sense of structure (Stock Whitaker 1995), in this work we are trusting both our knowledge of dramatic processes and methods to engage with our instinctual, spontaneous approach to the work combined with our long history of co-facilitating together and thereby being mindful of our trust and sensitivity to the leadership qualities and experience of the other. In this way, we model a cohesive working alliance, which implicitly is what we believe to be healthy role modelling to the patients, whom we have suggested often have little or no reference for good enough parenting in their own histories (Bowlby in Gross 2005; Gerhardt 2008).

A session

With regards to the start of the intensive victim empathy dramatherapy workshop, one focus group participant commented '. . . So you don't know what's going to come next, there could be a bang.' Despite the group being approximately 12 months into their process, the first morning of the intensive victim empathy dramatherapy workshop bears a resemblance to the first day of the initial group, where the patients are '. . . gathered together into a room . . .' – seated in a circle – with the expectation that the facilitators will '. . . do or say something to get the group started' (Stock Whitaker 1995: 245). Nervousness, anxiety, suspicion and a certain amount of paranoia are often present at this point. There are a number of factors which relate to these feelings, including the mythology that has grown around this work by patients who have previously undergone the violent offenders programme.

A start is offered by way of an invitation to hear the thoughts, anxieties, fears and expectations of the patients regarding the work that is to follow. It is often a tense opening and our focus as facilitators is placed on enabling patients to feel heard, by actively listening to them and thinking about the process that we may introduce them to. Basic watching of the group at the early stage of its development is essential, and we are constantly checking in with our own feelings at this part of the workshop in order to elicit what may be present in the unsaid communications from the patients and support facilitators. We remain open to receiving the feelings that may be sublimated, split off, denied by the patients. These protective defences against intimacy and vulnerability can so often be very present when working with severely damaged individuals, for '. . . one's own feelings can be indicators of or guides to appreciating the feelings of others and understanding certain total-group phenomena' (Stock Whitaker 1995: 216).

This open, non-directive discussion, acts both as a grounding and a risk assessment, where we aim to identify both individual needs and group themes, expressed verbally and non-verbally. We are also noting the shape of the group, the needs of our support facilitators, and thinking of creative ideas based on individual patient's narratives at this time. We aim to gain a sense of the individual's process, psychologically and emotionally at this point in the group's life. We can then respond spontaneously, attempting to meet the needs being presented in the here and now of each workshop session.

Frequent comments at the start of the work include 'What are you going to do to me?' 'I don't want to act out my offence', 'I don't want to look stupid', 'Will I be made to disclose something I have kept secret from the group?' Reference to both like and dislike of drama at school is usually mentioned along with fears of being 'made' to 'do things'. We return to these opening comments throughout the workshop, placing them in a different context, that of violence, particularly in cases such as armed robbery or burglary, where victims were 'made to do things' under the threat of violence. We do however reassure the patients that the workshop is based on their being in control of their own actions, responsibility and decision making and that the choice to participate is always with them. Encouragement from all the staff members in the group is employed many times during this process in order to support a patient's ambivalence regarding participation in a particular exercise or discussion.

A sense of intrigue about the victim empathy work is also present amidst the anxiety as the workshop begins. With significant time given to a check-in discussion, individual group members begin to articulate their hopes, fears and expectations, expressing desires to understand something more of their own behaviour in relation to the victims in their own narratives. Some suggest or articulate being unwilling or unable to see their victims as individuals and/or that their victims deserved what they got. This is commonly found in cases where the violent offence was committed against perpetrators of their own victimhood. Others may see themselves as victims as a way of justifying the offence they committed. It may seem for some, in the interests of their psychological skin, to 'rubbish' their victims in some way, to give them faults, accuse them of being in the wrong place at the wrong time. In this way, the guilt and shame that is within them remains consciously unacknowledged.

As the check-in discussion progresses, there is a notable increase in confidence, seen in the opening of previously closed body postures. An increase in eye contact, which until now has been reserved for the programme's ongoing facilitators, seemingly seeking out reassurance and safety.

The check-in discussion comes to a close and we invite the patients to begin working creatively, initially through the movement and stillness of their physical selves, engaging both the body and mind in whole group exercises. The aim of this transition from discussion to action is to assess the group's needs, engender cohesive working alliances and boundary setting for using physical contact, listening and responding to instructions. We employ energy release/control exercises, games to engage cognition and encourage concentration and focus, those that enable individuality to be seen in the group environment and methods which unite the group in problem solving. Rarely do we engage in competitive play at the start of the workshop, but will as the session develops, introduce exercises which enable the group to explore more self-preserving roles – both on a team and individual level.

The 'warm-up' is a well-used phrase in drama and dramatherapy and it can be employed in many different ways. In this particular workshop it refers to the initial process of body and mind working together, both intra-personally and inter-personally, i.e. awareness of the physical and mental, both in self and other. Working with the body and mind in this way sets the scene for the workshop sessions that are to follow over the coming days, where patients will be involved mostly in an embodied way, playing various roles in their own and others' real-life dramas, engaging in group exercises which explore the group's ongoing dynamic and the concept of victim empathy. Each day ends with a whole group verbal reflection by way of grounding and closing the work ready for '. . . re-entry into the world waiting beyond the stage door' (Andersen-Warren and Grainger 2000: 24).

Clinical vignette: Bill

In the following section we give a brief account of one patient's progress, and process, through the intensive victim empathy dramatherapy workshop, starting off with his initial presentation – before moving to a vignette of his 'personalised drama' segment and then exploring his reflections. We have named the patient Bill.

During the opening discussion of the workshop Bill had spoken of his 'problem with authority'. He appeared to maintain an invisible guard, on the lookout for any facilitator comment or action which may draw attention to him in what he saw as a negative way (i.e. making him 'look stupid'). We sensed an aggression and defensiveness in the quality of Bill's voice and his overall presentation, which appeared to defend against what he perceived as potential for an attack on his fragile ego.

Bill was quick to ask for clarification on instructions, sometimes even whilst the instructions were still being given. This behavioural theme suggested an anxiety at being 'caught out' on some level. Being 'caught out' is a feature in his offending history, inevitably meaning the difference between freedom and incarceration. Bill's vocal tone had an edge of sarcasm about this self-protection. It seemed that Bill wanted to partici-pate as fully as he could in the work, and was keen to 'enjoy' the drama exercises, yet he wanted to do this by pre-empting what might be expected of him, to not be 'caught out'. Again here we can see a parallel to his offending history, one which involved taking things that did not belong to him. It was as if Bill was searching for the 'correct' way to be in the group and, without it he would experience a devastating feeling of failure. Further thinking was around his membership of a severely dysfunctional family, in which he had experienced an abusive early life. This self-protection had developed over time into the contradiction between being anti-authoritarian, yet wanting and needing to be complicit, gaining attention and rewards, triumphing in the group's dynamic as a strong leader.

In this leadership role, Bill was supportive to other group members yet cold and emotionally absent towards the facilitators, ergo the authority. Indeed the group that Bill belonged to displayed an amazing level of group cohesion and trust, which had built up over the previous 12 months of the group working together. Bill's feeling of coldness, led us to wonder about his capacity to truly empathise on an immediate level, with fellow group members in this shared lived experience. Moreover, we wondered about his ability to feel and convey empathy towards the multiple victims of his offences through working in an 'as if' paradigm, with people who were not physically present.

Bill spoke about his victims from a very detached position, as if they were not really human to him. The sense that he conveyed was that these people represented obstacles which he needed to overcome in order to achieve his ultimate goal – taking possessions – thereby meeting his perceived needs. The feeling conveyed was of people as inanimate objects, devoid of history, intelligence, feeling or purpose of their own. Bill described the time he spent prolifically offending, as his most destructive.

During the second day of the workshop, Bill was invited to participate in a 'work segment'. With the room arranged like a mini theatre with both an acting and audience space and all group members seated in the audience area, Bill was invited to sit on the 'stage' and be interviewed by Emma, focusing on one of his offences. He was asked to remember the events of the offence, from its antecedents to his actions following the crime. Whilst the interview took place Mario, listening closely to the details being shared by Bill, began to devise a bespoke work segment for him, in the form of a piece of drama, to look at this offence in some dramatic detail which would require other group members to take on characters.

Following the disclosure of the offence Bill and Emma left the room, whist the remainder of the group were briefed by Mario on the roles they had volunteered themselves to undertake on Bill's return. Group members who were not involved in the action were nevertheless completely involved in the role of 'active witness'. For the person engaged in a drama-therapy enactment, 'the experience of being witnessed . . . can be experienced as being acknowledged or supported' (Jones 1996: 111). For those in the role of active witness, he '. . . can develop the "audience" aspect of themselves towards their experience, enhancing the capability to engage differently with themselves and life events' (ibid 111).

One patient volunteered to become a masked character, wearing a neutral full-face mask, which is designed to appear expressionless. The mask is intended to be a representation of the victim that Bill had identified and talked about during his witness's interview. The masked character was asked to stand on the stage area and adopt an equally neutral physical position. He is informed that when he begins to feel like a real person, then he can take the mask off and look towards Bill.

Bill re-enters onto the stage area and is asked by Mario to look at the masked figure and think about what it might represent. He quickly guesses that the figure might represent one of his own victims. He is playing with his hands, with a smile on his face, hoping, it would seem by his affectation, to elicit some humourous reaction from group members. He cannot easily pre-empt what might be the 'correct' thing to do. He is alone, with the rest of the group watching him. He appears anxious, hiding behind his anti-authoritarian defence. Only he can decide whether to take the risk with what is asked of him or to rubbish it through his defences, making little or no emotional connection with what is trying to be achieved with him.

Bill is asked by Mario to focus on the offence in more detail. He indicates quickly that he has done so and is informed that the masked character is representing the primary victim of the offence. Bill is then asked to begin creating an identity for this victim by first giving a name, followed by an age, height, eye colour. Then a history, relationships with friends and family, a personality with likes and dislikes, thoughts and feelings.

Bill's defence was to become literal. With a sense of triumphant refusal to enter into an 'as if' framework he said that he did not know the name of the victim. Encouragingly Mario re-emphasises the focus of the work: that it not to describe a real person, the real victim, but to engage in a creative and imaginative process whereby the representation, the mask, is given status and authenticity, a human-ness rather than the human-less projections towards his real victim. Bill's anxiety, shown previously in his humour, has now changed to anger. He continues to attempt to self-sabotage the work by refusing to answer any more 'as if' questions about the victim. The masked figure remains standing, neutral, facing Bill. However, Bill can see the eyes through the mask and may not be seeing a neutral pose, but maybe a menacing and blaming figure, reminding him of the crime he is attempting to distance himself from.

The feeling of shame appears to be present. Bill is trying to avoid connecting with the uncomfortable and painful feelings inside of himself, under his defences. Bill is asked what it would mean for him to make his victim a real person. He does not answer the question, but instead gives the figure a name. He then populates the figure with an identity, a life, a purpose, answering the questions he has already been asked, at his pace, under his control.

There is a sense that Bill wants to leave the room, but he does not. He gives brief answers to questions and his controlled anger is visible. Yet he stays on the stage area and continues with the work. The figure remains masked. He attempts to show that he is not affected by the work. However he is communicating that he has made a connection to the masked figure. The exercise is stopped after some time and the character remains masked. He has not felt like a real person behind his mask. The scene is de-roled by Emma who has been in the role of witness during the enactment. The masked character is asked to unmask and connect with their real selves, saying their name and something about themselves, whilst looking directly towards Emma. He will be asked for their input in a short while, but first Bill will be re-interviewed in front of the group. The main aim of the second interview is to reflectively explore feelings and thoughts about the experience as well as to ground Bill from this work and prepare him to re-enter the group who will engage in a whole group exercise and subsequent reflection towards the end of the day. Bill is able to talk about what occurred and his angry presentation is noted and explored. The active witnesses are invited to comment on what they saw and they offer insightful and personal connections about their own feelings and experiences of seeing Bill at work. The patient who was masked is also asked to talk of how it felt to be behind the mask and inevitably connections are made to other offences committed by group members. For the remainder of the workshop Bill is notably quieter and a little withdrawn during the group exercise.

In the next day's group reflection Bill spoke of his awareness of seeing his victims as real people. He commented that he had not done this at all during his long incarceration. He reflected upon his desire and ability to control his surroundings and of his fear of being out of control. He appeared at this time, to take a significant risk with this vulnerable part of himself, a part that is lacking, a failing to form empathic connections with people for whom he has caused pain and trauma.

Whilst Bill's work segment did not reach its hoped for conclusion – the un-masking of the neutral character through feeling humanised by Bill's description – it did stir in him deep feelings of his own life–drama connection; the realisation that he has not seen these people as real, as victims, but as objects for his own gain. Bill appeared to convey a deep longing in search of making a different kind of connection with humanity.

In this case study Bill presents as being in conflict with himself and with others, displaying on the one hand a need to belong and on the other a defence against this very theme. Bill was not able to humanise the masked character in the work segment and in so doing cut off the feelings of attaching to this figure on an emotional level. What we were able to experience and feedback to him through witnessing the dramatic exchange and the life–drama connection was something of his vulnerability in wanting to belong – versus his need to control and to distance himself from a sense of belonging.

Reflection and ending

Reflection and ending sessions are fundamental components of any therapeutic intervention. In dramatherapy, reflection takes on both verbal and non-verbal forms. In this way, ideas and thoughts that may be abstract and hard to explore verbally can be witnessed and held in mind by group members and therapists. As one colleague in the focus group noted, 'I sometimes think some things just can't be described by words, it can't be experienced with language, and I think dramatherapy gets into that really unspoken stuff.'

As Langley notes in the following quotation, there is value in closing sessions as a group and connecting with the shared experience. She says that

'coming together as a group for a general discussion . . . is the final stage before closure. Although it is ostensibly an opportunity to look objectively at the process of the session, group members often share with the whole group personal feelings they have already imparted in pairs or small groups. Having once described their experience, individuals can repeat their story with more distance and further reflect on it, maybe finding other group members have had similar insights. It is also an opportunity to obtain further witnesses to a private episode, and in doing so, feel less isolated' (Langley 2006: 100).

Earlier in this chapter we referred to some of the opening statements of the workshop and now we share the frequent comments offered during the final afternoon's reflective feedback session, which we leave usually around 45 minutes for:

- 'I wish I'd done this years ago'
- 'I think everyone should be made to do this'
- 'I didn't think I would but I really liked doing all the drama stuff'
- 'I found it hard but feel I got something from it'
- 'I've never done anything like this before it's so powerful'
- 'It's not what I expected, I thought I was going to be made to be a tree'

Patients invariably express a need to thank us for working with them, remarking on the use of physical contact and their appreciation of its presence, despite initial fear, resistance and anxiety over being touched. Touch is '. . . a powerful positive communication . . .' (Ramsden *et al.* 2006: 163) when used with safe boundaries and healthy intentions. It is vital to the healthy developmental growth of the infant. Touching in the workshop is both literal and metaphorical. Being touched is being seen and heard and acknowledged on some basic human level. As the work has developed over time, we have recognised its inclusion as a fundamental part of the process.

The being seen and heard is also felt by patients towards each other and group members acknowledge working together as a team and supporting each other. A desire to acknowledge the work of others in an empathic way is also present. For example a patient remarked 'I really felt for "Steve" when he had to play the role of his victim's husband. It was great that he stuck with it'. Also a desire to acknowledge reconnecting with painful feelings cut off at the time of offences being committed, yet somatically and unconsciously remembered. Rarely do patients leave the workshop part way through, but it has occurred, along with a few sleeping patients caused by factors such as medication or self intention or both.

At the end of the work, living through their anxieties and fears and having undertaken the challenges they have been invited to engage with, there is often more of a sense of group cohesion, openness, confidence, thoughtfulness and empathy between patients. As Yalom states '. . . the sense of cohesiveness [is] a major therapeutic factor . . .' that it '. . . – develops, and patients often derive enormous benefit from the experience of being a valued member of an ongoing, stable group' (Yalom 1995: 458). Over time we have seen these feelings of empathy have a life beyond the workshop, hearing feedback from support facilitators about the reflection on the overall group process when the end of programme approaches. We have also been invited to participate in the final session some months later, when patients are celebrating their completion success.

Let us turn now to the focus group held with our colleagues to hear a little more about their perceptions of the process and experiences of the work.

The focus group

Over our time of facilitating this work, we have been interested in exploring experiences of patients and colleagues. In keeping with an open multidisciplinary approach, the two-hour focus group was facilitated with Phil Jones. We invited five colleagues to participate in the discussion, which was structured around a series of open questions. The questions related to their perceptions and observations of the work and of being in a dramatherapy framework. The focus group participants had all been involved in at least two victim empathy dramatherapy intensive workshops over the past six years. They represented the disciplines of psychology, nurse therapy and music therapy.

We found the focus group to be a moving exchange of thoughts, feelings and experiences and noted the recurrent themes of action and experiencing, the uses of touch, cohesiveness of the group and desire to confront in the patients, the sorrow felt in the staff team about the life journeys they witnessed and the choices and decisions taken at times of stress, distress, isolation, vulnerability, fear and revenge. We would like to acknowledge the dedicated and wise practice of our colleagues and their sensitivity, patience, ability and skill to facilitate the process of this group work programme for violent offenders.

One of our colleagues reflected on the importance of '. . . re-creating life or what goes on for them, how they are in that space . . .', further adding that the work enables a particular kinds of encounter . . . 're-creating it so that everything, not just the act but the emotion, . . . and everything that goes with it' is engaged with. Another colleague remarked 'I sometimes think some things just can't be described by words, it can't be experienced with language, and I think dramatherapy gets into that really unspoken stuff.' We have spoken of the focus we place on the life–drama connection, enabling thoughts, action and emotion to be experienced in the lived moment of the work. The cognitive-affective position – that is the seeing and feeling the world as another person of empathy is developed into embodied empathy – connecting with the somatic experiences, that is the bodily feelings and sensations, of the patients – feeling through the action methods, the experiential nature of the work (Cooper 2001). Both our and our colleagues' capacity to work with empathy in the victim empathy intensive workshops is deepened by the invitation to participate on a bodily level in many of the exercises.

Further quotations taken from the focus group transcript, highlight this dominant theme of working with action methods – using physical embodiment – to enable heightened emotional connections for patients through the exploration of their own life stories. One focus group participant commented that the patients' stories become less like 'learnt scripts'; the process '. . . is a way of reconnecting and getting close to the feelings states' of the time of the offence. The word power was mentioned many times during the discussion, in relation to the power of the drama. It was noted that 'there's something in dramatherapy that I've seen helps connect with the reality of the situation in a much more powerful way than talking about it does ... there's something about scenarios ... actually you're in the room and you're feeling it, you're feeling what it would be like being in that situation. You're there and there's no hiding away that this is what that person did, and this is what it can make people feel like ... I think that's very powerful'. Also referred to is sitting with the unknown nature of the process at the start of the workshop '... questions around for patients are around what are we going to do with them, and we can never be very clear with them about what will happen because we don't know ... and that's the way that you work. It's about enabling them to sit with not knowing ...'

The focus group participants expressed with some certainty that drama-therapy is relevant to the needs of the forensic patient because of the difficulty the patient has in making connections with thought, action and emotion and the need for them to emphasise the link with reality – the life–drama connection – yet recognise that the process is '... really difficult to put into words ... what happens and what that powerful experience is about.' When briefly exploring being in the focus group one observation was that 'It's been nice to reflect actually, and I agree about how much do we know about dramatherapy and do we know the words to explain, I don't. I feel like the patient who doesn't know a couple of words to explain their emotions really. I couldn't tell you what the techniques were but it just works. I couldn't describe it, but I've really valued this part of the group.'

Reflection on theory and method

Energy and the body

Creative methods and physical dramatic work help release energy (Barker 1989). In the workshop we take the notion of the lived experience via dra-matic expression and work in a style which we refer to as 'spontaneous dra-matic action'. One definition of spontaneity suggests it is 'A moment of explosion; a free moment of self-expression' (Spolin 1998: 392). For many incarcerated individuals of violent offences, expending energy in life has been damaging and destructive. It is a known experience which has been a painful, yet familiar expression in the past of pent up feelings. In the workshop, we invite the patients to participate in methods and work segments with little or no room for contemplation or seeming choice to engage or participate. In truth, we are constantly reading what is written on the body and intuitively seeking consent. As one of our colleagues commented when talking about the differences working verbally and physically: 'There's something about the physicality of [dramatherapy], its directness, not necessarily relying on words ... these patients what they've done is physical ... They've done physical acts, so it's a language they are familiar with.'

Perspective

Along with our attention to working spontaneously, with the body and this dramatherapeutic theory, we work in a psychodynamic arena and this is particularly notable during the long periods of verbal reflection, in the form of open circle discussions, which occur, as mentioned above, at the start and end of each workshop day. The aim of these discussions is to provide unguided space for any thoughts, feelings and connections to be made between the external action of the 'doing' with the internal narrative of the 'being'. It is not therefore left in the drama as may be the case when working with a more theatrical or forum style (Boal 1979). To allow time for feelings to surface, we give importance to silence. This is an opportunity for group members to make connections for themselves with the material they have experienced and to listen to and witness each other's words.

We have experience of working with patients on a long-term basis, both individually and in groups, with interventions running for up to five or more years. The patients' capacity for 'destruction' from different perspectives is ever present. Thinking psychodynamically about our work has been an essential factor in looking at the underlying dynamics that exist in forensic patients. The patients' psychotic functioning results in quite primitive and unconscious destructive impulses (Klein 1997).

We have often experienced the unconscious attack on linking and thinking by the patients (Bion 1967). They can display both overt (external) and covert (internal) destructive behaviour within the work. For example, attacking the link between the drama and reality, by making negative statements about what is happening, choosing not to make connections between themselves and the scenes being portrayed, or by focusing on the 'fun' in the creative work, missing the depth of connection with the material to their experiences.

We think that it is crucial to help the patient to be able to make links with the drama and reality in an overt way and for the patient to feel supported that they will not be overwhelmed and consumed by connecting with their emotional world. Nevertheless, the work is powerful and can resonate deeply, leaving lasting images. As Bill, one group member commented 'I won't easily forget what has happened here in the past few days. It has been hard'. To expect a forensic patient to make links on their own would be to risk the patient splitting off the drama from the reality and therefore destroying the therapeutic intent. As Jones emphasised when referring to dramatherapeutic process of the life–drama connection: 'If the connection did not exist then the client might be able to create and maintain a separate dramatherapy world. This would be counter-therapeutic' (1996: 117).

Jennings, writing in 1992 about the potential benefits of dramatherapy in forensic psychiatry, recalls there being two trained dramatherapists working in the field. Of dramatherapy in this environment she says '. . . it is possible for people to "re-work" their experience . . . through the dramatic distance of the drama . . . it can re-shape affective material and integrate it in new and constructive ways . . . it can expand and develop role repertoire and replace unhelpful and destructive roles with more socially-acceptable and life-enhancing roles' (Jennings 1992a: 244). These suggestions have certainly been borne out in our work in the victim empathy workshop.

We encourage patients to take risks with their personal material, whilst offering a safe and contained space with dramatic methods with which to explore these risks, thus enabling the life–drama connection to be present in the work. Through the use of distancing we are hoping to maintain a safe space where deeply traumatic events are remembered in the living body and witnessed in the room by the strength and holding of the group and their history of working together therapeutically. In terms of dramatherapy processes, the vignette documented in this chapter could be experienced as provocative and harsh. Within the context of the work however, it is the opposite. Change and shifts occur when we undertake this work. There are many more stories of positive affective change we could document which we have witnessed in this work and in patients' post-workshop development.

The patient mythology that surrounds the intensive victim empathy dramatherapy workshop grows stronger with each new group. It is a living part of the process of being at this hospital and as such must have value placed on it for it to be discussed in this way. We are not suggesting that this brief intervention 'cures' the patients. For many, their severely damaged sense of self requires ongoing and intensive further work before release from secure services is possible. For some, release will not happen but value remains in working through trauma towards a more peaceful existence. What the workshop seems to offer and achieve is an opportunity to play and be creative with others, whilst also reaching into oneself and being responsible and having the choice to look at some of the significant damage that has been caused by the individual in the role of perpetrator. Also it provides a chance to listen to and hear the duality of the lost voice of the victim that exists within this same body.

We consider this work to be essential to providing meaningful methods of expression for these patients. We cannot prove that it works in an empirical sense, but from a qualitative perspective, there are many changes to the life quality of the patients which are captured in the final three-month phase of the group and on the post-group assessment tools which take the form of in-depth interviews with the outreach team from the specialist therapy unit. The 'feel good' factor at the end of groups and an improvement in self-esteem, both of which we have mentioned above, is something that Jennings *et al.* also note following a pilot group in the same high secure setting more than a decade ago (Jennings *et al.* 1997).

'Theatre and drama . . . has the ability to make both easily accessible and deeply resonant pictures out of often difficult emotional and intellectual information and constructs and can often provide the vital key to opening up channels of communication that may otherwise remain closed' (Hewish

1992: 219). In the victim empathy work patients are invited to access drama '. . . as a dynamic means of stimulating change within the individual; to challenge offenders to examine their own behaviour and to act out new approaches to change' (ibid 1992: 218).

Conclusion

In summary, within this chapter we have tried to show the journey of the victim empathy work with male offenders, its history within the high secure hospital that we have positioned it as well as described this client group and identified some of the main themes of this work. We have aimed to show both the patient's perspective and our own thoughts, along with those of our colleagues by way of quotations from the focus group. We believe this work is highly beneficial when undertaken by experienced clinicians supported by a group work programme. Whilst we have no direct experience of offering such a programme to female patients, we would suggest that would also be possible and worthwhile.

Throughout the workshop, and in Bill's drama, we see how the core processes, particularly interactive audience and witnessing, embodiment and life–drama connection, are brought to 'life'. Perhaps it is the patients who are in role as audience/witnesses that silently supports Bill in being able to tolerate the scene. Alternatively he did not want to be seen to be giving up and therefore failing in front of them. Bill uses the audience as a defence by 'entertaining' them through his jokes. The presence of the audience/witnesses undoubtedly has a powerful effect on him. The audience/witnesses becomes active by moving to 'actor' during the re-enactment of Bill's offence. As witnesses to a drama that has as its inspiration the powerful real-life events of all the patients in the room will cause strong emotions which we see in the faces and bodies of the patients. It is the embodiment, the here and now of the drama, that captures imagination and engagement of both the 'actors' and the witnessing audience. As Jones states: 'In Dramatherapy this physicalised knowing and being within a dramatic representation of a problem or issue makes a crucial difference to the verbal recounting or description of a client's material' (Jones 1996: 113).

Since Jennings made reference to having knowledge in 1992 of two trained dramatherapists in forensic services, we add that this field is ever expanding with arts therapies departments in a range of settings of varying security from low to high. The dramatherapists in high secure services can be counted on half of one hand, but there is great respect for the intervention of dramatherapy in these services and it is our hope that this chapter will contribute to the evidence base for our field, engaging the passions of other dramatherapists who may explore this way of working in their own setting.

9 Dramatherapy, learning disabilities and acute mental health

Naomi Gardner-Hynd

Box 9.1

Questions about practice

- How can dramatherapy be effective in work with clients with learning disabilities and mental health problems?
- How is the role of therapy connected to social exclusion?
- How is creativity related to dramatherapy?

Research perspective

- Dramatic work as evaluation
- Case study
- Staff questionnaires on the impact of dramatherapy

Client perspective sample

In the final session I asked clients to create a group sculpt reflecting how they had experienced the group. Frank took a chair, sat on it and positioned himself as if he was rowing with an oar. Peter took up a similar position with a chair on the other side. Oliver took some blue and yellow cloth and laid it on the floor; he then stood in front of the two chairs and positioned himself as if he was looking through binoculars. Gary stood next to Oliver, pretending to be fishing. (Description of dramatic work as evaluation.)

Introduction

The following chapter explores dramatherapy in an NHS context and consists of a case study of dramatherapy with a group of clients with learning disabilities and mental health problems. Using the creativity cycle as the conceptual basis of the work, clinical vignettes will aid discussion of some of the core processes at work in dramatherapy and group work in general. An introduction to the setting and background to the group sets the stage for discussion of key issues such as socio-economics, working within a medical model and use of a developmental framework.

Contexts

Fletcher argues that in the past, many professionals assumed that people with learning disabilities did not experience emotional problems, stress and psychiatric disorder (Fletcher 1993). However, professionals are increasingly recognising that individuals with learning disabilities have higher rates of psychiatric disorders compared with the general population. The 1995 Welsh Health Survey (Welsh Office 1995) found that individuals with a learning difficulty had a higher rate of psychiatric illness (32.2 per cent) in comparison to the general population (11.2 per cent). More recently, the second Dutch National Survey of General Practice reported that individuals with learning disabilities made 1.7 times more visits to their GP, than the general population, in regards to mental health problems. (Straetmans, Van Schrojenstein Lantman-de Valk, Schellevis *et al.* 2007). They also presented a different morbidity pattern and received four times as many repeated prescriptions than those without learning disabilities. Richards *et al.* (2001) found that learning disability was associated with a four-fold increase in the risk of affective disorder. The affective spectrum is a grouping of related psychiatric and medical disorders which may accompany bipolar, unipolar and schizoaffective disorders at statistically higher rates than would normally be expected. Psychiatric disorders may be an important, perhaps even a primary factor, limiting the functioning of people with learning disabilities, their quality of life and their adaptation to life in the community.

A report carried out by the Royal College of Psychiatrists in March 2004, confirmed the need for greater psychotherapeutic input for people with learning disabilities. Adaptation and flexibility of therapeutic approach was described as essential for this client group. Eighty-three per cent of psychiatrists surveyed indicated that there was a high demand for psychotherapy for people with learning disabilities. The particular vulnerability of this client group to sexual abuse, loss, psychiatric disorder and consequences of institutional care were cited as reasons for this demand. Government policy also seems to be emphasising the particular needs of individuals with learning disabilities. *Valuing People: A New Strategy for Learning Disability in the 21st Century* states clearly that the National Service Framework (NSF) for Mental Health applies as much to people with learning disabilities as to other patients. A person with a learning disability is now entitled to access mainstream mental health services and should be treated the same any other individual. The four key principles outlined are rights, independence, choice and inclusion. I work for a growing Arts Therapies team based in a large NHS Trust. The team comprises art, music and dramatherapists who work into different specialities and directorates. Working on three adult learning disabilities mental health wards, I offer short-term groups, long term one-to-one sessions, and some community-based work. Two of the three wards are adult male and all three have 15 beds. Having previously been a specialist learning disabilities trust, clients are referred from all areas of the country and originate from diverse ethnic and religious backgrounds. The mental health wards admit clients with acute mental health problems and on occasion, clients with behavioural difficulties, whose problems appear to have a psychological basis.

Clients are generally referred for dramatherapy through the consultant psychiatrist, ward managers and multidisciplinary team. Working in a psychosocial framework, the MDT meets weekly to discuss individual patients and make appropriate referrals based on their formulations. A psychosocial approach integrates cognitive, cognitive-behavioural, behavioural techniques and psychotherapy and offers a range of supportive interventions to relieve psychological distress. These can include patient education, interventions aimed at aiding relaxation, developing self-esteem and encouraging peer support. Formulation is the summation and integration of the knowledge that is acquired through extensive examination of case history, notes and other assessments. Once referred, clients are immediately given an assessment interview to consider their interest in and capacity to engage with dramatherapy. Individuals are then invited to a 'taster session' to establish their suitability for group or individual sessions.

Social and familial circumstances, as well as illicit drug use, have been shown to be precursors of mental ill-health (Sass 2000). Johnstone (1994) cites lower socio-economic class as a fundamental cause of schizophrenia and other disabling mental health problems. Margai and Henry (2003) have shown that individuals with learning disabilities are more likely to have a lower socio-economic status and may therefore be more vulnerable to mental ill-health. Stressful life events, such as family breakdown, bereavement, moving house or work related problems have been shown to precipitate mental health problems or engender a relapse. The impact of such factors has also been shown to be even greater on individuals with learning disabilities, which increases their vulnerability to mental health problems even further (Margai and Henry 2003) The reasons for this increased impact are connected to difficulty with processing the reasons for these types of life events (e.g. family breakdown), often attributing responsibility to themselves rather than others which can lead to low self-esteem and depression. Society's view of individuals with learning difficulties can often be unhelpful, which further undermines the creativity and independence of these individuals. Mindell, one of the few leading psychotherapists currently addressing social and political issues in their work, describes rank as 'the sum of a person's privileges' (Mindell 1995: 28). In this society very few differences are neutral with respect to power and rank. Gender, sexuality, class, ethnicity, income, age, disability – all carry with them enormous implications for perceived and experienced rank and . . . power. Rank is 'both perceived and experienced . . . the automatic . . . power and authority' that is within the therapeutic relationship, often unconsciously, but reflecting the social divisions and power relationships within society (Totton 2008: 149–150).

The role of therapist is undoubtedly affected by these wider socio-cultural issues. Initially one member of the group made a joke about my being 'posh'. All of the clients had strong Geordie accents but having been to drama school my accent had almost disappeared. This also seemed to be a reflection of power within the group. The client seemed to be communicating anxieties about whether the therapist would reinforce these social differences, but also raising an awareness of what it was to be different. In fact this client had created in me, feelings which he himself must have held. After all, I was the only 'posh' one in the group. These issues also became apparent in relation to what I was wearing, emphasising that I was the only female and therefore also looked different. The group seemed to have reversed the situation which they habitually face. I was led to experience being on the outskirts and 'different' while they were able to experience being part of the majority. Working through this issue was important for establishing trust. It felt almost as if I had been through some form of initiation to test my capacity to hold the group and relate to their current situation. Sensitivity to these types of issues seems critical when working with client groups which are traditionally marginalised by society.

Description of the work

Referral

Four, adult males in their twenties, with a diagnosis of schizophrenia, were identified as being suitable for group dramatherapy. All of the individuals were from low-income families and had experienced bullying, due to being learning disabled, and had a history of drug involvement. They exhibited difficulties interacting socially and had impaired communication skills. Two had been excluded from school. Each client had recently experienced stressful life events such as break up of parents, bereavement or onset of illness in a close family member. The four males visibly acted out their angry feelings and described finding it difficult to trust people or form meaningful attachments. Most had experienced loss and abandonment. Margai and Henry (2003) note that these types of life events can have a greater impact on individuals with learning disabilities. The four clients all described themselves as being on the outskirts of society, not belonging and feeling isolated. The report from the Royal College of Psychiatrists (March 2004) had found that it is harder for people with learning disabilities to access bereavement or counselling services mainly because of communication barriers. Bullying and exclusion further undermine the individual's confidence, communication and ability to seek help. Many of my previous clients had come to expect bullying as a 'norm'. A recent MENCAP survey (2007) revealed eight out of ten (82 per cent) children with a learning disability are bullied while eight out of ten (79 per cent) are also scared to go out because they are frightened they might be bullied. Dame Jo Williams, MENCAP's chief executive, said: 'These shocking findings show how big a problem bullying is for children with a learning disability. Bullying wrecks lives, making children scared to go out . . . children with a learning disability are missing out on opportunities to learn and make friends, socialise and play. If action is not taken to tackle bullying, children with a learning disability will face bullying and isolation all their lives' (MENCAP 2007).

The therapy room is off the ward in a separate building and thorough risk assessments were conducted to ensure the safety of the group. Working with this client group has challenged my perspectives and attitudes towards dramatherapy and learning disabilities. When reading ward notes and meeting with members of the multidisciplinary team, the therapist can often be left feeling 'hopeless', or that change is 'impossible'. One way of under-standing such a response is to see it as a reflection of negative stereotypes and prejudices that exist in society. These devalue individuals with learning disabilities and see them as incapable, or not of value, rather than as active agents in their own lives, capable of change and worth attention and value. It is important for the therapist to be aware of such negative dynamics and stereotypes, and to challenge them in their own, and in others' responses. A medical model of itself can often focus on what is wrong with a client to the exclusion of positives. This may represent a mirroring of society's attitudes towards this client group and sometimes the work of the dramatherapist is to encourage a more holistic picture of the individual at multidisciplinary meetings.

The taster session

The taster session took place on a Tuesday afternoon, the most suitable time for the ward and clients as there are no ward rounds and no other groups or activities. Opening circle provided an opportunity for the clients to voice anxieties and develop group awareness. Although the clients live on the same ward together, they are separated into two flats, with two of the clients living in each. It was evident from the outset that allegiances existed. Two clients from Flat 1 sat at the bottom of the room, while the remaining two sat at the opposite end. When asked to form a circle there was initial hesitancy; with encouragement however cushions were moved and with them new relation-ships initiated. To develop fun and facilitate movement a game of 'Anyone who' was initiated. This is often a productive and lively game which enables the group to learn about one another, while also using the space, instigating movement and creating different patterns of interaction. New friendships were forged after discovering that they all supported the same football team, liked snooker and hated being in hospital. Within five minutes the mood in the room was brighter, relaxed and laughter began to permeate the walls.

For initial assessment purposes I usually use Chesner's (1995) Dramatherapy Tree which helps to determine which levels the group are able to work at. Clients can then feel comfortable with the activities and are more likely to attend sessions. Focusing on what the clients can do automatically helps to develop self-esteem and ownership of the group. Ball games and object work demonstrated that clients were comfortable working at root and trunk levels. Developing trust and positive relationships was a central aim of the group. It was decided that working at these levels would be appropriate for the first phase of therapy.

Box 9.2

The Dramatherapy Tree can be used as an assessment tool to determine at what level clients are functioning and what activities will be suitable. For example clients with profound learning disabilities may only be able to work at root level, where basic movement of specific body parts or exploring boundaries and personal space may be appropriate. Clients with less severe communication, intellectual or physical disability may be able to work with more complex structures such as role play, storytelling or mask work and the progression up the tree from root to leaf can be used as part of formative assessment to determine progress in therapy. Whatever the client group or level of abilities, working with root level activities, such as ball games and trust work should always be the starting point.

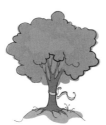

The creativity cycle

The creativity cycle influences the way my sessions are structured and provides insight into the therapeutic process. The following diagram represents the creativity cycle in relation to dramatherapy session structure which is based on a model by Payne (1993) used in dance movement therapy.

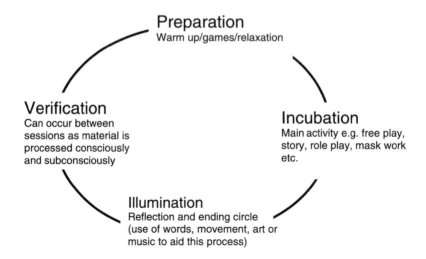

Figure 9.1 Dramatherapy and the creativity cycle (Gardner-Hynd 2008).

Hadamard (1945) and Poincaré (1952) were the first to maintain that creativity occurs within a set process. This process is cyclical and has four stages, which are, preparation (warm-up/games/relaxation), incubation (main activity e.g. free play/story/role play/mask work etc.), illumination (reflection and ending circle: use of words/movement/art or music to aid this process) and verification (can occur between sessions as material is processed consciously and subconsciously). The cycle happens both within a session and as part of the long term group process. Winnicott (1971) equates creativity with healthy functioning. He perceives creativity as an entity in itself that is present in *all* individuals. He argues that any simple act, even breathing, can be seen as creative, and that the notion of creativity is intricately and inextricably linked to our very sense of being. Winnicott also associates creativity with identity. Arieti (1980) argues that modern society has forgotten how to be creative and that this is a major contributor to psychopathology. May (1976) also believes that healing and creativity are intertwined. In terms of physiological processes he argues that creativity leads to physical healing and regeneration, while in emotional terms it consists of establishing, or creating, attitude changes. May perceives creativity as an emergence of new and valid synthesis of ideas which spring from the unconscious. Csikszentmihalyi (1992) argues that creativity in itself is a form of abreaction 'a magical synthesis of past and present, abolition of objective time, a healing through the reactivation of the former pain which can now be tolerated by the mature person.' (Csikszentmihalyi 1992: 23) The next section illustrates that the creativity cycle can also be seen as a framework for dramatherapy practice.

Preparation

The theme of new beginnings was evident from the first session. Client A announced that he was ready to begin. This had relevance on two levels. Sessions had started and the group was beginning to get to know one another, while each individual had made a commitment to the group and was beginning on a personal therapeutic journey. A variety of games were introduced to explore working in pairs and developing trust.

> ### Vignette: Trust walk
>
> Peter and Oliver lived in different flats but decided to work together. Peter decided to be 'A' and Oliver 'B'. Peter helped Oliver with the blindfold and began to lead him round the space. He warned him of any furniture in his path and guided him gently round the room. After five minutes they swapped roles with Oliver leading Peter. At first arms were held out in trepidation that they would be led into a wall or might hurt themselves. Peter assertively indicated to his partner that he was safe and that he wouldn't let him bump into anything. There was a moment of nervous excitement and apprehension when it seemed that both pairs might bump into each other. Both 'leaders' took their partners by the arm and indicated vocally that they should stop and move to opposite sides. In the next part of the exercise, the leader takes their partner on a 'magical journey' around the room. Peter took Oliver to the corner of the room and began describing a waterfall, cascading down the side of a mountain. The spray was cooling and refreshing. He then described a trail through some woods with leaves crunching under foot. It was dark in some areas but the sun provided warmth and light. Oliver commented that it had been scary at first. He admitted not trusting Peter and occasionally peeping through the blindfold. He likened the experience to when his illness was at its worst; not knowing what was happening and feeling completely helpless. The acknowledgement of these vulnerable feelings was enormously emotive for the group but also seemed to bring the group closer together.

Incubation

Session 3, the clients had all had a bad week and were feeling depressed. On entering the space they were very withdrawn and quiet. The group decided to explore emotions. Peter articulated that he was no longer able to express feelings and described being 'emotionless'. In 'magic shop', clients are asked to consider which emotions or characteristics they might need or like and those they may wish to have less of. Clients are invited to enter the shop individually or in pairs. For this shop the group decided to create the scenery and make the objects which were to be sold. They created a banner to hang over the door and laid out their objects in chairs and on tables. Peter was reticent about going into the shop unsure what to ask for. Frank took on role of shopkeeper and invited him into the shop. Having created a counter with tables and decorated a box for the till Frank asked Peter to explore the shop and choose an object. Each object had its own symbolism which was different for each client. Peter stood by the door unsure whether to go further into the shop. On one of the tables was a basket of stones, all of different shapes and sizes. Peter selected a large smooth stone. He noted that it was like the ones he used when spinning stones across the top of the river, attempting to get it to hop across the surface. He described these as happy times, free from worry and decided he would purchase the stone. It also symbolised strength. Peter bartered with Frank to buy the stone, Frank arguing that it was a precious stone and was therefore expensive. Peter wrote on a piece of paper 'negative thoughts', offered it as payment, which Frank accepted.

Clients with learning disabilities can often become institutionalised or deskilled, with decisions often being made by others. An aim of sessions is therefore to encourage clients to make decisions for themselves. I have also found that clients take greater ownership of the group and show greater willingness to engage when they are involved in session content. By session 4 clients were leading the physical warm-up and suggesting games. Gary suggested he lead the group in one of his favourite games from childhood – Simon Says. He got the group running around the space and the clients found this exhilarating and amusing. The group was then asked to think of a favourite toy from childhood, select it from objects provided and play/explore it for a few minutes. During this time, interaction between the clients was encouraged by inviting group play and sharing of objects. The clients were much freer in their movements compared to previous sessions and spontaneously used noises and laughter. Clients then introduced their toys to the group. The clients individually moved to a different part of the circle and were asked to 'become' their toys. The other clients could then ask questions about the toy.

Vignette: Bang bang

Oliver decided to become his old toy gun. As the toy, he described having been loaded and fired many times and that as a result he no longer worked properly. The group were encouraged to ask questions of Oliver, while in role as his toy gun. Peter asked if Oliver (as the gun) had been treated well by Oliver when he was younger. Oliver (as the gun) replied that he had been a good owner and had kept him close, even slept with him under his pillow at one stage. Gary asked if Oliver felt safe having him close. 'Yes', he replied, to keep away the Indians and attackers. Peter asked if he had been involved in any battles. 'Yes', he replied, sometimes he had been a hero and saved people from monsters, but occasionally he had been wounded and needed time in hospital to recover. Oliver described the gun as once being black and red, but that over the years the paint had come off and it was no longer 'shiny'. Gary asked if Oliver still had the gun. No, but sometimes I dream about it. After thoroughly de-roling Oliver described feeling powerful and 'in control'. Although not explicitly discussed or interpreted by the group, it was evident through the role of the gun, that Oliver had identified and made connections with aspects of his past and illness.

Illumination

The clients asked if they could re-enact being back at school. Acting as themselves, aged 16, they imagined a scene in the dinner hall. Gary had been severely bullied at school and was particularly nervous about engaging in this exercise. I reassured him he could sit out at any point, which he did after Peter asked him to 'pass the salt'. Gary later described how when at school, bullies, two years older than him, would empty salt over all his dinner. The clients spoke and interacted minimally throughout this scene. In the discussion later the clients described how this had been a particularly difficult time in their lives and a point at which for some of them, their illnesses had first emerged. The group were keen to explore roles. A picture of a wall with hand prints on was placed in the middle of the circle. The hand prints were of different sizes and colours. In the circle, the group discussed who could have made these prints. The clients were invited to create a character based on one of these hand prints. The clients agreed these characters would meet in a park. Peter became a character artist, drawing people's faces. Oliver became a business-man on his lunch, Gary a father with his young son, Frank a policeman. Frank approached Peter to ask if he had a licence for painting. Peter said that he didn't and so Frank gave him a formal warning and said next time he would be fined. Gary was in the play area with his son who had fallen and hurt himself. Oliver approached Gary and asked whether the boy was ok. Eventually the four characters came together around a park bench and these apparent strangers made introductions and shared their lunch. The group began to make connections with the roles they had chosen and related how they had been strangers at the start but were now close friends. Objects often allow clients to identify characteristics which they find difficult to express or talk about. By using objects these ideas can be given form.

Vignette: Broken record

Gary described how his family life was causing him great distress at the moment. His parents would cancel visits at the last moment or wouldn't contact him for weeks. The group asked to explore family relationships. In the warm-up game of 'fortunately unfortunately' the group was particularly attentive to the story that was unfolding. 'A man was walking along the street, unfortunately he fell down a hole, fortunately when he reached the very bottom there were people there to help him, unfortunately these people couldn't stay around for long, fortunately he wasn't badly hurt, unfortunately it was dark and he had to feel his way around, fortunately there was a light in the distance.' This story was full of potent imagery which the group acknowledged but chose not to discuss. The clients were asked to select five objects while thinking about family relationships. The objects were to represent the characteristics of the family member being referred to. A further object was chosen to represent themselves and the other objects were placed in relation to one another according to family dynamics. Gary chose a wine glass to represent his father and a broken record to represent his mother, a heart for his sister and toy wheelchair to represent his grandmother. The group was then asked to reorganise the objects according to how they would like their family dynamic to be. Gary chose to remove the wine glass and put a plastic bag over it and pushed it under a chair – saying it has disappeared. He then rearranged the other objects to physically support his object. Gary discussed how his father was an alcoholic and how his mother had always supported his father even when he had hit him, suggesting that he was to blame. Gary commented that he had never spoken openly about his father before and became tearful. The objects had evoked powerful feelings for the group generally and everyone acknowledged how difficult this had been for Gary to discuss. The openness of the clients was enormously emotive and I became aware of my own strong feelings of anger. In supervision it became apparent that a number of issues relating to the relationship I have with my own father had been evoked. In closing circle the clients decided to have a group hug. This action seemed to embody the loss which each had experienced but also the reparative and supportive nature of the group. Gary chose to share some of his feelings with his family, who were first annoyed but came to visit him a week later to discuss how their relationship could progress.

Verification

In the final session I asked clients to create a group sculpt reflecting how they had experienced the group. Frank took a chair, sat on it and positioned himself as if he was rowing with an oar. Peter took up a similar position with a chair on the other side. Oliver took some blue and yellow cloth and laid it on the floor; he then stood in front of the two chairs and positioned himself as if he was looking through binoculars. Gary stood next to Oliver, pretending to be fishing. Going round each of them, I asked how it felt being in this position. Frank described being strong and part of a team. Peter said he felt in control, Oliver described having direction and purpose and Gary described feeling relaxed and happy. The image of the boat with its 'crew' reminded me of the journey we had all been on over the previous months. We had experienced rough seas when everyone was depressed and couldn't see where to go next, to clearer waters where we had fun, relaxed and could see our destination. In reality although the sessions were ending the journey for each of the clients had just started. The group had provided the clients with a floating vessel, at times this had been a lifeboat, at others a submarine and at the end a rowing boat for fishing. In my opinion the group had given the clients an experience of how to stay afloat and demonstrated how sharing and team work can help steer them in the right direction.

Questionnaire feedback

Working as part of the Department of Psychological Therapies and Research assessment and evaluation of the work is conducted as standard, with feedback presented to the MDT and wider Trust. The department routinely uses a mixture of psychological quantitative evaluation measures such as CORE 10 (Clinical Outcomes in Routine Evaluation 2007), as well as a panoply of qualitative techniques. For dramatherapy this includes Jones' Scale of Dramatic Involvement (Jones 1996). Members of the MDT, ward staff and clients are routinely invited to fill in questionnaires, providing qualitative feedback on how the clients present after sessions and groups have finished as well as their impressions of the work we do. Information from these questionnaires has been collated and summarised as follows.

Analysis of main themes

1. Anxiety

- From staff about being involved in sessions – what their role is and feeling self-conscious.
- From clients about having to be good at drama, put on the spot or make a fool of themselves.

At presentations I routinely invite nursing staff and members of the MDT to write a word or sentence that comes to mind when they think of the word Drama. Responses invariably include, 'school', 'terrified', 'spotlight', 'feeling silly', 'Am Dram'.

Offering introductory workshops, providing extensive staff training and presentations has helped to overcome some of these issues. However underlying fears of drama and previous personal experiences of the staff undoubtedly permeate their expectations of the work we do.

2. Being childish

- Staff who have attended taster sessions have sometimes commented that passing a ball, doing role play etc. seems childish. They comment that it is fun, but can't necessarily equate more extensive benefits.
- Clients comment that although they enjoy the opportunity to play in a safe and contained environment they also feel pressurised to conform to certain cultural rules and expectations. They describe not wanting to do activities which make them appear 'childish' because they do not want to be perceived more generally in this way.

These ideas seem to stem not from the client directly, but from wider societal attitudes that adults (particularly those with learning disabilities) perhaps shouldn't play games or do activities which are associated with children. Clearly drama, art and movement are in themselves innate activities which humans of all ages enjoy and engage with. However within a hospital /institutionalised setting (particularly with learning disabled clients) such activities seem to arouse fears of historic methods of treating individuals and staff can sometimes seek to distance themselves from such interventions.

3. Bringing individuals together/developing communication

- Staff describe how dramatherapy groups naturally encourage and enhance group working and communication. Its greatest strength, they argue, is its ability to bring together individuals who would normally avoid (or cannot) communicate and directly explore relationships in a safe and playful environment. The Dramatherapy Tree enables clients to work at all levels (particularly at the common – root – level) within one space. The nature of the work facilitates clients to help each other, developing positive relationships and promoting self-esteem. They observe that dramatherapy groups 'encourage quieter individuals to speak while louder and more confident members learn to mediate their behaviour and listen'.
- Clients have similarly commented that dramatherapy is best at forging relationships, enhancing confidence and promoting verbal communication.

4. Diversity of techniques

*   Staff regularly enthuse about the array of techniques on offer, which they argue facilitates a wider attendance. They acknowledge that drama-therapy is not limited to 'acting' and that clients who may feel isolated or unable to express themselves using one medium are free to explore another.
*   Clients also describe enjoying the freedom to work with a panoply of activities and art forms, particularly those who feel specifically unable to draw, be musical, or do 'drama'. Many describe finding new skills within sessions that they had previously never known. For example, clients from dramatherapy groups have taken up learning instruments, joined drama groups in the community, joined a choir, started to perform on karaoke night or started attending the Arts Project. Linked closely with this, they acknowledge developing a renewed sense of identity, self-worth and purpose.

5. Role expansion and identity

*   MDT and ward staff invariably communicate how constructive drama-therapy sessions are in encouraging clients to revise how they picture themselves. They describe how clients previously constrained to feeling 'incapable', 'unlovable', 'non-creative' and limited by their perception of being 'someone with learning disabilities' is challenged. Exploration of different roles, situations and possibilities through group and individual sessions encourages clients to think differently about themselves and ultimately behave in new ways.
*   Clients describe feeling 'empowered', 'that life has possibilities' and that they have 'potential'. For individuals who are frequently viewed and treated by society as disempowered, this change is perhaps the most significant and beneficial.

Reflection on theory and method

Trust walk

Dramatherapy utilises a number of key psychotherapy principles. As the name of the vignette infers, trust is an essential part of any psychotherapy group. Without it, individuals are unlikely to feel safe exploring material or issues and the group would undoubtedly fail to achieve any of its aims. Establishing a safe, contained and boundaried space, where everyone feels they have the space to speak and be heard, should be the first aim for any dramatherapy group. In my experience the taster session allows clients to discuss anxieties about performing or 'doing drama'. Questions and concerns can be discussed and reassurance given. Clients who would undoubtedly never have ventured into the group are assured that they can 'sit out' when they want to. From qualitative feedback at the end of group, clients have commented that the taster session has reduced anxiety and shown them that the 'therapy' aspect of the group is just as much a result of having fun as discussing difficult issues. Although trust needs to be established at the start of the group, it must be maintained and continuously developed throughout the sessions. Clients need to feel that the therapist can hold the group particularly during the incubation stage, where there is often uncertainty about how and where sessions will progress. Trust walk is significant and symbolic on many levels. Exploring and discovering the space in which the therapy is about to take place is important. Individuals experience the space both from a leader and being led perspective. They are able to simultaneously experience feeling both the anxiety of the unknown as well as the control of leading someone else while also taking control of the space. In this exercise clients dictate how they explore the room and where they will take their partner. The next step is to take their partner on a magical journey around the space. This functions to heighten the sense of possibility of the space; the room can be used imaginatively and symbolically, hence, engendering within the client that the room has 'therapeutic possibility'. The client can also begin to feel some control over the environment, which is particularly important for individuals with learning disabilities. From the start of the group, these types of exercises encourage the clients to take control over their own therapeutic journey and provide them with opportunity to do so. Engendering trust for clients with learning disabilities can sometimes be the main focus of a group. Modern society still has many negative projections towards this client group which can undermine the individual's feeling of self-worth, acceptance and identity. The MENCAP report (2007) identified bullying as 'endemic' towards this client group. Dramatherapy groups can help to change distorted self images by offering a more open, welcoming and creative atmosphere.

Bang bang

In this vignette a number of key dramatherapy principles (Jones 1996, 2007) are elucidated. In this extract Oliver chooses to en-role as his toy gun. This is a particularly important part of the activity where the client is able to 'become' the object or person they are picturing. The process is aided by the presence of two chairs (one to represent 'the gun', the other to represent Oliver) so that the client can safely come out of role at any point. Clients must always be sensitively en-roled and de-roled at the end of the activity to ensure that the individual is back fully to being themselves and not left partially in role. For five minutes, while in this role, Oliver re-experienced a number of aspects of his life, ranging from his childhood to times in hospital. Role in itself employs 'aesthetic distance'. Having worked with Oliver, I am sure that if asked to discuss his childhood overtly he would have refused to do so and found the experience overwhelming. In role Oliver was in control of his memories. Speaking from the perspective of the 'toy gun' he was able to distance himself from painful feelings, but still discuss them and in some respects gain greater insight into how these were still affecting him in the present. This is reminiscent of Winnicott's (1971) 'potential' space, an inter-mediate area of experience that lies between the inner world, or internal psychic reality, and the actual or external reality. This space uses aesthetic distance, to facilitate thoughts and feelings being projected and explored (Jones 2007; Jennings 1994; Landy 1994). Role can be used in a number of different contexts. It can be used psychoeducationally where role play is more concrete and explores specific issues, such as assertiveness. Role can also function in more open and explorative ways. Goffman (1959) has argued that individuals are a composite of different roles. When asked what roles they play in their lives, clients that I have worked invariably respond with 'patient'. Institutionalisation and other factors enhance this belief and limit the cap-acity to progress and develop. The opportunity to explore other roles and work creatively with current roles has limitless potential. Discovering that they already play a number of roles, other than patient, such as friend or volunteer can of itself promote the individual to think differently about themselves. The significance of this discovery will often encourage and facili-tate further transformations within the client and group. Oliver may not have been able to change or delete his painful memories but by engaging with the image of the gun, he was able to internalise the characteristics of the gun which were useful to him. Out of role he made the analogy of how the gun had kept him safe. In terms of 'Illumination' Oliver seemed to have identified characteristics and strengths within himself that had become repressed and lost over the years in hospital. This new perspective and a renewed sense of his potential self was also useful in helping to challenge negative self beliefs and encourage development of new skills and confidence.

Broken record

Working with objects is particularly useful for this client group. From a sens-ory perspective the experience of touching, manipulating and exploring objects increases motor skills as well as enhancing coordination (Polatjko *et al.* 1991). Clients often inform me that they enjoy the tactile experience and that it heightens their awareness of the world around them. Objects also provide aesthetic distance and the opportunity to play. Csikszentmihalyi (1992) argues that play is the foundation of creativity and ultimately change and healing. Objects are often imbued with symbolic value for the individual and hold numerous memories. Gary chose to use the objects in a more literal way, the wine glass retaining its link to alcohol and drinking. However other members of the group used objects in a more lateral sense; for example Oliver chose a toy taxi to represent his father with whom he would go out for journeys in the car. Objects often have a powerful effect both on the indi-vidual and group. When clients discuss their objects the listener is often equally impacted. The audience aspect of dramatherapy is often just as therapeutic and involving as those actively engaged in an activity. Witnessing is therefore an essential aspect of group work, particularly when common themes are evoked.

Conclusion

In conclusion, dramatherapy continues to demonstrate its effectiveness in working with clients with learning disabilities and mental health problems. In my own work and experiences I have found dramatherapy to be effective with a wide range of clients, including those with physical limitations, challenging behaviour, communication difficulties and a variety of mental health problems. Dramatherapists are perhaps unique in being able to work with such a diversity of individuals and its flexibility of approach seems largely responsible for this. Dramatherapists also work closely with other professionals offering a multiplicity of interventions which can include groups addressing communication, relaxation, self-esteem, identity/role, emotional literacy and relationships. In this way dramatherapists can effectively adapt to changes and rise to the current challenges of working in the NHS.

10 Mind the gap: facilitating transformative witnessing amongst audiences

Nisha Sajnani

Box 10.1

Questions about practice

- How can dramatherapy inform work with the complexities and particularities of the experience of immigrant women of colour from West and South Asian Diasporas?
- What issues arise in practice with women experiencing violence from men?
- How can performance work bring together perspectives from Brecht, Boal and dramatherapy?

Research perspective

- Case study

Her (story) remains irreducibly foreign to Him. The man can't hear it the way she means it. He sees her as victim, as unfortunate object of hazard. 'her mind is confused,' he concludes. She views herself as the teller, the un-making subject . . . the moving force of the story.

(T. Minh-Ha Trinh 1989: 149)

For many of us engaged in theatre for social change, storytelling has been at the heart of our pedagogy. This chapter explores the opportunities for dialogue, coalition building and solidarity amongst witnesses to difficult stories; stories which emerge from dystopic, unsettled, disrupted and often violent realities in the context of public performance. I propose that when already marginalised experiences are staged for the general public's consumption, there is a risk of entrenching the margins and the centres of society especially when the gaze of the diverse individuals which comprise the audience is not noticed or engaged. This chapter presents the story of an interdisciplinary and community-based performance project developed in Montreal, Canada and its articulation of the core processes of witnessing and interactive audience in drama therapy (Jones 1996, 2007). The project, entitled Creating Safer Spaces invited newly arrived South Asian immigrants and refugee women to use various techniques within the Theatre of the Oppressed (Boal 1979) to collectively examine their experiences of dis/integration, and assimilation within Quebec, Canada. The purpose of presenting this project is to examine how performance oriented dramatherapy, situated as an interdisciplinary practice and a form of community organising, can create the conditions for meaningful dialogue amongst diverse audiences and lay the groundwork for social change. Women who participated in the project created an interactive performance that depicted several scenes involving women's encounters with structural violence (racism, classism, sexism) and intimate partner violence (emotional, economic and physical abuse). This performance was brought to various South Asian communities and then into the wider community, to women's centres, and neighbourhood health centres that had an immigrant population base as a part of a longer workshop promoting collective accountability for 'creating equal and healthy relationships' and galvanising a zero-tolerance response within communities to violence against women.

This is an investigation of the space between the listener and the teller in performances which purport to support a progressive change in the attitudes, beliefs or behaviours of those who watch and listen; the audience. As the opening quote suggests, the stories of the teller(s) risk becoming lost in translation when the listener(s) is not able to resonate, recognise or identify with the experience staged as a result of their differing social status and correlating social power. Without 'minding the gap' between the listener and the teller, the transgressive and transformative potential of the performance project risks impotency and may well result in an unintended affirmation of the status-quo. I believe that there are tremendous opportunities for radical empathy, solidarity and social change when this difference is attended to. I advance that dramatherapists who choose to engage in performance-oriented dramatherapy must contend with the audience in its diversity in order to effectively extend the therapeutic function of their work into the public domain and to avoid burdening those who risk performing their stories with increased cultural stigmatisation.

Witnessing and interactive audience: core processes in dramatherapy

This challenge is partially answered in Jones' articulation of witnessing and interactive audience as core processes, central to the therapeutic function of dramatherapy. He asserts that 'much consideration has gone into the dramatic work that occurs for those involved in the enactment, but much less has gone into the notion of audience in Dramatherapy' (1996: 110). Jones defines witnessing as an action that 'is an important aspect of the act of being an audience to others or to oneself in Dramatherapy' (2007: 102). He alternates the word 'witness' with 'audience' and stresses the multiple opportunities for the client in dramatherapy to en-role as an audience to the process of others, thereby supporting other group members in their expression of themes of concern. He also stresses the therapeutic function of witnessing, as being related to the process by which clients in dramatherapy develop their own internal capacity to be an audience for themselves through activities such as role-reversal or doubling towards gaining increased perspective on their own challenging situations. In this formulation, the audience is seen in two ways. One sees the 'witness' or 'audience' role as something that is internalised by an individual: this affects how they see themselves, for example, or how they act or interact with others. The other way of looking at the witness or audience role approaches it as fluid, changing and as being undertaken by group members at different points during the therapeutic process. In this second way people within dramatherapy shift from being an actor to a witness at different points within group work. The role is externalised without necessarily requiring a formal separation of actor and audience. Jones asserts that, where there is a formal demarcation between actor and audience, the act of witnessing is rendered increasingly visible (enhancing) the boundaries concerning being in and out of role or the enactment, (heightening) focus and concentration (and) the theatricality of a piece of work (2007: 111). The role of the public performance in dramatherapy is addressed by Emunah in her articulation of the nexus of theatre and therapy (1994). She writes of communities of people bound by a common struggle, be it to overcome drug abuse, sexual assault, homelessness or forced migration by staging their own realities 'that have been hidden from public domain . . . stories that have been kept secret . . . on stage [they] come out with their private identities and histories' (1994: 251). Emunah determines the therapeutic impact of performance to differ from and often supercede that of process-oriented dramatherapy in that it situates private experience in the public realm and in doing so, extends opportunities for public education about marginalised populations and suppressed realities. While her description and analysis of the process by which her company members, comprised of people who were living varied struggles, is thorough and engaging there is not much mention of the role of the audience, except in reference to its uniformly affirming applause at the end of their performance. The role of the witness or audience in performance-oriented dramatherapy does not deviate from Jones' original definition which situates its therapeutic function largely within the process leading up to the performance and remains problematically invoked as a homogeneous entity, uniform in its desire to affirm or challenge, irrespective of the diversity of witnesses gathered. This description of the 'audience' who bears witness in public performances depicting marginalised realities falls short of describing the process by which change amongst always already diverse audience members is achieved. Understandably, this invocation of the audience as a uniformly supportive entity is architectured to fulfil the therapeutic function of private therapy as public theatre. However, as I advanced in my original proposal, the utopian thrust of the social change project, with its ideas of participation, a tolerance for multiplicity, equity, a full integration of diverse lived realities and the dissolution of harmful marginalisation, is compromised within applied theatre practice[1] when the audience as a microcosm of society is given such a limited role.

I find further support for this assertion in the writings of cultural theorist and feminist, bell hooks, who argues that 'we need more written work and oral testimony documenting ways barriers are broken down, coalitions formed and solidarity shared' (1994: 110). She points out the ways in which groups will quickly seek mutual identification in an effort to preserve a sense, albeit a false sense, of harmony and cohesion. When we, as drama therapists, cultural pedagogues and conduits facilitate the staging of realities lived by those who have been excluded because of their 'race', legal status, class, age or sexual orientation (to name a few social locations), we risk the strong impulse the audience(s) and actor(s) may feel to obfuscate the tension, anxiety and related affect felt by both, thereby constraining the possibility for sustained solidarity. Towards this end, feminist activists and scholars have called for ways of creating equitable participation and pedagogies that recognise the inequalities of risk-taking faced by the teller(s) and the witness(es) as the former is traditionally tasked with revelation and the latter with reception (Razack 1998). Theatre and in particular popular theatre[2] and dramatherapy processes, offer useful methods of surfacing tension, conflict and contradiction constructively and creatively. As indicated by popular theatre theorists and practitioners, Selman and Prentki, our challenge is 'to create a radical kind of empathy, one that recognises the danger of storytelling and the inequality of risk in the storytelling process, one that creates spaces and relationships where stories are told and heard' (2003: 9). Our challenge is to create the conditions for transformative witnessing, wherein the multiple, multi-layered voices, experiences, attitudes and ideas of audience members can be engaged towards facilitating change outside the theatre.

---

1 Applied theatre comprises theatre practices that have an explicit intention to effect a change in the attitude, feelings or behavior of the audience and implies some form of audience participation (Ackroyd 2000).
2 Selman and Stewart (2003) describe popular theatre as encompassing community education, community organising and theatre making. It is chosen by people involved with education and development because of its participatory processes that recognise cultural forms, which engage body and mind, and which use specific stories to illuminate shared situations. It is a process of theatre making which involves specific communities in identifying issues of concern, analysing current conditions and causes of a situation, identifying potential points of change, and analysing how change could happen and/or contribute to the actions implied.

Facilitating transformative witnessing

The dramaturgical conditions that support transformative witnessing amongst audiences are presented by audience reception theorist, Bennett (1997). She emphasises the influence of playwright and theoretician Bertolt Brecht, whose ideas are 'important for any study of audience/play relations . . . his ideas for a theatre with the power to provoke social change, along with his attempts to reactivate the stage-audience exchange have had a profound impact on critical responses to plays and performance' (1997: 21). Brecht's objective was to provoke a critical yet entertained audience. His epic theatre rearticulated and politicised the relationship between the audience and the stage. The risk of sustaining the status-quo by forgetting or overly simplifying the function(s) of the audience is best summed by Brecht as he points out how contemporary practice constrained a direct relationship between audience and the stage: '[t]he theatre as we know it shows the structure of society [represented on stage] as incapable of being influenced by society [in the audi-torium]' (Willet 1964: 189). While the technologies of participation in society have changed and mobility has increased for some, Brecht's observations remain increasingly important today given the persistence of poverty and the differential access particular individuals and communities have to realising their full potential, based on their membership in particular social groups.[3]

At the time of writing this chapter, the first African-American president was sworn in. However, at the same time, a popular referendum, held in the state of California, revoked the right of homosexual couples to marry. In the project presented in this chapter, women who had recently migrated, by force or by choice, to Montreal lived with inconsistent access to health care and education as a result of their precarious legal status and experienced a constellation of anxious and depressive symptoms relating to the trauma of displacement and intimate partner violence. This reality, coupled with the racism, classism and sexism they faced outside their homes, rendered them increasingly vulnerable to violence within their homes. Fundamentally, people continue to need reminders that they can effect change, have opportunities to debate and realise differing visions of change, and to see themselves as complicit in the struggles and victories of one another.

Baz Kershaw, performance theorist, speaks to this necessity in his investigation of the conditions which give rise to an effective dialogue between the audience and the stage and what he terms 'performance efficacy'; that is to realise the 'potential that the immediate effects of performance may have to influence the community and the culture of the audience, a historical evolution of wider social and political realities' (1992: 257–258). He describes

3 A thorough analysis of social indicators such as health care, employment and education along with the interlocking impacts of racism, classism and sexism are beyond the scope of this chapter. Please see Himmani Bannerji (2000), Yasmin Jiwani (2001) and Sherene Razack (1998, 2008) for an informed analysis of present day inequalities.

the challenges of working amongst communities in which there are competing interests, a reality present in always already diverse audiences and advances the need for processes that forge a 'reinforcement of achieved commonalities' (1992: 245), constructing a basis for solidarity between differing individuals and community groups by identifying shared struggles.

There have been several practices that attempt to bridge the gap between the storyteller and witness that include dramaturgical and post-performance interventions ranging from non-traditional staging, feedback questionnaires and talk-back sessions to interactive improvisation with audience members. Beyond Brecht, perhaps the most well known is the work of Boal, originator of the Theatre of the Oppressed (1979). The Theatre of the Oppressed is a composite system of theatre-based techniques that include Image Theatre, Invisible Theatre, Legislative Theatre, Forum Theatre and Rainbow of Desire to address internalised, relational and systemic oppressions. Boal has defined the central thesis of his performance pedagogy to be the active participation of the audience who bears witness to injustices embodied and staged; the transformation of the passive spectator to the 'spect-actor', who is complicit in the co-creation of the realities we as a society sustain and support in their will to act upon injustice. Boal also emphasises the necessity of audience members to identify, resonate, or recognise the situations presented in order to establish the motivation to change the reality depicted (1995), an idea that is allied with Kershaw's indication to establish ideological compatibility with audiences.

The ideas proposed by Brecht, Boal and Kershaw are complemented by contemporary developments in ideas about social justice and social or cultural therapy. There is a growing trend in psychotherapy to challenge inequality and commit to social justice. This is evidenced by efforts to question the presumed neutrality of the therapist and to re-define the role of the therapist to include outreach, prevention and advocacy. Related ideas also include enlarging the therapeutic space to include community specific locations, usefully blurring the boundaries between the public and private by calling for public accountability, situating the encounter between therapist and client in sustainable partnerships and participatory practices, and in reformulating the purpose of therapy as facilitating an individual and/or group's capacities to identify, analyse and address the internalised, relational and systemic dynamics which limit the full arc of their desires (Thompson 2002; Vera and Speight 2003; Holzman and Mendez 2003; Fanon 2004; Toporek *et al.* 2006). Boal's and other practices that enable the agency of the witness will be explored and discussed in the context of the project presented.

Creating safer spaces with South Asian women: a violence prevention programme using the applied arts

The South Asian Women's Community Centre is an organisation with a twenty-five year history. It provides settlement and support services to immigrant and refugee women from India, Pakistan, Sri Lanka, Bangladesh and recently, Afghanistan. For many years it has tried different approaches to addressing the problem of violence against women within the many communities with which it works (Sajnani and Nadeau 2006). The centre has been hosting a community theatre project to address violence against immigrant seniors since 2003. This in turn inspired the centre coordinator to hire myself and dance-movement therapist, Denise Nadeau, to coordinate a women's group that would culminate in a community performance to raise awareness about the complexities of violence against South Asian women in Montreal amongst other South Asian communities.

Denise and I were both creative arts therapists with experience in addressing the impacts of violence on women. Both of us also had an interest in expanding the frame of therapy to include an engagement with the social and political context, which shaped the lives of those with whom we worked. With this in mind, we chose to develop a popular education process that would provide a scaffold for our group process, leading us and our group to a shared analysis of the relationship between intimate and structural violence and its psychological and social consequences. A popular education process emphasises reflecting on participants' shared experiences and incorporating new information in action (Arnold *et al.* 1991). We hoped to share authority with participants in the group and create a performance that would communicate the relationship between psychological distress and intimate and systemic trauma.

The centre's staff, comprised of women from India, Pakistan, Bangladesh, Sri Lanka and Afghanistan, would refer women who they were already working with to our program along five criteria:

1   their experiences of intimate and/or structural violence
2   their capacity to join a group of women from the centre in examining challenges and barriers to creating equal and healthy relationships
3   their interest in using the arts as a resource for self-care
4   a basic knowledge of English or French
5   and their willingness to commit to a ten-session process leading to a public performance(s) addressing the subject of violence against women.

This last criterion was enabled through the provision of childcare and transport services to ensure that women who wished to attend the group could attend and was in line with the centre's goals to encourage advocacy as part of the healing process. Our group was comprised of six to ten women who had recently immigrated to Montreal or who were seeking refugee status. They were variably in-between homes, jobs, countries, families and cultures. Their unstable realities were often the subject of our conversations and our group membership oscillated between six to ten members weekly; as some were called on for citizenship interviews, court hearings and other important appointments. However, amidst this instability, many of the women who participated in this program stated that they did so because it put them in contact with others, sustained their connection to the centre's staff who supported them in their integration process, allowed them to practise English or French and that it was a stress-release in their week. This was surprising to us at times given the severity of the realities each group member faced. However, it also confirmed what the centre's staff already knew; that a primary mediator of adverse situations faced by the new immigrants, forced migrants and refugees is the network of social support they have available to them (Punamäki *et al.* 2005).

Over our ten weeks together, women shared their experiences relating to a) the economic, political and interpersonal reasons for their move to Montreal through creative and verbal exchanges and b) the forms of violence that they or women they knew had encountered. From these stories, we were able to generate a collective analysis of the kinds of barriers immigrant women of colour encounter and expand our collective definition of violence to include both intimate and structural expressions. Drawing on their shared experiences, we created several short scenes depicting the violence immigrant women of colour face inside and outside their homes, and placed these scenes within a larger popular education workshop on violence against women. We toured our popular theatre workshop in various South Asian communities and then moved it into the wider community, to women's centres, and neighbourhood health centres that have an immigrant population base. Throughout the process we were assessing this approach in terms of its capacity to convey the particularities and complexities of a racialised immigrant woman's experience to our audiences as well on its impact on the participants.

Description of the work

The context

It is important to understand the interplay of the historical, social and political forces that shape the lived experience of individuals and groups we work with as they have a direct impact on mental health. In this section, I will outline the context within which the Creating Safer Spaces programme emerged. Montreal has a large Arab and Muslim population and the racial profiling that intensified against these populations before and since 9/11, throughout North America, has emerged in various ways in social and legal policies and practices (Razack 2008). In this way, we were working within a context that has further exacerbated what Bannerji, an anti-racist feminist theorist, describes as the fetishisation and essentialising of culture and the racialisation or ethnicisation of difference which has proliferated in a climate of state sponsored multiculturalism (2000).

Canada's celebrations of cultural diversity, in Bannerji's analysis, emerge as an impotent and patronising multicultural aesthetic designed to reinforce the modernity of white Canada and emphasise the backward religious and cultural traditions of all 'others.' This enables the construction of uncomplicated, diverse minority groups voided of any historical or social relations of power, while leaving the cultural, political, economic and representational apparatus of the dominant majority intact (Bannerji 2000).

This is the context in which the South Asian 'community', an ideological and imagined category of the state, has been constructed. This is further supported by Razack, another leading Canadian anti-racist feminist theorist, who emphasises how race, gender and class interlock within immigration, settlement and multicultural policies and procedures in the lives of women of colour who immigrate or seek refugee status to Canada (2008). This is central to understanding the kind of violence and oppression racialised women face inside and outside their homes. Under the political climate of organising difference around essentialised and static cultures, Canada's 'others' had, or have to base their cultural politics on their only grounds for eligibility; their visible differences from the average white Canadian. These cultural politics leave out problems of class and patriarchy and create an artificial division of the public and private sphere. It is assumed by both the state and media, as well as the legally endorsed, male representatives of these newly constructed so-called communities, that South Asians are essentially traditional and as such, patriarchy is a natural part of their cultural identity and therefore, violence is a natural part of their cultural identity and off limits. The result is that 'insiders' are reluctant to speak about it and 'outsiders' are reluctant to intervene.

Bannerji points to the risks involved in speaking out in a political climate where violence against immigrant and refugee women of colour is interpreted by the dominant society as the result of cultural practices. 'We are worried, understandably, to speak of "our" brutalities and shortcomings, because of not being even minimally in control of the public and political domains of speech and ideological construction' (2000: 136). In cases of domestic violence the media focus is often solely on physical acts of violence by the husband on a wife (the result of 'their culture and religion') and all other forms of intimate violence, as well as the structural factors and forms of violence that have made immigrant woman of colour vulnerable to intimate violence, are ignored (Jiwani 2001). As Denise and I have noted in another article on this project 'Violence against immigrant women of colour and Aboriginal women, as is violence against white women, is treated by the courts, medical and counselling systems as a psychological and individual problem rather than the result of structural violence which can only be remedied by structural and community solutions' (Sajnani and Nadeau 2006: 47). Experiences of intimate violence and the resulting hopelessness, anxiety, shame and isolation faced by racialised immigrant women must be understood in the context of living within a racist, classist and sexist society. In the following section, I will elaborate on the process we undertook with our group to emphasise the need for structural and community solutions to violence against women.

The process

As mentioned earlier, we chose to draw on a popular education model[4] that begins with participants' individual experiences as a basis for collective analysis and action to guide our group process. I will limit my analysis of this project to the efforts made to support transformative witnessing amongst audiences. Aside from the opening and closing rituals often co-facilitated by group participants incorporated into every group session, we generated a collective understanding of the realities lived by group members by asking them to communicate their experiences though a chosen visual or embodied process. We began, early in the group process, by asking our group to define what they considered to be violence both inside and outside their homes in order to examine the interplay of psychological, social and political factors which contributed to the reality of violence and to barriers to creating equal and healthy relationships. The women exchanged experiences in small groups and drew symbols and images depicting realities they had faced inside and outside their homes. What they shared was later incorporated into a handout that members of the group and the Centre's staff could use in the resulting performance or presentations (see Figure 10.1).

The handout we created was a power and control wheel that moved beyond the limitations of the widely used Duluth Minnesota Power and Control Wheel,[5] which is a diagram of a circle within a circle that depicts how 'power and control' are at the core of experiences of violence against women and best reflects the realities of violence against white middle-class women. Drawing on Jiwani's work, we created the structural power and control wheel that identifies the areas where immigrant women of colour experience racist and colonial violence.

As seen in the revised 'power and control wheel', immigrant women of colour are at risk in the area of education where women experience deskilling and a lack of accreditation, less access to adequate training and knowledge of dominant systems. In the area of health, women who come to Canada with the experience of the trauma of forced migration, sexual violence and the violence of war, are treated with the medicalisation of abuse and the obfuscation of social suffering, through assessments that do not take into account the role of context or the impact of structural violence in determining the origin of their symptoms. Within our legal system, women suffer from the criminalisation of racialised groups, wherein a person who looks Muslim is substantially more likely to be suspected of criminal activity than a white person (Razack 2008), and a potential lack of knowledge regarding their

---

4 See Freire. P. (1970) *Pedagogy of the Oppressed* for more information on popular education.

5 The Power and Control Wheel was developed by battered women in Duluth who had been abused by their male partners and were attending women's education groups sponsored by the women's shelter. See www.theduluthmodel.org for more information. We also developed a brochure detailing 'culturally safe' municipal resources.

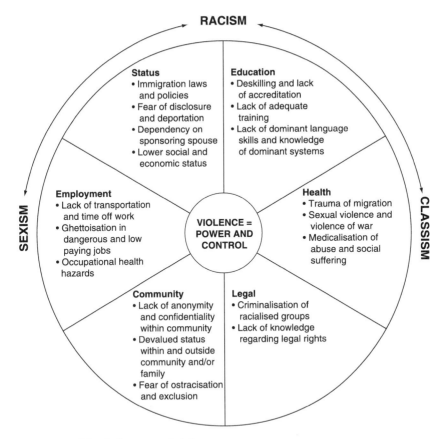

Figure 10.1 Wheel of structural violence.

Structural Violence Against Immigrant and Refugee Women of Colour, Nisha Sajnani and Denise Nadeau 2005. Adapted from *Intersecting Inequalities: Immigrant Women of Colour, Violence, and Health Care* by Yasmin Jiwani, FREDA, 2001

legal rights. In the area of employment, women experience difficulty with transportation as well as ghettoisation in dangerous and low-paying jobs in industrial and garment factories, in addition to occupational health hazards. Within their 'communities', or relational groups, women can also experience a lack of anonymity and confidentiality, resulting in a potentially devalued status in and/or outside the community and/or family and potential ostracisation and exclusion, should they speak out against their treatment. In the area of status, immigration policies and procedures position women as an appendage of her male counterpart, leaving her dependent on her sponsoring spouse; she may also fear that disclosure could result in deportation. Immigrant women of colour also experience a lower social and economic status. Isolated and excluded through all these forms of structural violence and a lack of language skills in both English and/or French (in Quebec), the immigrant woman of colour is in a condition of higher risk of intimate forms of violence. In accordance with Razack (2008), these areas of exclusion and violence are the daily lived experience for these women of interlocking of racism, classism and sexism.

Another aspect of our approach was to stress the resilience and resistance of immigrant women of colour in the face of violence. Drawing on the work of Traci West (1999) we supported participants in the trainings to name the ways they survived and resisted violence, and in what ways their differing faith traditions had provided them with comfort, if any, despite the suffering caused by forced migration and ongoing exclusion in Canada. This analysis, which moved beyond the individual immigrant victim story to a social suffering and a resilience framework, informed the therapeutic activities we chose over our ten week series, how we facilitated the performances and then how we animated the discussions in the community workshops. Our performances needed to represent the strengths of survival as well as the complexities of the many forms of violence to which the women were exposed. This framework provided the basis for a guideline that informed our performances – challenging any representation that reinforced the individualisation of women's experiences of violence. We wanted to avoid the trap of painting the immigrant husband as a one dimensional patriarchal transmitter of his culture. We wanted to expose the context he was living in, including loss of status, employment, and increased racial profiling after 9/11. These facters narrowed his options and reduced his sphere of power to the home, the basis for a guideline that informed our performances. With each audience member, our intention was to present the multiple violences that immigrant women of colour experience as a collective problem that required collective solutions. We also intended to reinforce the strengths of the women who would witness these performances as part of the process of encouraging receptivity and strengthening the resilience of audience members as they performed their collective attention to this issue.

Performance and pedagogy

The first community performance we created was in the form of Forum Theatre, albeit highly adapted. Forum Theatre is a type of popular theatre found within the repetoire of Boal's Theatre of the Oppressed, a collection of theatre forms and techniques inspired by the processes of conscientisation described by Freire (1970). In Forum Theatre, a group of interested individuals or community members are shown a scene, usually created by or with them, which depicts an issue(s) that is of concern to them. After the scene has been played once, it is repeated with an invitation to the audience to intervene when they have suggestions as to how the situation of the 'oppressed' might be improved. The play is mediated by a facilitator known as the joker who explains the rules of engagement and guides the interaction between the audience and the stage. This dialogic and embodied interaction between the audience and the actors is intended to stimulate a lively and urgent search for solutions to their own challenges.[6]

The scene created was developed out of the many stories shared by group members about the violence they faced inside and outside their homes. After some experimentation and scene development within the group depicting both individual and amalgamated stories, we collectively determined the outline of a brief, silent scene that we hoped would demonstrate the link between intimate and structural violence amongst our audiences. In the scene, a woman wearing a hijab, a scarf covering her head potentially marking her as Muslim, was subtly mistreated at a job interview where her obviously substantial experience, as depicted by a thick curriculum vitae, was barely glanced at by the prospective employer. We next see this same women return home and appear dejected as she presumably narrates her disappointment to someone over the phone. Her spouse returns home, slams the doors and moves towards her. She checks her watch and begins to scurry about the kitchen trying to prepare a meal. Her spouse becomes increasingly angry, presumably at not being served on time and begins to berate her while moving closer to her in a threatening manner, again in silence. She begins to weep. Her spouse leaves in frustration.

We had reservations about using this form of popular theatre as it ran the risk of reducing the characters to a simplistic oppressor and oppressed binary, reinforcing an audience's view of the woman as victim and the man's behaviour towards her as another proof of a 'backward' culture'. This has been a common reservation in using Forum Theatre (Spry cited in Cohen-Cruz 1993). At first reading, the scene portrayed a South Asian woman unable to find work and later abused by her husband. Unchallenged, this initial reading would relegate the character of the woman/wife to that of victim and her husband to that of oppressor. Our challenge lay in developing a Forum Theatre workshop and performance that did not reproduce these dominant and overly simplified representations of power, or reinforce powerlessness. We wanted to highlight the complexities and the potential for agency both amongst the women performing and our varied audiences.

Another challenge lay in how to create amongst the audience a sense of collective responsibility and willingness to act as a group within the medium of Forum Theatre, which has traditionally focused on individual protagonists and individual interventions from audience members. One of the first things we did was to create a community workshop around the theatre piece so that the performance was part of a larger process. We began by spending some

---

6 Forum Theatre has been used by hundreds of popular theatre practitioners and interested groups world wide to address a wide range of social and political, and most recently, psychological forms of oppression. It has also been used specifically to encourage a critical race consciousness in Canada (Goulet and Linds 2005; Sajnani and Nadeau 2006).

time in introductions with the audience. We asked participants, often mostly women, (though once all men) to break into groups of three, introduce themselves and share what are the resources or strengths they have and what languages they speak. We did this to check for the necessity of translation and to affirm the strength of speaking so many languages. Often we had women in the audience who could speak as many as five languages, for example Urdu, Bengali, Hindi, English and French. Given the many testimonies of deskilling and shame experienced by women in our group, one of our goals was to remind women of their strengths and affirm their resources before we even started the play.

We introduced the play as 'A Day in the Life of One Woman' and conducted the forum. The play itself was done in silence. Not only did this help us with the thorny challenges of presenting to multilingual audiences but it also enabled a multiplicity of interpretations of gestures, postures and roles. The silent performance not only deprivileges English as the dominant language but also draws attention to the silence surrounding the issue of violence against women in immigrant and refugee communities of colour; a silence that can only be broken through a collective response of zero tolerance. The animation of the workshop prior to, during and after the performance was done in English and/or French and was translated through whisper translation or, with the help of a co-animator, translated into the preferred language or dialects of the audience.

In the case of our play, we did not immediately move to the replay of the scene with an invitation to intervene, but, instead, we spent time laying the groundwork for collective action by decoding the scene, inviting multiple opportunities for audience members to identify with the situations presented and establishing the reasons why this scene needs to be changed. The first intervention, after the presentation of the brief scenario, is to go back and freeze moments from the first scene and use what are traditionally called 'rehearsal techniques' within the repertoire of the Theatre of the Oppressed, in order to critically engage the audience with the scene. We first asked audience members to identify who the characters are and if they or the situation depicted was recognisable to them by asking, 'Has anything like this happened to you or a woman you know?' We then ask what the characters are thinking and feeling, (i.e. what is going on inside their head). We then ask what options exist for women in this situation. The first scene, dealing with racism in employment practices often resulted in individualistic intervention ideas, such as suggestions that the woman take assertiveness training or become more confident as I mentioned earlier. Usually there was someone in the audience who would challenge that. One or two audience members mentioned human rights appeals or anti-racism training and we would intervene ourselves, at times, with these structural options if they were not mentioned, though it is here that it is harder to name alternatives. After this the joker would ask: 'How are the two scenes linked?' Most of our audiences, comprised largely of other South Asian women's community groups, would identify how the discrimination faced by the woman in the first scene further limits her options in the second scene as she became dependent on her husband's income to support herself and/or her children, thereby leaving her increasingly vulnerable to violence in the home.

In order to support collective action amongst our audience and to dislocate the characters presented from being easily situated as oppressor or oppressed, we also began to use a 'zoom out' technique in the second scene. At a performance for centre staff and board members, I stood first behind the 'man' and then the woman, and asked, 'if we had a zoom lens camera and could "zoom out" behind what you see here in this man, what are the larger social forces we would see at play behind this character, what are the messages he may have received that inform the behaviour that you see here today?' To this question, one person, for example, said, 'he is not able to find work', to which another added, 'he can't find work because his education isn't recognised and this is really frustrating.' This allowed the audience to name the context in which South Asian men and women live and to add structural dimensions to this seemingly isolated act. We wanted to avoid the trap of painting the immigrant husband as a one-dimensional patriarchal transmitter of his culture, thus avoiding exposing the context he was living in, the contexts articulated by the women in our group and in our audiences, including his loss of status, employment and increased racial profiling after 9/11; all which narrowed his options and reduce his sphere of power to the home. If culture and religion are mentioned, and there are patriarchal aspects to all cultures and religions, we make sure to ask more specific questions so it is not 'the culture' or 'the religion' that is blamed, but aspects of them that are being challenged. This was particularly poignant at a performance held at an Italian Women's Centre. In the interests of forging solidarity across community groups and women's centres towards combating intimate and structural violence against women, we decided to take our play outside the South Asian community. During the decoding process wherein the joker asks what each character is thinking and feeling, an elderly Italian woman in the audience stated that the woman in the play must be upset at 'how she is treated as a servant in her culture'. The woman playing the role of the wife in the play broke out of role and stated that she was more upset about how her 'husband' treated her. This scenario incited the joker to quickly return to the audience to see if they could identify with or recognise the experience depicted in the scene as a reality which existed in their own communities, to establish a 'community of interest', so they would see themselves in the struggle portrayed rather than dismissing it as the product of a uniquely violent culture.

Not all audience members could readily identify or admit to recognising the abusive scenes. There may have been several reasons for this, including the risks audience members may have refrained from taking by admitting to living in a violent situation amongst her own family or religious community members. Our goal was not to have them risk their own safety by disclosing more than they wished, but to provide an avenue to rehearse options for action together. Towards this end, we included the character of a bystander. This character, who would be standing stage left – again silent and listening with her ear against the wall – served to embody the false division between the public and private sphere. When we asked audiences to identify this character, they provided multiple options saying that it could be a stranger, a mother-in-law, a neighbour, a friend or a child. This character provided aesthetic distance from the violence in the scene, and yet remained a part of it. Audiences were drawn to replacing and discussing the bystander during the forum leading us to assume that this was the character where the audience could most readily identify itself. We also used a technique of asking the entire audience to play the bystander, asking them to consider what they might do together if they were all to take stage in the place of this character. This character, more than any other, was key in opening up new possibilities for hope and change towards promoting collective agency amongst audiences to this play.

After these interventions, the play is run again and audience members are invited to stop the action in the second scene to propose a way in which the 'dignity and respect of the character chosen can be better protected'. In this way, we chose not to limit the interventions to changes in the protagonist, but invited any intervention, including adding characters to the scene, that might aid us in our established desire to collectively promote the dignity and respect of any and all of the characters. For example, in one performance a woman stood up to take the stage as the bystander, with an offer to go over to the 'wife's' house after the 'husband' had left and to comfort her and develop a safety plan together should he become more violent. In another performance, the joker asked, 'who has the most power to change this scene?' This invitation brought out offers amongst audience members to play religious leaders and legal authorities. This is also a good example of how the joker's choices affect what analyses surfaced over the course of a performance.

After each intervention, the joker asks the one who made the suggestion whether they got what they wanted, and then returns to the audience and inquires as to the feasibility of the suggested action in their own contexts. At times, the joker would return to the actors to ask them if something changed for their character during that intervention. These questions tended to promote more dialogue and verbal investigation into the scenario. For example, the woman who played the wife in one performance stated that having the 'neighbour' stop in to let her know that she was in a difficult situation and to offer her help provided a sense of relief. At times, this would allow the complexity of the relationship between structural and intimate violence to surface and yet, in other instances, leaving the analysis to emerge from the audience through verbal discussions alone resulted in the deep entrenchment of opposing views and a resistance to continue with the embodied process of exploration and examination. An example of this emerged during the one performance we held with a group of men at a local Indian community centre. One man stopped the scene and asked to replace the 'wife'. Once on stage he commented, 'I have to get home on time in order to have supper ready.' Then, he looked at his watch, prepared the meal and had it ready for the 'husband' upon his arrival. Once he had completed his intended intervention he reiterated his actions for the audience, 'if she had better time management, she could avoid an argument with her husband.' Upon hearing this, a woman in the audience said, 'she doesn't need to have better time management, what a bad thing to say!' The two of them continued to argue despite the attempts made by the animator to bring the discussion back to the larger audience and to the group of women performing. The audience declined to demonstrate further interventions and the discussion soon became polarised and options for action increasingly limited. We debriefed this performance for some time in our group as a few women recognised the prescription for action offered by that man as an indication of what they have been up against in trying to make a change in their own interpersonal relationships. This experience provided an opportunity to notice if they had other responses to a message that they had heard all too often, namely, that they were to blame for the violence they experienced.

We added a new technique after a challenging session with an Ismaili Afghani group of older women who did not speak English or French, and had come from a background where women had not been allowed to be educated. We had used a variation of this play with an angry father not letting his daughter out and shouting at his wife about the daughter. At one point it seemed no one saw anything wrong with the scene, that it was good that the girl was not allowed out with a 'Canadian' boy. It was very difficult to get anyone to stop the play and suggest alternatives. As a final intervention, we asked someone to come up and either play or reshape/sculpt the actors into an image of the ideal scene. This somehow broke the audience resistance and when we talked in small groups after the play – during our evaluation process – several women said they wanted their daughters to get an education and/or higher education, and thus, did not want this pursuit to become compromised by the 'Western' culture of dating. This particular experience revealed to us not only the importance of showing the ideal, but also the challenges of playing to audiences that are deeply invested in maintaining the fixity of gender roles and resistant to complicating these roles amongst their own community members and in the wider public sphere. Finally, we spend time in evaluation with each audience, asking them what they remembered most about the play, what is one thing they might do alone or with others to help a woman facing similar difficulties, and what questions, and/or concerns they still may have.

Conclusion

The Creating Safer Spaces project presents a wide range of strategies designed to facilitate engaged, attuned witnessing amongst audiences. Through the use of Forum Theatre, audience members are invited to directly participate in an embodied search for solutions to a collective problem of intimate and structural violence against women, specifically women of colour who are new immigrants or refugees in Canada. The purpose, of course, is to generate multiple options for action, and not just actions that individual characters can take, but actions everyone in a community can take. Rather than presenting an individual woman's private domestic experience, this performance linked race, gender and sexual violence in a scenario that shows the cumulative and collective nature of the trauma many new immigrants experience. Our political claim is that we were encouraging the community not to look away from the structural violence operating in this reality. Their collective gaze, performing attention to what is normally perceived to be a private violence, is itself a political act.

Drama therapists are not necessarily encouraged, however, to only use techniques associated with Forum Theatre in their attempts to bridge the gap between the audience and the stage. The case study presented reveals several considerations that may be conducive to facilitating transformative witnessing amongst audiences:

- Alliances: This project began as a partnership between creative arts therapists and a local community organisation already dedicated to ongoing public education about violence against women. In this way, this program was situated as part of a larger community organising strategy. In addition to their clinical and logistical support, they also provided suggestions for community organisations that might be receptive to the workshop and provided multiple opportunities for women to stay involved with the Centre beyond the existence of this project. The audience was not 'off the hook' after the performance but invited to participate in an ongoing and allied effort.

- Interdisciplinarity: This program evolved out of an interdisciplinary approach to group facilitation drawing on our skills as dance and drama therapists as well as popular educators. This, in my opinion, provided a conceptual framework for attending to the needs of the group as well as the social objectives of the performance. Further, it situated group participants as collaborators and advocates rather than passive clients. With regard to facilitating transformative witnessing, we facilitated introductions and encounters amongst audience members connected to the themes of the performance to prepare them to bear witness and as a means of getting to know who was in the room.

- Proximity: The recognition of the situation staged and opportunities to see oneself as implicated in the outcome, or seen as 'insiders' to a situation, was a pre-requisite for action. In the forum piece, the role of the bystander invites this proximity as it compelled the audience to see themselves as implicated in the outcome. What is key is that the audience is invited to actively consider and have opportunities to reveal their relationship to the issues staged. Further, opportunities for audiences members to encounter one another throughout the performance through small-group interactions to share their stories relating to what has been staged is also a way to establish proximity, receptivity and a willingness to share one's perspectives even if they differ from expected social norms. In this way, the risk associated with telling one's story is circulated and the responsibilities associated with having heard the story are made available to dialogue. Transformative witnessing is also reliant on processes that facilitate awareness and the naming of the social, historical and political forces on the stories that are staged in performance-oriented dramatherapy. Further, transformative witnessing emerges from opportunities for audience members to reflect together with each other and with the 'actors' on the implications of what has been shared in their own lives. Having opportunities for audience members to interact together prior to the performance as well as after the performance provide additional avenues for exchange and relationship.

Familiar ways of conceptualising our practice are no longer effective when faced with the ongoing struggle to create inclusive communities that can better attend to the needs of those who are most readily excluded in present day society. I began this chapter with a call to drama therapists who engage in performance-oriented dramatherapy to mind the gap that exists between the tellers and the listeners in order to attend to the ways in which our social locations and their associated and intersecting privileges limit audience receptivity and, in this way, constrain possibilities for sustained change. Indeed, the uneasy isolation associated with the traumatic events that give rise to socially engaged performance is amplified when the audience is uniformly cast in the role of a silent bystander. Inviting the audience into proximity with another's experiences can facilitate the re/integration of previously splintered moments of human experiencing towards a mutual sharing of loss resulting in a restored and radical empathy.

11 Embodying difference: to join or not to join the dance

Ditty Dokter

Box 11.1

Questions about practice

- How do clients experience the different arts therapies?
- What are psychodynamic ways of approaching dramatherapy in a mental health context?
- How do factors such as culture, class and gender relate to client experiences of dramatherapy?

Research perspective

- Evaluation questionnaires
- Individual semi-structured interviews
- Post-session focus groups
- Ethnographic case study
- Participant observation

Client perspective sample

'Useful: It was a good laugh, working as a group, kicking the ball, it brought up a lot of feeling, using movement to change how I was feeling, helping others, being able to move to show feeling and to get in touch with feeling. Unhelpful: need more people to join in, more people, especially staff who can not be bothered to come in, need bigger room, more people needed, people sitting in the coffee room!' (From written evaluation.)

Introduction

Dramatherapy is one of the arts therapies modalities that can choose between embodiment, projection and role in its interventions. This chapter focuses on embodiment in group work and compares the effect of embodiment in art therapy, dance movement therapy and dramatherapy. Feedback from clients and therapists about the helpful and hindering aspects of therapy will be used to explain why, for example, different genders experience the impact of embodiment differently. This chapter will discuss cultural, diagnostic, class and gender factors influencing that difference, providing case studies from practice. The role of witness will be discussed as an important interacting factor with the client background variables.

The findings of this chapter are based on a research project studying arts therapies groups in a young people's psychiatric service. The aim of the research was to identify client and therapist perception of helping and hindering processes in arts therapies group treatment. The other aim was to study variables in background and treatment affecting that perception.

Contexts

The young people's service provided outpatient and day-patient treatment: outpatients were seen individually, while day patients received group treatment. The day-patient unit was run along therapeutic community lines for a client group of twelve young people, aged 16 to 25 years old. Their average expected stay was two years. Within the young people's unit the arts therapies groups were part of the group programme attended by all clients. The co-worker in the arts therapies group was an identified unit worker. The author joined the groups as researcher/participant observer for one and a half years; 18 young people attended the unit during that time. Three out of seven staff members also left and were replaced.

The arts therapies groups formed one day in the group programme. The morning group combined dance movement therapy (DMT) and dramatherapy (DT) interventions, with an emphasis on embodiment. It took place after the community meeting (a daily start of the programme) and was facilitated by the dance movement therapist and a unit-based dramatherapist. The afternoon group was facilitated by the art therapist and a unit-based nurse therapist as an art therapy (AT) group. Each group lasted one and a half hours and took the format of discussion, followed by action. In DMT/DT this was usually group-interactive, movement-based work, while in AT it tended to involve individual image making, followed by a sharing of the images. The dance movement therapist and art therapist were attached to the trust wide arts therapies department, comprising art, music, drama and dance movement therapists. They provided individual and group therapy to young people's, adult and elderly psychiatry in both outpatient and inpatient contexts. The clients were referred from both the wider rural region and the city.

Description of the work

The client group

The diagnosis and treatment history of the young people who attended the day-treatment programme was complex. The analysis of the diagnoses shows that 45 per cent (8 out of 18) clients had a diagnosis of personality disorder, of which six were borderline. The five cases of adjustment disorder fell in these diagnostic categories too, a high 45 per cent. Fifty per cent of clients also suffered depression and 50 per cent self-harmed. The co-morbidity with addiction was 45 per cent; 8 out of 18 abused alcohol, drugs or food. The smaller diagnostic groups were obsessive compulsive disorder, 11 per cent (2 out of 18), bipolar affective disorder 11 per cent (2 out of 18) and two diagnoses were not available in the medical file.

The main identified stressors in clients' lives were parental separation and death (8 out of 18), bullying at school (7 out of 18) and sexual abuse (4 out of 18). Certain diagnoses such as personality disorder, obsessive compulsive disorder and bipolar disorder are associated with higher dropout rates from therapy (Roth and Fonagy 2005), as does co-morbidity. Co-morbidity was present for 60 per cent of clients (10 out of 18), single diagnosis for 40 per cent of clients (8 out of 18).

Many clients received previous treatment before coming to the young people's psychiatric service. Previous treatment indicates repeated episodes, chronicity and severity of problems (Roth and Fonagy 2005), another factor influencing engagement with therapy. Previous treatment might involve treatment from the child and adolescent psychiatric service, or previous admissions in the acute adult psychiatric service. For some clients these continued during treatment at the young people's service, usually due to self-harm incidents. Research indicates that 40 to 60 per cent of clients drop out of psychotherapy treatment in the early stages (Lambert 2004). There are no specific arts therapies figures. The clients showed 33.3 per cent attrition within the first four months, while 66.6 per cent of clients remained in therapy. Studying the cultural background, class and gender factors that might influence client and therapist perception of the arts therapies groups, the following differences were identified. There are differences in cultural diversity between the urban and countryside population; 2 per cent of clients from visible minorities receive treatment in the trust with a locality city population of 2.1 per cent of visible minorities. The therapists are all white. One member of staff and one client in the sample are from visible minorities; a classification used by National Office for Statistics to indicate non-white minorities. The rural communities (clustered in villages and small towns) have a much smaller percentage of 0.3 per cent visible minorities. Migration history in the trust over three generations is high though: first generation migrants amongst the staff are 25 per cent in comparison with the 8.65 per cent in the city and 3.32 per cent in the rural region. When two further generations are incorporated, staff migration history amounts to 55 per cent while clients total 35 per cent.

Religion as a cultural diversifier was present. The religious affiliation of staff is similar to that of the city (totalling 65 per cent and 60 per cent), but lower than the rural population (75 per cent). The clients in the sample have higher rates of no religious affiliation (50 per cent) than the staff, local and adult trust populations. In relation to class, both staff and clients are downwardly mobile (Office for National Statistics 2008) in relation to their parents. For the clients this is due to a combination of their age and mental health difficulties, for the arts therapists their choice of career is potentially due to other factors than those of socio-economic class (Gilroy and Lee 1995; Grainger 1999).

The young people included ten female clients and eight male clients. The arts therapists at the time of the research were two men (one also a unit-staff arts therapist) and ten women. The unit-staff sample included a male arts therapist, two male nurse therapists, a female nurse therapist (an additional female replacing the arts therapist later in the year) and a male consultant. The other arts therapists in the department were female.

Client and therapist evaluations of the therapy

I used evaluation questionnaires completed by clients and therapists at the end of each session, as well as individual semi-structured interviews and post-session focus groups to ascertain what clients and therapists found helpful and hindering in sessions.

I found that an overall picture emerged about similarities and differences in perception. The following tables compare these similarities (consonance C) and differences (dissonance D) in perception.

Table 11.1 Art Therapy client–therapist consonance and dissonance

Useful C	Unhelpful C
Art is central Contact between people	Absences

Useful D	Unhelpful D
Enough time to paint and talk – therapist	Feeling obliged to draw something meaningful – clients
Arts as distraction – clients	Feelings left unaddressed – therapist

Table 11.2 Dance Movement Therapy/Dramatherapy client–therapist consonance and dissonance

Useful C	Unhelpful C
Group contact Use of certain structures Having fun/play	Absences

Useful D	Unhelpful D
Client self directedness – therapists	Use of particular structures – clients People not joining in – clients Being too tired/session too long – clients Unexpressed feelings – therapists

Comparing the perceptions in art therapy and drama/dance movement therapy, the following picture emerged:

- Consonant themes identifiable for art therapy and dance movement/drama therapy are as follows:
  ◦ DMT/ DT: group contact, having fun/playing and the use of certain structures are useful. Absences are unhelpful.
  ◦ AT: art being central, expressive and 'for real', as well as contact between people are useful. Absences are unhelpful.
- Dissonant themes identifiable for art therapy and dance movement/drama therapy areas are as follows:
  ◦ DMT/DT: clients not joining in the movement as a useful choice or an attack on the group and whether the use of humour is the same as play and the symbolic nature of the movement.
  ◦ AT: art as distraction of genuine therapeutic value (clients) or as defensive (therapists). The role of humour here can be useful or unhelpful as a lack of focus. Across AT and DMT/DT relevant themes are: the symbolism in the art or movement, the use of interpretation and an emphasis on boundaries and containment.

The individual interviews showed differences in perception between clients and therapists about the problem they were trying to address in therapy and how helpful they found the sessions in addressing that problem. I will now discuss two case studies of a male and female client Ted and Belle, who started treatment simultaneously and experienced the same unit and group dynamics. Their experience of embodiment within the arts therapies groups was different. These differences were related to culture, gender and diagnosis/problems. An alternative way of understanding dissonance may be that of resistance. The psychodynamic concept of resistance is defined as the client being unwilling/unable to become conscious of unconscious motivations (Segal 1982). This alternative psychodynamic understanding will be considered in parallel with that of cultural difference affecting dissonance.

Case study: Ted

Ted was 23 years old when he joined the community and remained in treatment for three years. He joined in the research period of initial observation at the same time as Belle. He had been referred for depression and panic attacks. The unit assessment did not identify any other stressors, although staff saw his problems as related to his childhood. His dominant mother had been replaced by his dominant girlfriend and Ted suffered from low self-esteem. Ted himself said that his depression and panic attacks were caused by doing what other people wanted him to do, while he himself did not know what he wanted. He left school after his GCSEs and became a car mechanic. His father was an electrician and his mother a housewife. A few years ago he moved out of the parental home to live with his girlfriend. She was still working as a hairdresser, but he had been off work for three years, becoming increasingly withdrawn and housebound. This meant that he lost his job. Ted had lived and grown up in the same small village, where he was still living with his girlfriend, near his parents. His treatment prior to coming to the community consisted only of drug treatment.

When Ted was asked how he felt treatment could address his problems he described that having a structure to his day, talking about his problems, finding solutions and a change in medication, had all been efficacious. He felt that DMT/DT gave him confidence by doing things seriously with other people. He could not say what he found useful in art therapy. The unit staff, including the dramatherapist, identified movement as particularly useful to him, because they saw him channel his frustrations non-verbally. The art therapist felt it was useful for him to express his dissatisfaction and anger in words but also felt that his use of the art medium changed over time. Initially he could not relate his feelings to the image, but over time he was more able to do so. Ted felt he had changed during treatment. He had relaxed more and was more able to communicate with people. His aim for treatment was growing independence and re-employment.

Ted's ethnic and cultural background were both self-identified as English. Both his parents and grandparents were British born and he grew up in a rural community. Neither he nor his parents had a religious affiliation. Ted completed his statutory education, but did not enrol in higher education. Within his peer group that made him one of the 50 percent in a lower socio-economic class than the therapists and other clients. Unlike the majority of clients and therapists, he was neither upwardly nor downwardly mobile. Ted attended 85.5 per cent of the dance movement therapy group and 80 per cent of the art therapy group. This was a higher than average attendance of the clients.

In the session-evaluation questionnaires, clients were asked to grade a session between one and five, from unhelpful to very helpful and to comment on their choice. Ted graded sessions higher than his peers. He also graded higher than the therapists. When the art was expressive and for real and there was contact between people, he found art therapy sessions useful. This meant for him, that people created an image and were able to discuss in the reflective closure of the session, how the image connected to what they were feeling; thus expressing 'real' emotions. When there were absences and/or the session felt too long, it was unhelpful. Additional useful focus group themes for him, were that a session was relaxing, and that there was enough time to paint and talk. Art as a distraction was also felt to be useful. Absences were not mentioned in the focus group, but other themes were identified to make a session unhelpful: a lack of group connection; timing being problematic (often related to the balance between talking and action, i.e. too much talking made the sessions feel too long); feeling obliged to draw something meaningful; over interpretation and a dislike of staff and fellow clients. In dance movement/drama therapy he provided a greater variety of themes to qualify his grading. Useful factors were again connecting with other people in the group, expressing feelings through talking or movement, having fun and using certain structures such as kicking the ball 'to let off steam'. Hindering factors were a lack of structure and/or direction, balls being out of control, absences and people not joining in. Additionally, unhelpful factors were that feelings were blocked or the physical space was too small. This was related to various sessions where he kicked the ball around the room, where it caused damage to light fittings and scared some other group members. In the focus group he added that it was useful if clients could initiate and 'move to get rid of stress'. As in art therapy, unhelpful factors were more varied and identified with greater frequency in the focus groups. The fact that other people could mention things he could agree with, helped him. Additional factors thus identified were a lack of connection between movement and talking. Repeated in a group context were the use of certain structures, i.e. the ball being out of control, absences and dislike of staff and fellow clients. The movement group often started by members discussing how they felt, followed by a therapist intervention suggesting a way of embodying what they had talked about. If Ted experienced this as connected, he liked it, if it did not; he felt the talking went on too long. He was also very sensitive to people sitting out of the movement watching; it really felt that he wanted everyone to move and paint together.

Ted attended five per cent more DMT/DT than AT sessions. Over time it showed that the issues concerning timing (sessions too long, needing a break) were raised nearer the beginning of the treatment. The absence of people was felt later. Ted gave more detail in his comments on the DMT group throughout the year. The art therapy low-grade comments had question marks, indicating that it seemed difficult for him to articulate the reasons for finding a session unhelpful.

Table 11.3 Ted's questionnaire grades and the comments in his own words

Art Therapy

Grade	Comments
1	Ok, don't know
2	Ok? Sitting down for 1.5 hours, need a coffee break and time in loo
3	Ok, but a bit too long
4	Not too bad
5	Ok (ten times), very well (three times), very sexy (once). Comments: being able to talk and show how I was feeling, explained how I felt in pictures, seeing tits, showed how I felt using art, drawing what was on my mind, using art to show how I was feeling (five times), working together as a group. More people? (three times), not seeing penis.

Dance Movement / Drama Therapy

Grade	Comments
1	It did not go well, dick all useful, like shit. Reasons: Having a wanker have a go at me, the group being one and a half hours too long, what is the point of this group, Belle being in hospital.
2	Not used.
3	? Ok, not being able to hit someone.
4	Ok, moving fast and as a group, breaking the light. The length of the group unhelpful, sitting down for half an hour, could use video or keep fit tapes to help come up with ideas.
5	Ok (five times), very well (six times). Useful: It was a good laugh, working as a group, kicking the ball, it brought up a lot of feeling, using movement to change how I was feeling, helping others, being able to move to show feeling and to get in touch with feeling. Unhelpful: need more people to join in, more people, especially staff who can not be bothered to come in, need bigger room, more people needed, people sitting in the coffee room!

Case study Belle

Belle was a 20-year-old young woman who arrived at the unit at the same time as Ted and stayed for two and a half years. She was referred for depression, self-harming and an eating disorder. Other stressors the unit identified in their assessment were sexual, emotional and physical abuse in her birth family, as well as being fostered in adolescence. Belle received previous treatment in child and adolescent inpatient psychiatry, in acute inpatient psychiatry and was still receiving drug treatment. In the interview, when asked why she was in the unit, she said after six months that people 'piss her off' and she is too wound up to sleep. Initially she said the problems started aged 14, but would rather not say why. Later she stated 'people say it is the abuse from childhood.' The unit staff, including the drama therapist, articulated the abuse by her brother and her subsequent period in the inpatient adolescent unit as precipitating factors. They felt this had affected her ability to trust and to make sense of her experiences. The dance movement therapist cited her difficult relationship with her parents, two family members abusing her. The art therapist cited family relationships as problematic. The three arts therapists mentioned her acting out as part of Belle's way of relating to people, particularly the self-harming incidents.

Belle said that she 'really does not have a clue' what type of treatment might be useful to her. She found the individual time with her key worker most useful. This clashed with the dance movement and drama therapists' emphasis on the usefulness of group therapy. The art therapist felt that Belle's ability to come back to the unit after acting out and hospitalisation, was really useful to her. When talking about the arts therapies as part of her treatment Belle said that she hated it in the beginning. After six months of treatment she preferred art therapy; she did not like to get up and do things in DMT/DT: 'in art everyone gets on with their own things.' The fact that in DMT/DT clients would sit out of the action as an audience to those who did move and 'get up to do things' was very inhibiting for Belle. In the follow up interview later, she felt that the expectation to do something, to express what she felt, further inhibited her. It reinforced her feeling unable to express herself. She felt she enjoyed it more now she was able to relax. Belle could not see any aims for her life, she said that she had become used to the way her life was now and could not see the possibility of change.

When referring to her ethnic and cultural background Belle referred to her birth family. She self-identified ethnically and culturally as English. She identified her mother as Irish born, when she was asked where her parents and grandparents were born (one set of grandparents were born and resident in Ireland). This had, however, not influenced Belle's self-identification. The language spoken at home was English; the home was urban without a significant Irish neighbourhood to identify with. She was raised a Roman Catholic, with a Roman Catholic mother and Methodist father.

Her father was a factory worker, her mother a receptionist. She herself had worked as a waitress in the past, but was now unemployed. She had not completed her statutory education, fairly common for clients with her longstanding history of mental health problems. This placed her, with Ted and half the clients, in a lower socio-economic class than the therapists and other clients. Belle attended 51 per cent of the dance movement therapy group and 59 per cent of the art therapy group. This was a lower than average attendance. This was due to several periods of absence from the unit after overdoses and hospital admissions. She graded lower than her peers, lower than the dance movement therapist and higher than the art therapist.

In AT, the art being expressive and real and contact between people in the group made a session useful to her, while absences and problematic interpretation made a session unhelpful. She mentioned in the focus groups that relaxing was useful; having enough time to paint or talk was felt to have contributed to the usefulness of the session. Hindering, on more than one occasion, were a lack of group connection, over interpretation and a dislike of self and others. A lack of focus and feeling obliged to draw something meaningful were an occasional hindrance. In DMT/DT Belle found connecting with other people in the group, being able to sleep in a session and the use of certain structures as useful. The structures she found useful were going for a walk and gathering material outside to give shape within the session, more diversion than conscious expression. Unhelpful were the use of other structures (after talking in chairs getting up to move was very difficult; interventions where she was watched moving on her own), absences, people not joining in (difficulties about being watched again) and the blame game. Expressing feelings, clients being able to initiate, having fun and moving to get rid of stress were added in the focus groups. One of the structures she really liked was suggesting group games that they had played as a child; it removed Belle's self-consciousness and the fact that the whole group participated meant she felt appreciated without being watched. In unhelpful factors; a lack of structure and a lack of connection between movement and talking were added. Like Ted, the absences were mentioned in the questionnaires, not in the group.

Belle attended eight per cent more AT sessions than DMT/DT. In AT the strong dislike of staff and self, as expressed in blaming others, occurred on one

Table 11.4 Belle's questionnaire grades and comments in her own words

Art Therapy

Grade	Comment
1	Crap, art therapist is a knob, hating art.
2	Not used.
3	People being open, having ideas suggested, having a laugh, anger at co-therapist for sexual interpretation of image.
4	Being able to prat around, express myself, relaxing, therapist is a prat.
5	Relaxed, having fun, doing what I wanted.

Dance Movement/Drama Therapy

Grade	Comment
1	Load of shit, crap. I feel like shit, unhelpable and a miserable cow. Therapist and co-therapist are prats.
2	I was in an arsy mood and could not be bothered.
3	Everyone joining in and trying. Balls being out of control. Kicking /hitting the ball and letting out frustration.
4	Enjoyed it, a lot of activity. Pace gained speed and everyone joined in. People missing. Sleeping for ten minutes at the end, walking with my eyes shut, relaxing.
5	Al and Jack away, having an idea that people liked, people sulking and not joining in (otherwise enjoyable session).

occasion before an overdose and period of hospitalisation, but that was not repeated during the second time this happened. In DMT/DT more dislike of other clients and the therapist was expressed via the 'blame game' throughout.

Case study discussion: comparing Ted and Belle's experience

Ted's relationship with Belle occasionally affected his relationship with the therapist and the group. He was upset when she was admitted to hospital and when he felt she 'had a go' at him early in group therapy. This 'pairing' (Bion 1967) was more prevalent in the first six months. 'Pairing' in this case refers to the formation of a defensive relationship, forming an alliance that excludes the ability to relate to others. His attachment in the second six months was more general to the group. He frequently expressed a wish for more people to be present and actively involved, especially in DMT. He blamed particular clients for Belle's readmission to hospital after another overdose. One factor, which influenced Ted's dissonance with the arts therapists was the absence and leaving of co-therapists. Ted regularly commented on the absence of people (peers and staff) and once stated that 'staff not bothering to come in' felt an unhelpful aspect of the session. The absence of people was much more frequently articulated in relation to the dance movement/dramatherapy group.

The role of the medium influenced Ted psychodynamically. Resistance may be a possible explanation for Ted's difficulty with certain interpretations. His frustration with too much talking and too little movement could be considered a resistance to thought; the movement a mere acting out/abreaction. 'Abreaction' meaning that he used action to distance himself from emotion, rather than using the action to express and reflect on what he was feeling. However, the more direct irritation with the art therapist seems to be connected to not understanding; the question marks a sign of confusion, rather than resistance. The question marks were more frequent in art therapy and directly linked to low grades. The divergent understandings between him and the art therapist about how he uses the art may affect his relationship with the therapist. Ted preferred DMT/DT to AT. Linking this to the medium, he seemed to find it more difficult to give meaning to images and found DMT/DT a better way to channel his frustrations. Given how he understood his diagnosis and identified problems, the more direct physical expression in dance and movement may have facilitated easier expression in a direct, rather than metaphorical, form. The movement has a functional effect on his stress levels and as such is useful to him, rather than that it provides a symbolic expression of underlying internal conflict. He expressed difficulty with the issue of interpretation and frustration with the lack of action in DMT/DT and with the interpretation of images in AT. He valued being able to express what he felt through the images. His emphasis was more on expression than understanding. The greater emphasis on group interaction in DMT/DT may have been experienced by him as more directly useful; he valued everyone joining in and doing things together.

The interacting factors influencing dissonance for Belle are her diagnosis and treatment history, as well as cultural background variables such as her Catholic religion and second-generation Irish migration history. These client variables interact with setting and group dynamics, cross-gender relationships and absences in particular, as well as treatment interruptions. Belle had many treatment interruptions; sometimes they were due to the setting, therapist and co-therapist absences for example, but they were also due to her overdosing incidents resulting in admission to hospital. Her long and frequent absences from the group meant that she maintained better contact with her peers (who often saw her outside the community and visited her in hospital) than with the arts therapists, who would not see her if she did not attend the groups. However, disagreements and conflicts with her peers might have been an issue affecting Belle's relationship with the therapist. In the questionnaires and focus groups she mentioned Al and Jack as an inhibiting factor in DMT/DT (as they watched and did not join in). Excepting Ted, Belle was mostly dissonant with other male clients.

The psychodynamic understanding of Belle's problems relate to early abuse and consequent problems in forming trusting relationships. The latter would be problematic with peers as well as authority figures, as both father and brother were active in the abuse. Her dissonance with male peers can, in a psychodynamic framework, be explained by her history. Being watched by people who do not participate, especially male (she does not mention it when female peers sit out and watch) can be understood as an objectified watching by a male. She is angry with the male co-therapist when he interprets sexual imagery may be a reflection of this same dynamic. The self-hate is common in abuse survivors, who tend to blame themselves for the abuse having occurred. Her cutting and eating disordered behaviour may be a reflection of hating her body, which would make an arts medium that requires embodiment more difficult than one with an external form of expression. The difficult feelings could be projected on others, such as male clients and co-therapists. In addition to these intrapsychic ways of understanding Belle's difficulties, the political level of women taking the guilt for male misogyny needs to be considered. When looking at dynamics such as these both the cultural, intrapsychic, political and interpersonal levels need to taken into consideration (Blackwell 2005). The interpersonal aspect of the conflict can be seen when absences of therapists evoke anger. This seems to indicate some form of attachment despite therapy interruptions. Nevertheless, absences could negatively influence forming a trusting relationship. Her ambivalence, as expressed in contradictory grading and comments, may be a further expression of this.

In the interview Belle said about the arts therapies treatment that she hated it initially. After six months of treatment she preferred art therapy to dance movement therapy. She linked the reason for this to the medium. She did not like to get up and do things in DMT; in AT everyone got on with their own things (more individual in the group than group-as-a-whole orientation). In the follow up interview she felt that the expectation to do something, to express what she felt was really inhibiting, as it reinforced her inability to express herself.

Both therapists and the client shared the view that traumatic familial relationships affected Belle's ability to relate. She said that people 'piss her off', but she could not tell them. It is interesting to note that in the December focus group (16 months into her treatment) she reported having missed the art therapist 'as she would be able to shout at her.' The arts therapists (AT and DMT) felt that her acting-out behaviour was her way of relating to people and that she found it hard to trust. Efficacy of the overall treatment for Belle would have been that she found it easier to go out and have friends. Belle could not say what would be appropriate treatment for her difficulties, but felt individual time was most effective for her. This might conflict with the dance movement and drama therapists' stress on the importance of group therapy. The stronger group orientation and the embodiment nature of DMT/DT might have influenced the greater client–therapist dissonance.

Belle's sense of alienation and distrust can be psychodynamically explained by past experience, but it is interesting to note that she came from a mixed-cultural background which remains unrecognised. She may be more comfortable as the daughter of a first-generation migrant with the first-generation migrant art therapist. A minority religion and lack of identification with one side of her cultural heritage, as a potential alternative to the abusive one, does not seem to have been open to her. Her sense of self-loathing diffusely connects to many factors that cannot be causally linked, although culture as a contributing factor to a problematic identity formation could be argued. This could be expressed as dissonance in the form of scapegoating of difference as expressed towards the art therapist and Sam, a client from a visible ethnic minority, whose taste in music and clothes was derided by her. On the other hand this allows for a greater capacity of articulating anger towards people, one of her stated problems. In articulating missing the art therapist she values the fact that she is able to express anger towards her. Difference may provoke scapegoating, but also a greater ability to relate; the ambivalence about the own difference leading to a greater ability to express both negative and positive emotion in the attachment relationship. As mentioned earlier, an understanding how the political (gender politics concerning abuse), cultural, intrapsychic and interpersonal factors interact is crucial. This is in contrast with Ted, who identified more with the arts therapist from a similar background to his own. Ted's differences in cultural background were in nationality, religion and language with the art therapist. These variables were the same for him and the dance movement therapist. I wonder whether these differences may be particularly relevant for a client who identifies as English for several generations and whose contact experience with people of a different background may be limited (rurally based in one place throughout his life, in a community with little diversity). The irritation with interpretation may be due to a difference in perception of underlying causes; the emphasis on relationships with people in general is congruent.

Reflection on theory and method

The therapist role and psychodynamic approaches

The findings show that in their nature the arts are an active medium, which rely on therapist intervention to influence the form in which they are offered.

Therapist determined structuring can be in contradiction to the process orientation of arts therapies groups (McNeilly 2006; Skaife and Huet 1998; Davies and Richards 2002; Holden 1990). The process orientation expects a non-directive stance from the therapist (Burlingame *et al.* 2004), where the clients are expected to initiate the arts expression in the session. An example is a client suggesting playing childhood movement games in a DMT session, or clients suggesting group rather than individual painting in an AT session. If the therapist waits for the clients and they for her, it may explain Ted's suggestion that a more directive 'keep fit' would help give them ideas. The literature shows a theoretical dilemma about dependency and authority issues in the group. If the therapist 'leads' the group, the clients will maintain that expectation and not take the initiative themselves; if the therapist initiates, the group members remain dependent on the authority figure. Related dilemmas are whether the symbolic meaning takes precedence over the working through of feelings through the artistic medium. The clients say that they are happy to paint, but do not want to interpret their imagery: 'It is only a pretty picture and does not mean anything.' Some therapists feel that this leaves too much in the unconscious and means that the clients are not able to make use of this work in their lives. Other therapists emphasise that, over time, the clients will themselves recognise patterns and themes that have meaning for them. A related issue is that verbal interaction can start to dominate over art making (Skaife and Huet 1998); clients commenting on the session being too much 'blah blah' seems to indicate that they agree. The group interactive form of structuring in the arts therapies may influence client preferences for a particular medium. The movement tends to be interactive – people moving together or are seen by others when they move on their own. Individual art making can remain private and not seen, if the clients choose not to show or discuss the image. A second factor influencing the preference for the medium is its possibility for direct or symbolic expression. The literature shows a discussion in the arts therapies about the symbolic communication through the arts form. Images may be considered indirect communications about the way clients construe the relationships in the therapy session (Springham 1998), whether diagrammatic or embodied (Schaverien 2000). As shown in the case studies, the client wish for direct expression can clash with the therapist emphasis on symbolic meaning of the image representing internal conflict. When Ted wants to move to let out feeling, this clashes with the therapist's emphasis that his movement reflects underlying conflict. She may be correct, but it is wrong for Ted at that time and inhibits his ability to use the movement for abreaction. Belle struggles with the interpretation of her imagery. Again this can be seen as resistance. It can also be seen as a lack of psychological mindedness, often considered a pre-requisite for being able to use psychological therapies. However, both these clients go on to use the treatment, including arts therapies, after their initial year to good effect. Maybe arts therapies are a good way of facilitating the development of psychological mindedness. The generalisability across the arts modalities may be open to debate here. There may be a difference for performance arts modalities like dance, drama and music from visual art. This is an area that needs further research. However, as an implication for practice, I propose that all arts therapists consider the possibility of arts as direct expression as well as arts as symbol. The findings of this research show that the potential for inaccurate or mistimed interpretations is increased when client and therapist diverge in their perceptions of the arts as symbol or index.

Structuring connects to a therapist expectation of directive or non-directive interventions, often combined with a group process approach that aims to facilitate client independence. If the therapist keeps waiting for client initiatives while they feel very stuck, it can be counter-therapeutic. The findings of this research are that a more directive structure is useful to clients, if it leads to a sense of safety and containment. A non-directive approach can be experienced as empowering, in being able to initiate and 'do your own thing'. Client–therapist dissonance occurs through a lack of safety in a directive structure, or a lack of focus in a non-directive one. The arts therapies' current trend towards flexibility (Carr and Vandiver 2003) eclecticism (Karkou and Sanderson 2006) and adaptation to the clients' needs (Huet 1997; Skaife and Huet 1998) can allow for adaptation to stages of treatment and client variables such as cultural differences, diagnosis, stage of treatment and gender.

Another aspect of structuring is the balance between talking and the arts expression. Clients and therapists were consonant about the importance of arts expression and talking in an arts therapies session. I found that dissonance occurs in the balance between the two. A lack of connection between talking and moving or too much talking, creates dissonance. If there is not enough time to talk, the therapists perceive that feelings remain unexpressed or blocked. However, the clients perceive the talking as blocking their ability to use the medium as a distraction. Clients value distraction as it allows them to relax and 'get away from their problems'.

A psychodynamic understanding of resistance may lead the therapist to reinforce an interpretation that the clients are not ready to hear. As defined earlier, the psychodynamic concept of resistance is understood as the client being unwilling/unable to become conscious of unconscious motivations (Segal 1982). As stated earlier, Skaife and Huet quote McNeilly (1983) when considering that increased structuring by the therapist may be transference avoidance. This means that the therapist does not look at the recurrence of a client's childhood relationship patterns in the present therapy relationships. However, this emphasis on theoretical orientation does not allow for consideration of the clients' perspective beyond resistance/transference. The findings of this and other research emphasise the value of play and fun in the arts therapies (Amir 1999; Casson 2003). This can counteract the view of distraction as resistance. The therapeutic value of play (Winnicott 1997) provides an alternative conceptual arts therapies framework which, in inter-action with stage of treatment and client diagnosis, provides a more flexible therapist response.

I hypothesise that a history of sexual abuse can create greater dissonance with the dance movement medium, especially in a group interactive mixed-gender context. It would be useful to see further research undertaken in the (dis)advantages of mixed-gender group therapy. The women's therapy centre, for example, has facilitated interesting work in this area. When there is an expectation of group-as-a-whole interaction, the impact of non-participating members as an audience can lead to greater peer dissonance and self-consciousness on the part of the clients who are being watched. A therapist orientation of client autonomy may see the sitting out as clients exercising choice, or see it in terms of resistance. It may be that the effect of audience on a performance based arts medium needs further consideration beyond these two explanations. This study has shown that gender dynamics and previous life stressors impact on the effect of audience. Jones (2005) discusses the concept of the active witness in the arts therapies, to stand apart and be a part/involved at the same time (Grainger 1999; Schaverien 1992; Aldridge 1996). In addition, the experience for those witnessing in a group context can be therapeutically important (Jones 2005, 2007). Jones views this as therapeutically positive. The possibility of 'malignant mirroring' in a group dynamic sense (Nitsun 1996) needs to be further researched as a phenomenon in arts therapies groups. Jones' core process of witnessing may need to incorporate this destructive possibility, in addition to the helpful aspects of witnessing identified.

Conclusion

Having listened to clients' perception of helpful and hindering processes around group art, drama and dance movement therapy different influencing factors emerge. These include: group-as-a-whole or individual-in-the-group structuring, the effect of the audience or witness, the freedom to play and client preference for direct rather than symbolic expression. These all affect a client's ability and willingness to 'join the dance'. Embodiment is present in all arts modalities, but being witnessed in the embodiment is most strongly present in dance movement and dramatherapy, where there are no images or instruments to distract the attention. When we ask a client to use P(rojection), this may be useful to consider as part of the development of therapy. E(mbodiment) and R(ole) involve a more direct experience of the body being witnessed. When using projective work the therapist needs to heed the risk of over interpretation of symbolism.

12 Cinderella: the role fights back

Clare Powis

Box 12.1

Questions about practice

- How can individual dramatherapy be offered within a child and adolescent mental health service?
- What remains after the closure of the therapy?
- Does the therapeutic relationship exist in isolation?

Research perspective

- Case study
- Structured questionnaire
- Semi-structured client interview

Client perspective sample

Clare: (referring to the list): Now, there was a boyfriend. In fact, there were a couple of boyfriends . . . (Jenny squeals): weren't there? That came and went in those dramas . . .

Jenny: Kane and Stephen.

Clare: What do you remember about them?

Jenny: Well, they kept swapping places. Like, well, they kept sleeping with Sabrina and Kelly, like, so Kelly kept sleeping with Ruby's boyfriend and then Ruby kept sleeping with Kelly's boyfriend, and it was getting really mixed up.

Jenny: (looking at the list): Can we skip to the dog?

Clare: We've got the prince and the dog left.

Jenny: I don't want to do the prince.

Clare: You don't want to do the prince?

> *Jenny:*   No. Because he's ugly . . . The dog was very funny.
>
> Evaluation interview

Introduction

When engaging in a dramatherapy session the therapist and the patient(s) or client(s) are entering into uncharted lands. How far they travel will depend on how far each of them is prepared to open up their creative and psychodynamic processes. The risks can seem great for our often emotionally damaged patients and clients – and for the therapist. In the dramatherapy session we have the potential to open ourselves up to the worlds in our imaginations. Invited – and uninvited – characters may want to join in our play. In addition, before therapist and patient can enter those worlds of imagination in the dramatherapy session, there will be influences outside the therapy room that affect how, or indeed whether, a patient might do so. This chapter explores such issues within a reflection on a case study of one-to-one work conducted over forty-seven sessions.

Contexts

One of the many factors affecting engagement in dramatherapy can be the patient's preconceptions of the experience of being 'in therapy'. Previous experience of appointments with health and social service professionals, for example, may have an impact on his or her feelings about therapy. Perhaps a child may make up a reason for missing school so they can attend a therapy session without being teased or bullied. On entering a clinic, a patient who uses a wheelchair or who does not use verbal language as a primary form of communication may feel at an immediate disadvantage in a supposedly, 'therapeutic environment' if he or she is surrounded by ambulant, verbally articulate professionals. Some patients may be dependent on a relative, carer or support worker to bring them to a therapy appointment. The escort's attitude to the appointment is crucial to the patient's experience of his or her therapy. All of these factors, outside of the immediate dramatherapy space and encounter can feature in the patient's experiences of the therapy. It may be that the realities of the patient's and dramatherapist's worlds differ greatly in terms of age, gender, mental and physical health and functioning, social, political and educational factors. It is likely that therapist and patient match each other in shared experience in only a few of these areas. It may be worth acknowledging that any characters emerging from the dramatherapy patient's creative process are likely, at least initially, to reflect roles within his or her world with which he or she is familiar: an overbearing parent; a dominant step-brother; an aged teacher; an alcoholic neighbour. In many different ways the therapist may not share the same reference points. This extends to other differences: of culture, race, gender, disability, sexuality, age and class. How (the patient, his or her family and friends might think), given such differences, can the therapist possibly be of any help? Haugh and Paul (2008) have commented on this area in relation to cultural contexts and power. They link such areas to one of the central acts within the process of therapy: the creation of empathy and a supportive environment. Drawing on research, they suggest that a key aspect of effective therapy involves the therapist's capacity 'to understand and experience, as deeply as possible, the world of the other as they experience it', linking this to the 'context of our lives ... ethnicity, gender, sexuality, physical abilities or class' (2008: 43). They argue that therapy has not concerned itself with such issues of 'difference' and that it is crucial for the therapist and patient to be able to connect across and within such differences. Totton has argued that if the act of therapy takes place with such areas unacknowledged they can be counter-therapeutic:

> Experiences of difference in social interaction are a potent source of the emotional wounds which people bring to therapy. They can also easily be re-enacted and re-inforced in the therapeutic relationship ... A key feature of mainstream culture and values is that they tend to be invisible to their holders ...
>
> (Totton 2008: 149)

Dramatherapy offers a particularly potent route within these issues via the worlds of imagination and play. As described previously, the experiences of patient and therapist are likely to be different. In drama and play, however, the feelings behind and within the patient's experiences can be shared and, in Totton's framework, made visible and explored. The dramatherapist aims to tune into those feelings and experiences which can be identified, explored, understood and owned in the mutuality of the shared space of the play or drama.

A measure of therapeutic movement and the patient's developing ego strength is surely reflected in his or her use of characters and role in any dramas created in the session. I wonder if the characters therein become invested – perhaps as part of the patient's unconscious processing of material – with the patient's burgeoning ego-strength which takes its baby steps hiding under the apron of the role. Through the safety of an emerging character or role created in the dramatherapy session the dysfunctional and damaging aspects of him or herself and others, as experienced by the patient in his or her world, can be challenged. It is the use of role in the patient's therapeutic process in dramatherapy that prompted the writing of this chapter. I will be exploring the idea that the role adds a third party to the therapeutic alliance of patient and therapist in one-to-one dramatherapy.

Case study: Jenny

Reasons for referral

The dramatherapy intervention I shall be referring to in this chapter took place over 18 months consisting of a total of 47, once-weekly, hour-long individual sessions. Jenny had been referred to her local child and adolescent mental health service (CAMHS) team by her GP because she was finding it difficult to form 'lasting and appropriate relationships with her peers'. At the time of referral Jenny was nine years old. She lived with her mother, and had no contact with her father. This fact was to become a significant issue in her dramatherapy, as it is in my experience of CAMHS work in general. I sense the issue of absent fathers is a reflection of the breakdown in the structure of the family over the past five or so decades. For at least Jenny's lifetime the concept of relationships with fathers, grandfathers, uncles, boyfriends and husbands is in flux. Jenny attended a local day school near to her home in a council estate on the outskirts of town. She was the only child living at home with her mother. I understood that she did not often play out with friends after school or at weekends, and she rarely went to classes or social events outside school hours.

The CAMHS team was based at a local out-patient clinic. At the time of Jenny's referral the team was made up of community psychiatric nurses, most of whom specialised in child and family mental health; primary mental health workers; a psychologist, consultant psychiatrists, an occupational therapist, two art psychotherapists and myself, a dramatherapist. At the time, I worked for this team for two days per week. Other professional involvement included the consultant community paediatrician, a family support practitioner from the local family support team and a special educational needs coordinator (SENCO). Jenny was referred for dramatherapy by a specialist nurse from the clinic, who had done an initial assessment following the child's referral to CAMHS.

The nurse had done some individual work with Jenny, but she felt that Jenny avoided engaging with an approach that depended, to a large extent, on verbal interaction. Meetings with her specialist nurse, her case notes, and subsequent conversations with Jenny's mother led me to believe that Jenny's external world was chaotic: disputes with neighbours, which included the front door of the house being kicked down; yelling matches and name-calling; disruptive loud music being played; objects being thrown over the fence into her garden.

At the time of Jenny's referral, a dramatherapy student was on placement with the CAMHS team. She and I were setting up a ten-week creative drama group with children between 9–12 years old. The specialist nurse (CAMHS) asked me to consider Jenny for the group.

As the ten weeks of the group passed it became apparent to me that Jenny could benefit from individual dramatherapy. Jenny's work in the group had highlighted significant attachment issues. Individual dramatherapy sessions were negotiated with Jenny, her mother, the referring nurse and Jenny's form teacher at school.

Description of the work

Following the referral for one-to-one dramatherapy I met with Jenny and her mother to discuss expectations and aims of the intervention. At this stage the aim of the dramatherapy was to work towards identifying reasons behind Jenny's difficulty making and sustaining positive relationships with her peers and teachers at school. When Jenny had been in the dramatherapy group at the clinic, prior to her being considered for one-to-one dramatherapy, I had noted that, in her eagerness to be friends with other children in the group, she tended to alienate them by not reading the 'rules' of social interaction and play, such as turn-taking and sharing; allowing others to express and try out their own ideas; not imposing oneself on others' space or task. Aims would be reviewed during the course of the one-to-one therapy when Jenny, her mother and I would meet for regular reviews.

Jenny was brought to sessions by her mother and, on occasion, a family friend. For the first few times her mother stayed in the waiting room for the duration of Jenny's session. After about a dozen sessions she would drop her off and return to pick her up. I would make time to speak to her mother before and/or after Jenny's session. During these pre- and post-session chats I soon became aware that issues to do with Jenny's mother's own parenting were having an impact on Jenny's therapeutic process in the session. I came to understand this in the light of the improvisations Jenny created. I felt it was helpful to me, as a therapist, to be able to relate the mother I saw outside the therapy room to the 'mum' I saw Jenny bring into the therapy arena. Jenny brought a lot of her mother's issues into the therapy room. She (Jenny) seemed to be sorting out her mother's issues; which had, over their years together, merged with hers. I hope to illustrate, below, some examples of how this blurring and confusion was expressed in Jenny's dramatherapy. I believe Jenny needed to understand the issues that impacted on her mother's relationship with her; and I feel she was trying to sort them out for her mother because she, Jenny, needed her 'mum' back: i.e. a parent who could help Jenny manage her own feelings. On many occasions Jenny would put the baby-daughter character she had devised to one side in order to take on the role of 'mum' in her improvisations and create situations that echoed her mother's story. My dramatherapy reports on the work with Jenny would recommend that Jenny's mother seek her own mental health support through adult services. I was aware that Jenny's mother would often turn down any counselling intervention offered to her by the adult mental health service.

However, I was also aware that Jenny's dramatherapy referral came loaded with supposition and assumptions. Jenny's file was thick with notes from the many professional involvements. The assumption that the family was 'difficult' to work with was grounded in the professionals' past experience. Jenny's case notes described an instance when Jenny's mother and uncle had been to the clinic to demand that Jenny be diagnosed with Attention Deficit Hyperactivity Disorder, and be given the 'necessary' prescribed medication. According to certain clinicians some family members were not always co-operative with health or social services; on occasion refusing intervention unless it was on their terms. I am conscious that the clinicians in CAMHS are used to being the ones who are informed (at least about aspects of mental health/social care). In being so, they will have some authority. Jenny's family was, relatively, uninformed. By going into the consultant's office and demanding a diagnosis Jenny's mother and uncle were, perhaps, trying to make a stand – albeit in what was experienced as a socially clumsy and threatening manner – to retain a sense of control over Jenny's intervention. The potential for confrontation between those with authority and those without is always present. Certainly, the interpersonal dynamics being played out between clinicians and family, and family and Jenny seemed a reflection of what was happening in Jenny's unfolding story in the therapy room. Parental 'authority' became a major issue to come out of Jenny's drama-therapy work.

Jenny attended her dramatherapy sessions regularly. I was encouraged by her mother's commitment to bring her. Jenny's attendance was also dependent on her teachers giving her time off to attend sessions at the clinic in school time. At the beginning of her therapy Jenny presented as a sweet, obliging girl. She was keen to impress upon me that everything was really OK, and that she was coping. She said she liked coming to 'drama' because 'it's fun doing drama with you.' I was quickly aware of how uncomfortably this 'sweet girl' image sat on Jenny's shoulders; and of how hard she worked at trying to hold her up there. I sensed Jenny was fearful of confronting the confusion, tension and terror that would emerge in the improvisations and in the thera-peutic relationship between us. Despite her early attempts to avoid engaging with me Jenny seemed more comfortable to do so through the drama; gradually developing a cast of characters which became central to a series of weekly improvisations.

I was curious as to why Jenny was drawn to the theatre style of improvisa-tion; as opposed to other forms of drama or projective play such as the sand tray, puppets, or dolls' house play. What led her to make this choice? Perhaps the choice was made by an impulse from her unconscious, which was responding to and recognising an opportunity of being given possibilities of a shape and a voice through the characters in the improvised play between herself and me, the dramatherapist. I sense that at this stage in her thera-peutic process Jenny needed to include me – the therapist – in her play. In this way she could relate to me in a manner she felt comfortable with. In her usual everyday contact with adults she rarely felt in control. Through impro-visation she could relate to me, Clare; a real-life therapist, via a character she could feel in control of – to a certain extent – by engaging in devices such as freezing the action; saying what happens next in the drama; giving the character specific words to speak or reactions to play. This relates to issues concerning verbal and non-verbal communication as described by Cox and Theilgaard:

> the patient's story may be so disturbing that it is repressed and thus banished beyond the possibility of verbal access. Indeed, it is often the impact of repressed experience which leads to that story which is so disturbing that the patient seeks the opportunity to tell it; so that he can learn his own life-story at first hand.

(1987: 3)

Improvisation can be one of the most challenging and risky forms of creating drama; not least because the actors involved are allowing – inviting, even – spontaneity, uninhibited play and free association into what Read Johnson calls the 'play space'. He describes the 'playspace [as] an enhanced space, where the imagination infuses the ordinary' (1992: 112). I suggest that in this context the actor becomes vulnerable – or as vulnerable as his or her defences allow. Paradoxically, it can be that through 'pretend' reality may be seen. Disguise may also reveal. In Jenny's case, improvisation gave her permission to take off the 'sweet girl' mask.

In the following section I list the cast of characters that developed over Jenny's sessions: I believe that many served the function for Jenny of holding or expressing parts of herself or projections of aspects of herself or her life:

- Kelly: young girl: (8–16?). Hides her wishes from her mother. She even hides her friends away from being discovered by her mother. Engineers situations where mum and dad get together. Generally tries to create and maintain peace in the household.
- Sabrina: Friend of Kelly. Same age as Kelly (8–16?): she is allowed out – to stay with friends and have sleepovers. She is often the one to get into trouble. She is usually looked after by Kelly, who is protective of her.
- Aislene and Ruby: other girl friends who make up the numbers for sleepovers, school class, etc.
- Kane and Stephen: boyfriends of Kelly and Sabrina; Aislene and Ruby. Confusion about who is whose boyfriend.
- Mother: usually Kelly's mother, but interchangeable with Sabrina's mother. She is often getting ready to go out dancing. She offers Kelly new clothes, trips out, but often retracts her offer at the last minute. She is jealous of Kelly's new clothes, friends and boyfriends, and she may try to take them from her. Mother continually rejects Father when he turns up in the scene.
- Mother's boyfriend: more confusion about whether he's mother's or Kelly's boyfriend.
- Father: father often appears in the scene to try and get back with Mother,

and move into the family home. He wants to be with his daughter. His attempts at wooing Mother are always foiled.
- Grandpa and Nan: make occasional appearances.
- Teacher, policewoman, doctor, paramedic: witnesses to Kelly's frequent fainting/collapsing episodes. Authority figures; rescuers, challengers.
- Cinderella: wants to go to the ball and be with the prince who has declared his love to her.
- Prince: falls in love with Cinderella the moment he sees her, and asks her to marry him. When the ugly sister tells him to marry her instead he agrees, and he rejects Cinderella.
- Ugly sister: tells the prince to marry her instead of Cinderella.
- Dog: Kelly's confidante, helper.

Jenny had established the central characters: Kelly/Sabrina, mother and boy-friend/father. She had also identified the core situation or context wherein improvisations started out: Mother promises Kelly a birthday party/new clothes/trip out only to withdraw her offer and leave Kelly to fend for herself/complete a household task while she goes out dancing. Jenny and I played all these roles. She usually played Kelly and she cast me in the adult roles; though sometimes she cast me as Sabrina. A role could also be projected onto an empty chair, a puppet, or a toy dog. (Often this is a necessary facility when the cast list is larger than the number of actors available.) Because the use of role was a regular feature of the sessions it was important to establish a convention of taking a role on and off. In the early sessions I introduced a procedure whereby, after identifying who was playing which role, and explaining that Jenny and Clare would 'wait for us' while we played, I would count 'one, two, three.' Jenny and I would take our place in a defined play area, in role. Once we were in the drama we would sometimes forgo the precedent whereby we counted ourselves in and out of a change of role. I was reminded of the fluidity of children's play in the school playground. There seemed to be an unspoken understanding and acceptance of this 'rule' of fluid, almost stream-of-consciousness play that allowed us to move in and out of roles without losing spontaneity, and the impetus of the drama's intention. Landy tells us that, 'the dramatherapist does not, and cannot, remain permanently over-distanced if she is to effectively enter into the one-on-one drama . . . the dramatherapist must not only be able to shift from one role to another, but from one level to another. Thus the role safety of remaining in control and super-rational becomes difficult to sustain' (1994: 101). Indeed, I was struck by the intensity of the dramas, and the depth of characterisation. I became aware of how readily and powerfully her and my unconscious inhabited the characters. Read Johnson writes that 'the playspace is summoned merely by the creation of the illusion of an alternative reality, without necessarily establishing with clarity what the roles are. In this sense the playspace is a form of trance' (1992: 113). Sure enough, it felt as though we were being driven by a powerful force; the force of unconscious processing, I believe. And by staying with this force – surrendering to it, perhaps? – I feel unconscious material found its way through. However, it was important for the therapist-me to be aware of this potential to surrender to the play. Landy draws our attention to the power of the role to seduce the therapist-in-role into acting out his or her own unconscious material, 'this [seduction] occurs unconsciously and needs to be monitored by the dramatherapist in her supervision and/or in her ability to develop an internal supervisor, an observer part of herself that stands by in the wings during each moment of role-enactment' (1992: 106). One of the implications of this is that I, the therapist, must become a witness to my own actor. I need to ask myself 'What is this character telling me?'

One of the most noticeable features of Jenny's dramas, as mentioned above, was the blurring of boundaries between the mother and the daughter characters. Sometimes, I – the therapist-in-role – would stop the drama so I – (and, I think, Jenny too) – could clarify who was who. Indeed, it was hard to keep track of who was who without the means to stop the drama; a facility we both became familiar with. Moreover, as the associated confusion and tension of 'who is who's mother, and who am I?' infused the dramas I needed to allow this projected material to inform my understanding and consequent responses as a therapist – and also as an actor. It felt important that any new understanding I reached was reflected, as and when appropriate, with Jenny; not only to check out my understanding with her, but also to let her know that, together, we were trying to make sense of what was confusing. Consequently, by stopping or freezing the drama we were able to come out of role to acknowledge and reflect on how we felt. Confusion can often cause a 'blanking', lack of momentum and, as in Jenny's case, a sticking point where an alternative action or outcome is inhibited. In reflection, Jenny was able to relate Kelly, Sabrina or father's confusion to her own situation; for example, who was looking after whom?

Once established, Jenny played and re-played her 'script'. Although, over the weeks, there were a number of minor changes – (the nature of the task or the type of 'gift' that was ultimately withheld from Kelly) – we wouldn't get beyond the point where the father and the mother are going to get married. Inevitably, the wedding was never allowed to take place. The drama was becoming stuck and repetitive. I understood the importance of staying with this impasse; to attend to it. What did it tell me about Jenny's internal world? How was Jenny's unconscious process influencing the improvisation – and the actors therein? And yes, I needed to keep a check on my restlessness to 'do' and 'create drama'. Yet I also understood the importance of being aware of the feeling of helplessness that I was picking up; and of my role as a guide to Jenny's therapeutic process. It was in session 16 that I noted an association between the situation and characters of Jenny's improvisation and a well-known fairy tale. Once again, Kelly had been promised a night out dancing. She had been given a beautiful new dress by her mother for the occasion. Before she was allowed to go, she had to sweep the kitchen floor, do the washing-up and hang out the washing. Kelly's mother said she was just 'nipping out' and would be back to fetch her. However, when she returned, her mother changed her mind and refused to let Kelly go dancing with her boyfriend.

Later, when Jenny and I were reflecting on the improvisation I told her I had noted a similarity between the improvisation and the Cinderella story. In her book *The Play's the Thing* Marina Jenkyns has observed that:

> The interventions of the dramatherapist are largely taken from the realm of the metaphor and symbolic action ... The dramatherapist is constantly allowing his or her associations and intuition to inform the therapy session and to help make the decision as to what structure to create for the work ... This is one of the ways that the dramatherapist's unconscious manifests its understanding of the client.
>
> (Jenkyns 1996: 53)

Reflecting together after the improvisation gave Jenny and me an opportunity to stand back from the intensity of the drama and look at what had been an expression of internal and unconscious processes. I suggested to Jenny that we could try acting some of the Cinderella story in the next session. Jenny's face lit up, and she happily agreed to this. At the beginning of the next session Jenny cast me as the ugly sister and herself as Cinderella. Before going into role Jenny instructed me to make the ugly sister taunt and tease Cinderella, and find ways to stop Cinderella going to the prince's ball. The story of Cinderella, and the character of the ugly sister, provided plenty of opportunity for teasing. I sensed there were several connections here with Jenny's reality outside the therapy room. Jenny had sometimes made a passing reference to herself as 'ugly'; and this word, used as a taunt, had often found its way into the improvisations with Kelly, mother and Sabrina. I had noticed, too, that Kelly would be promised beautiful dresses and trips out – only to have these promises withdrawn: more taunting.

Reflections on the therapy 1: different perspectives on change

In any reflection on the process of change in dramatherapy, in any evaluation, a number of different perspectives are naturally involved. The needs, demands and languages of the patient, those of the therapist and of his or her discipline, those of the multidisciplinary team and of the authority funding and supporting therapy can have parallels and differences. There can be useful differences that acknowledge and respond to the variety of different perspectives. However, there can also be tensions. Positive elements may include the ways in which less 'traditional' ways of evaluating change may be developed by the patient and dramatherapist together, prioritising the patient's meanings and perceptions. Tensions may exist between methods of describing and accounting for change that have been developed within general systems, and that do not easily engage with the kinds of complexity of specific languages which can occur within an arts therapy such as dramath-erapy. In many accounts of dramatherapy this is not acknowledged. The following explores different ways of understanding change in relation to Jenny's experiences.

In reflecting on the impact of dramatherapy a number of questions are crucial to consider. For example, what remains after the closure of the therapy? Does the therapeutic relationship exist in isolation? I saw something of how Jenny's family and family friends, school, peers, television, internet, etc. had impacted on her when she was referred to the clinic. What kind of impact will her experience of dramatherapy have on her family, school and social life? Once her dramatherapy is over can Jenny reconfigure her relation-ships with her family, friends, peers – and future partner(s) – for the better?

Reflections on the therapy 2: Jenny's perspective

Throughout Jenny's therapy I held reviews at regular intervals, usually every dozen or so sessions, or as needed. I had tried various ways of recording and evaluating Jenny's reflections on the sessions. One was a structured question-naire which asked her to identify:

- why she thought she had been referred
- what information she had been given about dramatherapy
- her expectations of dramatherapy
- whether she had found her sessions helpful; and if so whether she could describe why or how
- whether she had noticed any changes in herself, her friends or mother, and other family members since she had been in therapy: if she had, could she describe what these changes are?

I did not feel the feedback from this format was always reliable. For one thing, answers could seem – if read by someone who had not been party to the dramatherapy process – contradictory. For example, Jenny might assert that she enjoyed coming to her dramatherapy sessions, then qualify her statement by explaining that she enjoyed sessions because she got out of her maths class. This may have been true, but I came to realise that this feedback format did not allow for the complexity or ambiguity behind Jenny's state-ments. It was hard enough for her to express these qualities through her drama let alone via a set of written questions. I noted that even when given the time to complete a form Jenny would undertake the task as if she was doing a test. Interestingly, I sometimes sensed that any answers she chose to give – or not give – indicated how she felt about her therapy and about me, her therapist. So, in a way her answers could be seen as a true reflection of what was going on for her at the time. However, unless analysed as such by the therapist a reader of these feedback forms could easily have assumed Jenny's dramatherapy wasn't particularly effective.

I felt the most effective and reliable evaluation came through the drama and subsequent reflection – both in the session with Jenny and in clinical or peer supervision after the session. For example, I had noted that Jenny – and other clients/patients I have worked with – may repeat a (series of actions in a) scene over a number of sessions. Reflecting on this with Jenny towards the end of a session I acknowledged the 'block' in the development of the drama which, perhaps, reflected a block or unease in her understanding of a situation in her reality. Could we, I wondered, use the drama to find a way through the 'block'? As with many patients or clients a 'way through' may not be reached through verbal or cognitive reasoning. In such cases it is when – or sometimes if – the patient or client brings a new element to the scene that I get the clearest indication or feedback that there has been a shift in his or her therapeutic process. So it was with Jenny. In her sessions Jenny and I had been playing out the actions leading up to the moment when the mother character and the boyfriend/father character get married:

- Father (usually played by me) turns up unannounced at mother and Kelly's home.
- Father is reunited with Kelly (usually played by Jenny).
- Mother (usually played by me) buys Kelly a new dress.
- Mother announces she and father are going to get married.
- Mother wants the new dress back.
- Kelly gets things ready for the wedding: she books the church, the vicar, and the bride's car. Then she buys the wedding ring to give to father.
- Kelly drives the bride to the church.
- They arrive at the church too late. (The reason may vary from week to week.)
- Father has gone home.

For about five sessions the wedding never took place. In the sixth or seventh repeat of the wedding scenario Kelly (played by Jenny) decided to stay at home and look after her pet dog rather than drive mother to the church. On reflecting together about this change Jenny told me that the dog needed looking after. I decided not to analyse or interpret this change further with her at this point. I felt that it was enough for Jenny that she had instigated a change. She did not return to the scene again. Sometimes, I would consider initiating a change in the details of a drama that seemed to be 'stuck'. However, the decision to do this needs to be made with judgement. It would not have been appropriate to 'rush' Jenny's therapeutic process. Clinical and peer supervision was helpful in allowing me to check out my motivation for introducing an element of change to a drama. Usually, if my initiative – perhaps of introducing a new or archetypal character; a ringing telephone or doorbell – hadn't hit the mark for Jenny she might: a) respond briefly before returning to her 'script', or b) ignore it and carry on regardless. At worst she might be irritated by the perceived interruption to her script. Either way, I got the message: she wasn't ready to accept the therapeutic potential of a change. However, if my initiative did hit the spot the message was equally clear; as when Jenny's face lit up at my linking her play to the Cinderella story. To me, this was the most reliable feedback.

As part of the evaluation of the sessions, and as part of the writing for this chapter I interviewed Jenny four months after her final session. This was undertaken within the ethical protocols of the setting and with her full agreement. Jenny's interview throws light on her experience of dramatherapy sessions at the clinic. In her reflection she alludes to some of the themes in her work, as identified earlier. I structured questions which related to the process of the therapy, responding to Jenny's directions. I focused on key elements of the process over time and the key characters she developed. Firstly, I invited her to remember how she felt about coming to the clinic.

Clare: What do you remember about the clinic itself? What was your experience of . . .
Jenny: (interrupting and speaking over the end of Clare's question)
  It was scary when I first come . . .
Clare: (finishing sentence at same time)
  Coming to (repeating Jenny's answer) scary . . .
Jenny: And when I went . . .
Clare: Mmm Hmmm . . .
Jenny: When I . . . when it was the last day that I went . . . I didn't want to leave 'cause it was so much fun . . .

I note here Jenny's honesty about disclosing her feelings. On the occasion of our first meeting at the clinic I remember her coming across as being the nonchalant, apparently indifferent 'sweet girl'. This had been the mask protecting the vulnerable, scared Jenny I came to see in her sessions.

In the interview with Jenny I explained that I had made a list of characters, places, objects and events that had appeared in her dramas and improvisations, and invited her to comment on them. She began by talking about Kelly and Sabrina, the two roles she usually played.

Clare: So what do you remember about Kelly?
Jenny: She was bossy. And that's it. Well, she. . . . I don't know.
Clare: What do you think about her now?
Jenny: I miss her.
Clare: Do you miss her?
Jenny: Yeah.
Clare: Oh. (Pause, reading from the list) Sabrina. What do you remember about Sabrina?
Jenny: She was like . . . she was like . . . my favourite character.

Clare: Was she? How do you feel about Sabrina now?
Jenny: Miss her, as well.

I was curious to know what it was about Kelly and Sabrina that Jenny missed. Was it that she missed the freedom of self-expression these roles had given her? Or, perhaps she missed a sense of comradeship from their shared experience; as though the characters had been her playmates. I was aware that, at the time of her referral Jenny was unable to sustain friendships with her peers. She had been isolated from their shared play in the playground.

Although I invited Jenny to elaborate on her comments in the interview I did not feel it appropriate to push her. I had made a decision to hold back from my stance as an enquiring, 'wondering' therapist in order to preserve a distinction between my role as it had been in the therapy room and my role as interviewer. I was cautious, too, about re-visiting what may still be sensitive issues for Jenny without the immediate recourse to therapy sessions. I felt it best that Jenny regulate her own reminiscences of her therapy.

Jenny reads out the next name on the list.

Jenny: Cinderella.
Clare: Cinderella!
Jenny: You kept being the ugly step-sister (*Jenny's description*) and get me to do everything.
Clare and Jenny laugh.
Clare: 'Cause you played Cinderella, didn't you?
Jenny: Yeah.
Clare: What was it like playing Cinderella?
Jenny: Mmmm . . . alright . . .
Clare: Well how do you feel about her now?
Jenny: Um . . . I miss her. Because she was one of my favourite main characters.
Clare: OK, what about the Ugly Sister?
Jenny: Oh, she was bossy, weren't she?
Clare and Jenny laugh.

Later in the interview Jenny referred to the sense of confusion that had been a significant issue in her sessions.

Clare: (referring to the list) Now, there was a boyfriend. In fact, there were a couple of boyfriends . . .
Jenny squeals.
Clare: . . . weren't there? That came and went in those dramas . . .
Jenny: Kane and Stephen.
Clare: What do you remember about them?
Jenny: Well, they kept swapping places. Like, well, they kept sleeping with Sabrina and Kelly, like, so Kelly kept sleeping with Ruby's boyfriend

and then Ruby kept sleeping with Kelly's boyfriend, and it was getting really mixed up.

In the sessions I had understood that Jenny may have projected aspects of her father into the handsome prince character in her Cinderella play. Jenny's next reflection – or, rather, avoidance of reflection – about this character in her dramas caused me to consider that she still held some of the confusion she had felt about her absent father. Note how she makes light of her avoidance, and changes the subject.

Jenny   (looking at the list):   Can we skip to the dog?
Clare: We've got the prince and the dog left.
Jenny: I don't want to do the prince.
Clare: You don't want to do the prince?
Jenny: No. Because he's ugly . . . The dog was very funny.

Towards the end of the interview Jenny reflected on the dress which had featured prominently in the Kelly, Sabrina, mother, father/boyfriend scenes and the Cinderella improvisations.

Jenny gasps: she has seen the next item on the list of reminders.
Clare: This list shows . . .
Jenny: Oh, yes!
Clare: . . . some of the things that happened . . .
Jenny   (interrupting):   You know that purple dress . . . the new dress, remember?
Clare: Yeah . . .
Jenny: I kept wearing that. Is it still there?
Clare: The velvet one?
Jenny: Yeah.
Clare: With the beads, the shiny beads on . . .
Jenny   (overlapping):   No, the other one.
Clare: Ah yes, I do. The one that you kept saying was the 'beautiful dress'?
Jenny: Yeah. Yeah. OK.
Clare: Yes. It's still there.

During the Cinderella improvisations I had understood Jenny's wearing of the dress representing a state of transformation: a literal and a psychic change. I feel that Jenny's comments here highlight her sense of the experience as holding a lasting impression of awe and delight.

    I was grateful for the opportunity to carry out this meeting with Jenny. The intention of setting up the interview had been to invite Jenny to feed back her experiences of her dramatherapy sessions. She had responded to the invitation with an energy and enthusiasm that I found both touching and humbling. The interview also revealed the differences, acknowledged at the start of the chapter between my own language and concepts of what occurred within the dramatherapy, and those of Jenny. The interview reveals what Jenny remembered, wanted to say, and could talk about using words. The next section will draw on my perspective as therapist, looking at a variety of her expressions and experiences.

Reflections on the therapy 3: therapist's perspective

The next section will draw on the areas identified by Jenny as important, and upon my own reflections on aspects of the therapeutic work. What are we to make of the traditional Cinderella story in the context of Jenny's experience, for example? Through storytelling and storymaking the dramatherapist can work with the patient's concept of familial relationships. I note how Jenny finds what she needs within the story to explore her own experience. After all, the story of Cinderella contains obstacles (the ugly sister, the tasks, the poverty, the absent father) that Jenny recognises in her world. What, too, has become of the traditional happy-ever-after ending? Sometimes, for our patients/clients or service users the ending isn't always so prescribed or definitive. At some point in Jenny's dramatherapy I was made aware that Jenny had a half-sister who lived with her father. I wondered if Jenny felt rejected by her own father, and perhaps she felt she was (the) 'ugly' (unwanted sister). She may also have projected 'ugliness' onto her half-sister. I had been told that, at home, Jenny had been teasing her new pet dog. From discussions with her teachers I was aware that Jenny could bully other children. By taking on roles in her Kelly improvisations and in the Cinderella story, Jenny seemed to be expressing the anger and aggressive impulses that she would otherwise act out through her bullying and teasing behaviours at school and with her dog. The ugly sister did, indeed, taunt Cinderella. I, as witness, actor and therapist, was aware of the power and domination of this character. The ugly sister relished her power; so it came as a shock to her when Cinderella suddenly started throwing coals – hand puppets – from the 'scuttle' at her. Landy tells us: 'The client surprises as the therapist surprises, through a kind of dramatic transcendence – unrehearsed, unconscious. This occurs when the client transcends his everyday role . . . and accepts the challenge of the therapeutic stage – the permission to play' (1994: 102). At this point in the improvisation Jenny stopped the drama. We came out of role. Jenny wanted to comment on what was going on for her. This was the first time Jenny had initiated reflection or, indeed, acted on her own volition to step away from the role in order to do so. We noted together that Cinderella had been unable to find words to accompany her coal throwing. Jenny said this was why she had to stop the drama: because Cinderella was afraid how – not if, I (the therapist-me) noted – the ugly sister would retaliate to the 'coal' throwing attack. Jenny told me that Cinderella was afraid the ugly sister would hit her. I also wondered with Jenny if she was afraid that I, in role as the ugly sister, might have hit her. I wondered to myself whether the character of the ugly sister was so powerful

I – the therapist-as-protector – would actually be taken over by her. And once unleashed, would the ugly sister be all-consuming? I realised I, Clare, was afraid of this character. I needed to consider why I was picking up on this fear.

The issues that emerged and were worked with during Jenny's drama-therapy covered: attachment, fear of rejection, control, confusion and tension and the blurring of roles. Some of these issues had been suggested at a clinical, multidisciplinary team level. Yet I feel it was in the dramatherapy that these issues were experienced and verified by me in my role as a drama-therapist and in subsequent reflection with Jenny.

At the final review with Jenny and her mother we noted that:

- Jenny had become able to tolerate boundaries being imposed (by teachers, mum, etc.).
- Jenny said she has a more positive attitude in the way she manages situations that challenge her.
- Mother said she and Jenny were able to enjoy each other's company more.
- Jenny said she was more confident in relationships with her peers.
- Mother and Jenny claimed to be less angry (with each other); and more relaxed generally – so that unexpected or untoward events didn't seem to overwhelm them so much.

Reflections on theory and method

The above examples from Jenny's dramatherapy sessions illustrate seven of the nine core processes identified by Jones (1996: 99–100, 2007: 81–136).

Dramatic projection

Dramatic projection can be seen in the use of role to give shape to Jenny's thoughts, wishes, beliefs and experiences. I consider one of the pivotal moments of Jenny's dramatherapy, as described previously, happened when, in role as Cinderella, she threw the puppets (representing lumps of coal) at the ugly sister in retaliation at being taunted. Jenny used the safety of the distance afforded by the role of 'Cinderella' to direct her own anger at the 'ugly sister'. Even though she was confronting her fear of a negative reaction in doing so, both roles served several functions in reducing the risk to her. First, at one level, by being in role Jenny could still feel that the anger she expressed belonged to Cinderella, not to her. Jenny may have been afraid that the force of her own anger could have destroyed whoever the 'ugly sister' represented and/or me, the therapist. I suspect that without the role Jenny would not have been able to tolerate her anger at this time. Second, Jenny could project aspects of herself that she found difficult to own or manage into the character of Cinderella and, perhaps, the ugly sister.

Furthermore, the characters of Cinderella and the ugly sister inhabited the world of imagination as well as of pantomime where words and actions have permission to be as big and bold as the feelings experienced by the patient/ actor. Importantly, Jenny cast me to play the role of the 'ugly sister'. I suggest that she would not have done so if she had not felt confident that I, as therapist, would maintain the safe boundaries of play that had previously been set up between us. In addition I feel Jenny had, over the weeks, become assured that we could be 'tuned in' to each other during the play.

Therapeutic performance process

Improvisation became a core element of the sessions. As dramatherapist I could – nay, needed to – be both performer and audience at the same time. I consider that as soon as a role is entered into and invested with authenticity, and the drama happens in the 'play space' a performance is taking place. The notion of 'performance' provides a necessary complement to the reality of the 'here and now' of the dramatherapy session. Between the poles of reality and play/performance a shift in understanding can be managed.

For a while Jenny had inhabited the alternative, yet parallel, dimension of the character of Cinderella. This role, as conceived by Jenny, was allowed to be angry. It's as though by being the actor in charge of a character a patient can experience a greater degree of control and freedom. If there is an expectation that for a performance to take place at least one performer and an audience is required, can there be a performance element in one-to-one dramatherapy when patient and therapist are both in role, in the 'play space'? The dramatherapist can be therapist-as-actor as well as therapist-as-audience.

Dramatherapeutic empathy and distancing

As indicated elsewhere in this chapter I feel that in the experience of playing and creating drama together it is possible for the therapist and patient to share a sense of knowing each other at a deep and authentic level. When this happens the therapist is more likely to feel empathy towards his or her patient or patients. Such a feeling promotes a sensitivity and receptivity in the therapist. His or her skills of attending, playing and witnessing are primed. Furthermore, in my work with Jenny, as described previously, I came to understand more about her internal world through the process of projective identification; for example in recognising Cinderella's fear of being hit by the ugly sister.

Role and personification

One of the challenges of psychotherapeutic intervention for the patient is that there may be pressure from family, society, school or work, friends and from him or herself not to make a fuss; not to upset the boat. It is not unlikely that Jenny played a useful role in her family and social group; a role that held the anxiety, fears and frustrations of the group. When she acted out these fears in her disruptive behaviours at school and at home she was identified as the source of trouble. Amongst her peers at school she was scapegoated as the difficult and unsociable child in the group. At home she carried the weight of the projections of all that was dysfunctional within the family. So why didn't Jenny rebel against this role? Possibly because: a) she was unable to articulate her frustration and anger in a contained and safe way; and because b) her need to conform to others' expectations of her may have limited opportunities for expression of her genuine feelings. Her overriding wish was to be liked and accepted. In order to survive, then, Jenny chose to hide her frustration and anger behind the facade of 'sweet girl'. One of the uses of role in Jenny's dramatherapy was to create an emotionally safe distance between her and the reality that she otherwise repressed.

Personification

One of the central features of Jenny's improvisations was the sense of control and power that shifted between the roles. Jenny's cast list contained some archetypal roles, some of which may have personified control in various contexts.

Playing

I feel it is important that the therapist is able to be seen as playful by the patient. The expression of authentic feelings demands a degree of risk from patient and therapist. Having fun during play can be a welcome antidote to the seriousness of some of the subject matter.

Life–drama connection

In reflection of the session Jenny related the improvisation of Cinderella and the 'ugly sister' to her own situation; specifically in naming the fear of being hit by the 'ugly sister.' Following this session I advised the child protection officer at the clinic of my concerns for Jenny's safety.

Transformation

In Jenny's dramatherapy the improvisations with Kelly and Sabrina reached a point where the narrative became stuck and repeated week after week. I believe a moment of transformation occurred when Jenny's story was able to move on thanks to linking this improvisation with the story of Cinderella. A new perspective entered the 'play space'. This prompted an insightful moment when Jenny could name her fear: of her gift of – and need for – love, being rejected. At this moment I sense Jenny also identified the disappointment of losing her fantasy of the father who would come back to her.

These processes underpin the creative process that is an integral part of dramatherapy. Drama and play can access the unconscious processes of the patient, by making the unbearable more manageable. The drama allows therapist and patient to collude in pretending the story is pretend. In the initial stages of the therapy this can be crucial. When a patient is feeling vulnerable it might be too frightening for him or her to accept the essence of the story in the drama as their own truth. If asked to do so too early in the therapy, he or she might well emotionally close down. And yet, often – on a conscious, pre-conscious or unconscious level – the patient knows the truth; and may know the therapist knows it, too. There can be an understanding between therapist and patient that in the therapy space the story will at some point be made real. For this understanding to be a resource to the patient, rather than a threat, I believe a sense of humour and humanity are necessary qualities in the therapist. This is one reason why the relationship between the dramatherapist and the patient can hold an intensity that highlights the therapeutic potential.

Reflections on the role of Cinderella

Jenny's Cinderella improvisations became the essence of her exploration of feelings associated with being overwhelmed, unsupported, bullied, uncared-for, 'got at', useless and let down. Outside the dramatherapy sessions it was apparent that Jenny's mother was inclined to disengage with services. The likelihood of these very issues being acted out amongst and within the family and the professional group was apparent. Jenny found that her dramatherapy sessions had helped her name and, significantly, contain the fear that had kept her authentic feelings suppressed:

- First, she had discovered that she could make up a play which provided the framework within which she could explore some of the main anxieties in her reality.
- She was able to project and separate 'good' and 'bad' parts of herself – and others who were significant to her – into the roles of, for example, Kelly and Sabrina.

When the drama could not get beyond the point where Jenny's own life-script was 'stuck' (i.e. where she could not find a way out of the dysfunctional role she had been playing) I recognised a connection with the story of Cinderella.

This story provided a bridge which led to a shift in Jenny's therapeutic process: from a static place to a landscape where movement could take place. The creative (i.e. moving) process in dramatherapy provided the structure of that bridge between the two states.

The Cinderella story was not unknown terrain for Jenny. I remember here how her eyes lit up when the story was referred to in connection with her own (as seen previously):

- The known fairy tale offered the comfort of role types that Jenny recognised and understood.
- The story also offered distance through metaphor which could contain emotions that could have overwhelmed Jenny.
- Jenny and the therapist's creative use of improvisation and role made the story versatile enough to suit and adapt to Jenny's therapeutic needs.
- Jenny consciously realised in the moment when Cinderella threw coals at the ugly sister that she, Jenny, had been suppressing her own anger at feeling and fear of being rejected. Jenny both acted and witnessed the role of Cinderella rebelling against her script.
- As her therapy came to an end it was apparent that Jenny had developed internal resources to enable her to see her fear of rejection from a different perspective; and that, maybe, her fear wasn't likely to be realised.
- At the final review of her dramatherapy sessions both Jenny and her mother reported a positive change in their relationship.
- An insight into the dynamics of the conscious and unconscious interactions between and within the services and individuals concerned would seem helpful. The dramatherapist can play a useful role here.

Reflections on the politics of provision

During her time with the clinic many professionals were involved with Jenny and her family: paediatrician, primary mental health worker, consultant child and adolescent psychiatrist, psychiatric nurse specialist, child protection officer, special educational needs coordinator, social worker – and myself, dramatherapist. The 'eligibility criteria' for accessing social care and CAMHS services are currently being tightened. Unless it is obvious who's responsible for the care, it is common now for both services to pass a 'case' back and forth between them rather than accept responsibility for the work. For example, if a clinician recommends therapy input, there may be a dispute about which service provides the transport from the child's home and/ or an escort to accompany the child to his/her therapy session.

In addition to the reviews of Jenny's dramatherapy, which usually took place between myself, the referring specialist nurse, Jenny and her mother, several multidisciplinary reviews and meetings were called. These meetings were held on one of the three days I did not work for the clinic. Although I sometimes received the minutes of such meetings I missed out on the face-to-face dialogue which I feel can promote greater understanding between professionals. For example, I would have appreciated the opportunity to meet with teachers from Jenny's school, but my part-time hours did not allow for this.

Even within the child and adolescent community health team itself there could be a lack of communication. I was disappointed that I was not told that Jenny would be stopping her medication for Attention Deficit Hyperactivity Disorder (ADHD) for a trial period of two weeks. I was unaware at the time of any information regarding Jenny's change in medication being accessible either in her central file or on the computerised patient information system at the clinic. Many dramatherapists work part-time and/or as lone arts therapists. This can mean that in the workplace his or her professional profile is still on the margins of the multidisciplinary team. Is the patient who, in dramatherapy, has found a way to articulate his or her story similarly marginalised from the mainstream 'results table'?

I have noted, above, that Jenny's case was complex. I have been aware of how complex referrals often got passed onto the art psychotherapists and dramatherapist in the clinic. Many professionals were involved in areas concerning Jenny's housing, education, social care and mental health. Children with a history of being abandoned and neglected – at least once – may be re-exposed (re-traumatised, even) by their experience of social care, education and NHS services. I am referring here to the current trend in high staff turnover and staff cuts in these services. In times of crisis – such as the current severe cuts – these services can reflect the dysfunctional families they're supposed to be helping.

In the months following the Agenda for Change process I have become aware of fellow arts psychotherapists being asked by their employers to redefine what an arts psychotherapist can – and perhaps, 'should' – be doing in their job. For example, in my experience, specialist clinicians such as arts psychotherapists are being expected to do more generic work. In response, my art psychotherapy colleagues at the clinic and I considered offering (more) clinical supervision or consultancy to other clinicians in the team. This is a good way of promoting a greater understanding of our work within the team.

Conclusion

In writing about Jenny's dramatherapy I have tried to illustrate how, through her sessions, she found a way to give voice to the fears underlying her chaotic, defensive and avoidant behaviours. Contained within the therapeutic relationship and within the metaphors of dramatic play Jenny was motivated to identify and confront these fears. Dramatherapy made this possible by allowing Jenny to project her reality outside the therapy room into the 'play space', thereby making it more manageable. The description and analysis of the work give a sense of how Jenny and I tried, together, to work across and within our differences, and that the many roles she held internally, and within her life, were able to be made visible and explored within the dramatherapy space. Instead of reinforcing unhelpfully held roles we were able to create and use space and, crucially, time to explore them and their attendant dynamics between us.

As an organisation championing dramatherapy in the UK and abroad the British Association of Dramatherapists works to raise the profile of dramatherapy and dramatherapists nationally and internationally. On an individual and local level many dramatherapists are investing energy and commitment in promoting their work; perhaps through research, writing, meetings, training and audit. In effect, I sense, in my experience, a move towards an homogenisation of clinic staff; a result, perhaps, of the cost-cutting agenda of the NHS in 2008/2009. Is this a national trend? In the instant-fix, money saving, mindset of the NHS there is a sense that long-term therapy/psychotherapy is an indulgent and expensive intervention. This sense of want-it-now-and-want-it-quick-and-want-it-cheap intervention fails to recognise the complex, unpredictable and multi-layered nature of the present-ing issues in a child like Jenny. As we have seen, housing, education, poverty, family dynamics all have an impact on a child's internal world.

Dramatherapists need to consider how we/the profession of dramatherapy will respond to a changing NHS. It is possible there are positive aspects and opportunities to be considered; and I think the individual therapist and the profession are being challenged.

13 'The river of my life – where things can break and things can mend': Ruth's nine years' therapy programme at Family Futures and three sessions that stand out. An account by Ruth and her therapist

Jay Vaughan

Box 13.1

Questions about practice

- How can dramatherapy support long-term fostered or adopted children who have a history of early trauma and are struggling to settle in their families?
- How does legislation such as the UK's Children Act (1989), and cultural practices concerning child protection, impact on dramatherapy?
- What are children's perspectives on the therapy?

Research perspective

- Case study
- Retrospective interview with a former child client

Client perspective sample

This is my memory of the life story session. I don't know, not final it's like an ending. She's not as innocent as she portrays herself, my birth mother. I am not sure how it helped because in many ways I knew it already. It helps that was then and this is now sort of thing. It was the first time that I wasn't hiding it all or covering up for my birth mother. Like a weight had been lifted. I didn't actually call my adoptive mum 'mum'. I still don't call her mum but we have more of a mother and daughter feel to our relationship. I suppose that's

> when we started getting closer and like a real mother and daughter. The session was helpful.
>
> (Retrospective interview)

Introduction

Ruth and her adoptive mother were referred to Family Futures shortly into Ruth's placement with her prospective adoptive mother in 1996. It had become apparent in the early weeks of the placement how violent Ruth's behaviour was and what a challenge this was going to be to any parent. But before I go any further I should stress that Ruth is not her real name and that some of the facts have been changed to protect her identity. And most important of all, I wish to add that Ruth has read and agreed to everything that has been written here as well as adding her own comments. It is a collaborative piece of reflection between client and therapist.

Contexts

However, before beginning to 'tell the story' of the therapy it is important to set the scene. Family Futures, where I work as a dramatherapist, specialises in working with long-term fostered or adopted children who have a history of early trauma and are struggling to settle in their families. It is not unusual, from Family Futures point of view, to have a referral only months into placement. Perhaps what was unusual in this case was the extreme nature of the violence being inflicted on the adoptive mother. The initial assessment and treatment process involved myself, as a dramatherapist, as well as a social worker, parent-mentor and child and adolescent psychiatrist. The work offered a combination of parent sessions and twenty-four hour telephone support to the adoptive mother, as well as regular fortnightly half-day sessions with the mother and child. If Ruth was to have a diagnosis today that was helpful and would make sense it would probably be one of Development Trauma Disorder (van der Kolk 2005). Although it was only during the course of the therapy programme that the degree to which Ruth had been traumatised came to light.

Family Futures in its therapy programme usually focuses on three main areas, the child's early history of trauma, the need to help the child develop a more secure attachment relationship to their parent or parents and the need then to help the child make sense of their identity. This involves helping them integrate their past into a 'coherent narrative' and develop a positive sense of self. In the case of Ruth, perhaps the first key thing that was considered was about safety and how to keep everyone safe in the family and in the therapy sessions. Family Futures specialises in working with traumatised children and settling them in their long-term foster or adoptive families; however, the work with Ruth was just that bit different. In the early phase of the work it was quickly established that, if Ruth's adoptive placement did not work, then she would need to be placed in a secure unit. It was probably largely for this reason that the work was funded for the number of years it was. I think credit should be given to the local authority for their insightful funding of this work. Whilst lots of children and young people come to Family Futures for around three years of therapy, the therapy for Ruth stretched from aged 9 years old to when she was 18 years old and in some ways is still ongoing. We were, of course, not funded for all this time but careful management of the budget and some subsidy from Family Futures meant that the work has been sustained until the present day, and will continue to be so into the future.

It is important to see Ruth in the context of the children today who are removed from their birth families. Adoption is probably traditionally seen as babies being 'relinquished' for adoption whereas actually the picture today is very different. Today the children who are placed for adoption have been removed due to neglect and abuse from their birth families. However, in the UK since the Children Act 1989 it has been harder for local authorities to remove children and the tendency has been for children to be left for longer periods of time in neglectful and abusive families. It is sadly not unusual today for Family Futures to see children who were left for more than four years in neglectful and abusive situations. There is a belief around in the court system that children fare better if maintained in their birth families and lots of local authorities sadly still seem to be working on this principle. The consequence of this is that children are left in horrific situations for longer than they need to be and the cost to the child and society as a whole is huge as it is these children who without help end up populating our prisons and psychiatric hospitals. Ruth was at risk of being one such statistic.

Description of the work

When I asked Ruth in 2008, now aged 21 years, whether she would like to collaborate on a book chapter she was delighted. Ruth had always said she would like to write down her story. So we embarked upon this journey of recalling her life and our work together. I asked Ruth what she remembered about our therapy work together when she was nine years old. She immediately said the brown-paint session. She and I smiled. We both remembered the 'brown-paint session'. Ruth said that sometimes when she and her adoptive mother think about all their work at Family Futures her mother reminds her of that one session. So what is it about that session that sticks in all our minds?

Session 1: aged 9 years old – the beginning

And there it was brown paint everywhere. The paint was smeared all over Ruth, her adoptive mother, myself and my co-worker, quite apart from a liberal layer all over the cushions. It was funny, well sort of, or at least funny now we were at the end of it all. We were all breathing heavily recovering from the exertion of rolling in the paint.

So how did this happen? Well, it was a regular family therapy session to help Ruth and her adoptive mother attach to one another and address some of the difficulties that they had been having. Talking about their relationship was not an option, as Ruth did not talk about things. And anyway I am a dramatherapist, so approaching the situation using the arts was a familiar way of working. My co-worker and I thought that a family painting exercise would be a good way of helping them have fun together and think together, something they found hard to do, and a good way of helping them collaborate and negotiate.

Initially things went well and the usually uncooperative Ruth worked with her adoptive mother to roll out the paper, choose the paint colours to go in the paint palette and begin the large painting. The suggestion was that they drew around one another to create a life-sized body outline of them together and then paint the image. It began peaceably enough and then somehow – it seems very hard to recall how – the whole bottle of brown paint was grabbed by Ruth and brown paint began to be squeezed all over the image obliterating it. The brown paint poured gloriously onto the paper in satisfying globules. Ruth was delighted by the mess and the freedom to pour. But the pouring progressed to the outer edges of the paper, to her hands and arms, her clothes and her mother. Three adults scrabbled to intervene and get hold of the brown paint pot whose contents were by this point everywhere. In the middle of the paper covered and surrounded in brown paint sat Ruth. She smeared herself all over her adoptive mother and the two therapists. It was chaos.

The pleasure in what now looked more like smeared excrement moved rapidly to rage as Ruth grabbed handfuls of her adoptive mother's body and tore at her. The two therapists fought to stop anyone getting hurt as Ruth lashed out kicking, hitting, head-butting and biting. It was unclear which limb belonged to whom as four bodies wrestled, coated in brown paint on the cushions where they had somehow ended up. Is this therapy? It was certainly high drama, but in what way was this helpful?

Ruth fought and fought. The adults tried to keep themselves safe and contain the situation. Eventually exhausted Ruth calmed down and curled up a messy brown blob with her adoptive mother. All was calm and painty. Ruth's mother thanked the two therapists for their support. Ruth apologised to the two therapists for hurting them. The two therapists disentangled themselves and the paint-covered, sweaty four said their goodbyes at the front door.

During the next parent session Ruth's adoptive mother said how important it was for her that this sort of chaos, explosion, and violence was seen by the two therapists. How important it was for her that what she was struggling with all the time at home happens in the therapy too. And how important it had been for her that the two therapists had got messy trying to help.

Ruth's response

That is how I remember it. Brown paint was everywhere. It was good to use the paint – it's a way of expressing. It reminded me of all the mess I lived in with my birth mother and whilst in foster care – being made to eat cat and dog food whilst in foster care, dog shit being everywhere and being abused. I felt I calmed down afterwards – it was all about calming down.

How hysterical it was, the madness of it all. I suppose because of letting out of emotions. Maybe I showed how I was actually feeling as well. What was helpful about this session was the support. I remembered being held down but I don't know what could have been done differently. I did not like being held down. You could have left me be but then I would have run riot and stuff and caused harm to others and myself. I don't know why I remember this session – it was the chaos and that's maybe why it's so distinct, the brown paint. Why did we choose brown? I don't know why my adoptive mum remembers it. I've never asked her but I know she does, she brings it up in the car or anywhere.

Session 2: aged 12 years old – the middle

Now let us turn to a later session and another memory Ruth immediately had when asked of our therapy work. The second thing that Ruth remembered about her therapy work at Family Futures was making dens, which became a regular feature later in the middle phase of the therapy work.

Ruth had been asked to create a den out of the cushions for her and her adoptive mother to 'live in' together. Ruth had hold of a huge cushion, nearly as big as her, and she wrestled with it dragging it to one corner of the room. She was very strong and very determined. Her adoptive mother tried to help, but Ruth would not have it. She issued instructions but whatever her adoptive mother did somehow did not seem necessarily to be as she wanted. In this complex way the den was made. A triumphant pile of cushions was created, with a small crawl hole at the centre of it all. Ruth crawled into the hole and resided inside. She was delighted with her creation and curled up content for a while inside. Her adoptive mother offered to join Ruth in there or perhaps just to visit. Ruth weighed this up but seemed unsure. She then relented and allowed the visit, moving over to allow her to squeeze by. Ruth tolerated this visit but rapidly wanted her out and the cushion nest to herself.

And so the sessions progressed in this way – a repetitive pattern of den building and den visiting. There was comfort in the pattern for Ruth's adoptive mother, the therapists and Ruth as everyone knew the rules. Ruth was in charge of the process and the adults complied. Less high drama and more peace but was this therapy helpful?

Ruth's response

> That is how it begun but later in the sessions – towards the end, middle to end of the session – its like my adoptive mum and me went into a room and made the dens together rather than the instructing and stuff. It was good being able to do it over and over because it was my own comfort zone. The den building reminded me of a safe place, fun! This helped my relationship with my adoptive mum – I suppose it was an understanding between us. She had an understanding I suppose it's more of constructing something together and stuff, working as a team. I remember this session because I suppose it was a key part of my life, making dens in therapy. I made them at home with friends and stuff. It was also because I like designing my own stuff.

Session 3: aged 16 years old – the ending

Now let's move to much later in the long term therapy work with Ruth and her adoptive mother when Ruth was 16 years old. Ruth had changed a lot over the years of therapy and sessions in the last couple of years were less frequent as things were generally better. The work had progressed from fortnightly family sessions, plus extra emergency sessions when needed, to individual sessions with Ruth on her own with occasional family sessions. This was an extra family session, but a key one in my mind. This was the first session when Ruth was able to tolerate really thinking about her history and when Ruth for the first time was able to acknowledge pretty much all of her childhood abuse and neglect and the sheer horror of it all. Ruth herself had requested this opportunity to review her life story. Life-story work in adoption is very much the 'bread and butter' of therapeutic interventions. It had only taken us seven years to get here! In previous attempts at 'life-story work' Ruth had ripped up file information (luckily copied) and become physically aggressive so that the work had to stop. But now Ruth wanted to know, wanted to think about it all; and with her adoptive mother. She also accepted that I work with a male colleague for this family session as my previous co-workers were not around. She accepted this male colleague knowing that her history of sexual abuse would be part of the work and, whilst expressing anxiety about this, she did manage to tolerate the idea and the reality of his presence.

Ruth was clearly anxious at the beginning of the session but so much less so than in any previous therapy sessions. She wanted to have the file information read out to her and she sat and quietly listened to it all. She listened horrified as slowly she began to realise that her birth mother had even, at times, asked for Ruth to be removed from her care. Time after time when a new man entered her birth mother's life and she wanted to go out to the pub she asked for Ruth to be removed. It was the first time Ruth had allowed the thought to enter her head that her birth mother was not a victim of the system with her baby brutally removed but a woman, who more than not caring for her was party to her neglect, abuse and abandonment. There was a stillness and silence in the room as Ruth allowed all this information and a huge shift in her thinking, to sink in. Just before lunch it all got too much and she lashed out with her foot. A break was needed – she was letting us know.

After lunch Ruth agreed that she would like to create a visual image of her life – a timeline. She collaborated on this task and was thoughtful and engaged throughout. Ruth listened to an explanation about how in life threatening situations we all instinctively to survive do 'fight, flight or freeze'. She marked the paper thoughtfully. She said when she was very little and with her birth mother she took flight to the street often dirty and unkempt, wearing only a vest. She marked the timeline images to show when she was being sexually abused. She froze to survive it. She said 'I learnt to be frozen on the inside.' And with a knowing smile at her adoptive mother she marked her fight response on the paper. Depicting how, now safe with her adoptive mother, she has begun to fight to survive. Ruth knew herself and this way of managing well. She was flooded by feelings and memories as the timeline became more and more complex marking out all the major transitions in her life. But Ruth managed to contain all these feelings and keep thinking about what her life had been to date.

Together Ruth sat with her adoptive mother and looked at her life. As a title she chose to have written on the timeline 'In the river of my life – where things can break and things can mend'. She then added 'In the cycle of my life the beginning will never be repeated'. As her final image she chose to draw a heart. In this heart her adoptive mother wrote of her:

> I met Ruth and was immediately drawn to her strong, feisty, alive and independent and love warming spirit . . . that goes on and on.

Ruth wrote of her adoptive mother:

> She is a lovely warming and generous woman with the sun as her heart because I know that resource in her will never run out!

Ruth's response (after wiping away tears in her eyes)

> This is my memory of the life story session. I don't know, not final it's like an ending. She's not as innocent as she portrays herself, my birth mother. I am not sure how it helped because in many ways I knew it already. It helps that was then and this is now sort of thing. It was the first time that I wasn't hiding it all or covering up for my birth mother. Like a weight had been lifted. I didn't actually call my adoptive mum 'mum'. I still don't call her mum but we have more of a mother and daughter feel to our relationship. I suppose that's when we started getting

closer and like a real mother and daughter. The session was helpful. There is nothing I would have done differently.

And now?

And now Ruth is 21 years old, completing a three-year-degree course, engaged to be married and pregnant with her first baby. Ruth also has a good relationship with her adoptive mother and her extended adoptive family. When Ruth found out she was pregnant she wanted to have some more therapy at Family Futures. She felt that her history was likely to be triggered by having her own baby and she wanted to do her best to ensure the best for her baby. She has therefore, since becoming pregnant, had monthly one-to-one sessions with me once more. These sessions have been counselling sessions talking about how she is feeling, making links with her history and thinking about her future as a mother. Ruth is thoughtful, insightful and a pleasure to spend time with. Ruth said in a recent session that she is very aware that she did not have a good start in life and she wants to ensure by taking at least a year's maternity leave that she has the opportunity to bond with her baby. How wonderful is that?

So what was Ruth's story?

Ruth was asked if she would like to say this bit, but it was too painful for her so she agreed that I would write a brief account and then she would agree it was okay to be shared in this chapter.

Ruth was five years old when she was finally removed from the care of her birth mother. She rang the police herself. When the police arrived she was filthy, covered in bruises and with knife cuts to her face. She was trying to fry herself an egg; balanced on a stool. The egg was the only food in the filthy flat. The police photographed her and the flat and took her to the safety of a police station. Ruth was safe for the first time in her life. And yet her sad story was not over. Ruth had already during the first five years of her life come to the attention of local services but somehow or other despite numerous telephone calls from neighbours and even requests from her birth mother to place her in care she was not removed.

Following this removal from her birth mother Ruth was placed in foster care with local family friends, but within a short time the local authority decided that the filthy environment full of dog excrement was not suitable and she was moved to another family friend. And so it went on. Ruth's account of this phase in foster care was of being neglected as well as physically abused – all whilst in the supposed care of the local authority. And then finally Ruth was placed in a foster family (the first one outside of the family and friends network) where she was well cared for. Although even in this 'good' foster home her abuse by other children in the family continued. It was not until Ruth was nine years old that she was found a permanent placement with her now adoptive mother. Only now could this sad and lost child, neglected and abused in her birth family and in the care of the local authority, begin to let the adults around her really know how bad her experiences had been. It was now that Ruth could truly let go of all her fear, hurt and anger. It was in the midst of this whirlwind of emotions that her adoptive mother sought therapeutic help for Ruth to try to make sense of challenging behaviour.

The therapy journey for Ruth with Family Futures began when she was nine years old and now, aged 21 years, is in many ways ongoing. There was no formula for how this therapy programme should look, just as there is no formula that existed for how to parent Ruth, but the collaborative, flexible and creative approach meant that Ruth, her adoptive mother and the therapy team embarked upon a journey together to find ways to help. There are things that could have been done differently, better I am sure, but we all did our best to find a way forward. It is hugely significant that it was not until Ruth was in her late teens that she finally disclosed the depth of her abuse and in particular her sexual abuse. It took that long for her to trust. It was a long journey and one where really the credit lies with Ruth and her adoptive mother for whom I have absolute respect and admiration. They are remarkable people and this is really their story.

Reflections on the client experience

Ruth's thoughts and feelings about the therapy process are integrated into the main account of the three therapy sessions. However perhaps what is most significant is Ruth's response to the reflective process, which was to be moved once more to tears. Tears that she hardly shed during all her years in therapy – tears that are an absolutely appropriate way to respond when looking back on the river of her life and all her losses. Ruth is an adult now who fully understands her history and has in so many ways come to terms with her past and how it still impacts on her present. But when she truly thinks about it she is moved to tears. She has developed what is now known to be so crucial which is a coherent narrative. Yet, when thinking back, the sheer power of her story and the understandable depth of her feelings about what she has survived is still disturbing to her, and appropriately so.

Perhaps what stands out so powerfully for me is her final comment that 'there is nothing I would have done differently' and what I see in this is not really about the therapy but rather as a comment on her life; that there is nothing she would have done differently. Whilst at some level of course Ruth would have liked her life to have been different and not to have suffered such neglect and abuse, the dilemma for her, like so many adopted children, is that whilst they would in one way like to change the past they also know that if the past had been different they would not have the adoptive parents that they have and the good things that they have gained through the process of being adopted. For Ruth adoption means not just the horrors of her early years, but all the good things she has gained from being adopted by a mother who has truly attuned to her needs. Ruth is the lovely and thoughtful human being she is today not despite, but because of, her history.

Reflection on theory and method

Perhaps my overriding question is 'Is this dramatherapy?' Certainly there were points in the therapy when it did not feel like therapy – more like surviving and trying one's best to make sense of what did not seem to make sense. And yet now, looking back and reflecting on the process, it does seem to make more sense than it appeared at the time. Most important of all looking back and reflecting with Ruth highlighted just how much Ruth had grown and developed. Of course, therapy cannot take all the credit. It is Ruth who has managed to survive and make sense of her experiences, and it is her adoptive mother and her support network that have made that possible. But maybe the therapy did have some part to play in it all? In my view the very fact that all these years later I am sitting beside a young mother holding her precious new baby and thinking about our therapeutic relationship feels like a success. There is so much to potentially consider when reflecting on the process of nine years of therapy. I would like to consider it all but for the purposes of this chapter my focus will be on the dramatherapy process. In terms of adoption where the adoption rate for breakdown for later placed children (Rushton and Dance 2002) is one third, then Ruth is a success. Her history and her age at placement, quite apart from her extremely challenging behaviour would make a disruption from her adoptive placement a high risk. So when thinking of adoption Ruth's work was successful in securing her in an adoptive family.

I think what is most helpful is to consider four different ways in which the dramatherapy element in the therapy helped move the process forward and how that thinking informed the work and our understanding as a therapy team of the work. The four elements I am going to focus on are dramatic projection, witnessing, embodiment and non-verbal work. All are key elements in the therapy with Ruth and all elements are referred to by other dramatherapists in their practice work described in *Drama as Therapy. Theory, Practice and Research* (Jones 2007).

Dramatic projection

Ruth, in her throwing of paint in the first session, was externalising her inner conflicts. In this way Ruth was expert in her use of dramatic projection in the therapy (Jones 2007). The art forms introduced in the therapy, whilst not always used in the ways envisaged, became a way in which Ruth communicated her feelings and her experiences. Her inner states were clearly expressed and worked through using the dramatic form. In the painting session Ruth used the paint to convey information about her abusive early experiences. In the den-building second session Ruth used the dens to think initially about all her moves and then to begin to create a safe place to be with her adoptive mother where she could literally learn to let her in. In the third session described Ruth allowed her whole story to be pulled together in the timeline describing her life.

In Ruth's first session her dramatic projection was as extreme and potentially dangerous as her life had been. By the third session Ruth's dramatic projection, and the need for it to manage all her feelings, was minimal as she was able to use the art form to contain most of her feelings and not be activated into a 'fight, flight or freeze' response. Instead in this last session she was able to use her higher brain functioning to think about her bodily responses to the trauma and her feelings, thus making sense of her experience in quite a different way. In this way the dramatic projection enabled her to gain a perspective on her life and so gain insights about her need to enact what had happened to her.

Witnessing

Another vital aspect of the therapy programme with Ruth was the importance of her distress being witnessed. From the very first meeting with Ruth until the present day there has been the telling of her story by her and by her adoptive mother, until the story came together as one united and shared story. The storytelling happened in so many different ways and on so many different levels moving from an 'acting out' of the story as Ruth showed quite literally what it had been like for her to a re-telling of the story in a reflective way. Ruth needed to tell what had happened to her and have it witnessed by receptive and compassionate ears. As she said when reflecting on the last session 'it was like a weight had been lifted'.

As Stirling Twist stressed in *Drama as Therapy. Theory, Practice and Research* (Stirling Twist cited in Jones 2007: 106–108) young people need to be able to tell their story with all the nuances and unacknowledged truths so that the listener listens with their whole being to all aspects of the story. For Ruth it took nine years of telling her story before all the different aspects of her abusive early experiences were able to be fully shared. She really needed to know that her adoptive mother and myself, as therapist, were to be trusted and able to hear without judging her before she could tell it all. Another important aspect to stress here was the need for Ruth to tell her adoptive mother. Research has indicated that children who tell their adoptive parents in the first instance rather than their therapists fare better in terms of increasing their attachment to their adoptive family (Macaskill 1991).

Embodiment and non-verbal work

Ruth in the early stages of the therapy needed to 'act out' her story so that her body showed what had happened to her. What had happened was not expressible in words. It was always clear that for Ruth her experiences were in the beginning unsayable and language would not help her share her experiences from her own perspective. In this way the smearing of brown paint that looked like excrement and the creation of homes and then safe places was a vital first step in the therapy. It not only provided a way in which in therapy one could begin to try to make sense of her early experiences it provided a bridge between home and therapy, so that what was happening 24/7 could be understood. Ruth, as a little child, had no power over her neglectful and abusive carers and now she had found her power to create her experiences for others to witness. Ruth, understandably, wished to have control over her world and the ongoing dilemma for her adoptive mother, and for the therapy team, was how much to allow her reasonable control and how to intervene once this control got out of control and presented a danger to her and others. This delicate process forged the trust that finally enabled Ruth to disclose her sexual abuse.

Novy in *Drama as Therapy. Theory, Practice and Research* (Novy cited in Jones 2007: 124–131) explores this transformative quality of embodiment work and how both necessary and powerful this process is. Ruth very much embodied her early experiences for the first years of therapy, perhaps from aged 9 years to aged 16 years, so for seven years she found other ways of communicating her experiences. And the role of the therapist was to trust her process and believe that in time she would be able to communicate rather than act out her experiences. Another important part of the therapy was the way in which it 'acted out' for Ruth positive nurturing experiences within the safety of the therapy. So that, in the second session described, the den-building, thereby creating a safe space, was key. Later in the therapy more nurturing interaction between mother and child was encouraged and integrated into the therapy.

Finally I think that overall what I have learnt from Ruth is the importance as Rogers put it of being able to 'work from the hip' (Rogers cited in Jones 2007: 175) and being able to receive, hold and make sense of meanings that are conscious or unconscious communications. In many ways the therapy at Family Futures and the therapy for Ruth and her adoptive family was group work with the therapist as facilitator. Ruth needed a therapist who could hold all the chaos and the lack of coherent sense in mind and wait whilst the pieces of jigsaw puzzle fell into place. It was indeed working from the hip, to the point where Ruth concluded that: 'The river of my life – where things can break and things can mend.'

Conclusion

This account of the work with Ruth highlights a number of key issues, when thinking about working with severely traumatised adopted or long-term fostered children. Perhaps, first of all, most obviously, the work needs, in my view, to be long term. Children with a history of broken attachment relationships need to have a therapeutic response that is sustained and takes account of their need to develop more secure attachment relationships as well as to have help addressing their experiences of trauma and how this impacts on them. It should also involve the long-term foster or adoptive parents in the process as they are very much part of the solution to the problem. And as for the question what is dramatherapy? Dramatherapy in this context is the ability to trust the non-verbal process, to hear the story however and whenever it is told and to work creatively from the hip!

Finally I would like to thank Ruth for all that she has taught me and all that I have gained by knowing her!

14 Saisir les étoiles: fostering a sense of belonging with child survivors of war

Athena Madan

Box 14.1

Questions about practice

- How can dramatherapy help children traumatised by war?
- What is the relationship between dramatherapy and psychoeducational practices?
- What do feminist and post-colonial perspectives have to offer dramatherapy?

Research perspective

- Case study
- Interviews with parents
- Art and drama as evaluation

Client perspective sample

There was nothing beautiful about the war [in the home country]. I don't want to draw a picture of all the things I don't want to see. Sometimes I felt like they only wanted me to talk about what happened so that they, the [white people], could feel better.

Introduction

Arc-en-ciel 2: Saisir les étoiles (translated as 'Playing with Rainbows 2: Reach for the stars') was a twelve-week group programme conducted with child refugee war survivors (des enfants réfugiés témoins de la guerre) and their classmates at a French-speaking elementary school (École) in a major Canadian city. The group aimed to provide a space for the children to process their experiences of war trauma and mourn their multiple losses. It also aimed to address intercultural conflict resolution, with emphasis on the subjects of belonging, collaboration and safety in groups. The group ran for twelve weeks, meeting once weekly, for two hours: one hour focusing on individual projects, and another hour on collaborative group work. Three co-therapists facilitated the programme, with about six children each per group.

This chapter will look at trauma from a perspective that acknowledges the historical, cultural and racial assumptions relevant to these child survivors of war. I will also question the traditional way trauma seems to be framed in clinical mental health, as a system of symptoms and deficits, and suggest ways in which systemic contexts can be integrated in that frame. Last, I will focus on three vignettes illustrating the use of drama and art in these groups that help facilitate positive therapeutic outcome, and discuss my own reflections upon the processes of projection, symbol, metaphor, and witnessing inherent in the work.

Considering trauma in treatment

Post-traumatic stress disorder

Current best practice for trauma rests on diagnosis and treatment for post-traumatic stress disorder (PTSD) (American Psychiatric Association [APA] 1994, 2000), mainly because PTSD comprises the diagnostic language available. Theoretical, clinical and empirical support for various therapies in the treatment of PTSD are still emerging, many of which are shown to yield solid 'results' in PTSD treatment. Of these, and specific to this chapter, the use of dramatic play, symbolic processes and metaphor have been evaluated as 'supported/promising and acceptable treatment' in child post-traumatic stress and maltreatment (Saunders, Berliner, and Hanson 2003: 101–103).

Complex trauma

'Long term or chronic exposure to traumatic events extend beyond PTSD,' write Cook, Blaustein, Spinazzola, and van der Kolk (2003: 5); the PTSD qualifier of 'a traumatic event' (APA 2000: 219) seems an inaccurate framework for an individual who has witnessed a series of conflicts, lasting a number of years. As such, the diagnostic 'Complex Trauma' (C-PTSD; see van der Kolk 2003) has taken root to help provide context for understanding the impact of multiple traumatic events. The World Health Organisation (WHO 2004) and van der Kolk (2003) advocate that C-PTSD deficits are more severe, more prolonged and more interpersonal in nature that those seen in a singular traumatic episode qualifying PTSD. Also noted are more long-term, multiple or chronic stressors wherein the survivor is subjected to intentional control, force and humiliation. Our team thus found it relevant to consider C-PTSD as a construct in planning our programme and informing this research.

Feminist and post-colonial considerations

Trauma in the contexts of mass organised violence is hardly 'just' about war-trauma symptoms within a diagnostic framework. There are deeper, more systemic and ingrained long-term implications. Bracken, Giller, and Summerfield (1995, 1997) have highlighted a strong political referent in working with war survivors, and a racially charged history often rooted in post-colonial tensions. Madibbo describes the collective experience of subjugation that translates into a feeling of being 'less than human' (2005: 13). Also very relevant is a collective loss of safety, community, family, property, dignity and interpersonal rights, including rape and torture. For those who have fled the conflict, there are additional complexities. Blackwell (2003, 2005) and the WHO (2004) note these may include a loss of culture, home, and status, with the fear of perpetuating these losses under the threat of deportation; the threat of deportation from a system the individuals are still trying to trust; and stress from daily circumstances, which often include inadequate housing, a poor diet, financial instability and separation from/death of family and community of origin. Specific to relocating children, Revell (2001) and the National Institute of Mental Health (NIMH 2002) note that there can also be fears of abandonment due to the unavailability, disappearance, or death of family members; interruptions to schooling; difficulties with a potentially new language; and a general, sustained sense of uncertainty. Thus, while the diagnostic framework and reasons for referral in the case of war trauma may focus on a set of particular behaviours in a particular individual, there are a myriad of external, social factors that serve as very relevant points of departure. To ignore the impact of these would in fact perpetuate trauma instead of help assimilate it; especially because, and as feminist literature so strongly advocates, the political is felt so very personally.

Feminist contributions to and analysis of psychotherapy (Greenspan 1983; Brown 2007; Burman 2005) have been helpful in creating discourse around these respective subjectivities. Examinations of power and privilege, of race and difference and of the construction/perception of dominance have been possible largely because feminist research gave these ideas location. Feminist notions of participatory research, of power structure analysis and of non-conscious attitudes (Herman 1992) provide great understanding of the interpersonal influences in and out of therapy, and how these might unknowingly interact and perpetuate original dynamics of trauma. Specifically, feminist sensibilities of the political, as having direct bearing on the individual, and of social constructions, as having direct bearing on individual subjectivity, have helped create, define and contextualise a need for reframing therapeutic approaches.

Post-colonial perspectives further support the relevance of socio-political contexts in therapy. Important specific points to consider in war trauma include a legacy of feeling perpetually second-rate under the 'colonial blueprint' (Canadian Broadcasting Corporation [CBC] 2009; Shamsuddin

2009), a collectivist world view, and a response/ability to act in the com-memoration of loss (or, as is said in the case of the Rwandan genocide, 'le devoir de mémoire'). Post-colonial theory examines assumptions held by traditional psychotherapy that may in fact not be very neutral: its roots in Western European culture and patriarchy; a focus on the individual as the root of pathology; and a process of assessment that lacks multicultural norms. Not to consider these nuances, or to attribute them as attenuating, independent, or non-primary factors, limits the 'success' of any eventual outcome (Blake, Diamond, Foot, Gidley, Mayo and Yarnit 2008; Diallo and Lafreniere 2006).

Description of the work

Focus research

The programme described in this chapter was a follow-up programme to a programme called 'Arc-en-ciel/Playing with rainbows' (© YWCA by Revell, 2000) addressing the impact of war on direct survivors. This particular school, and a number of students in it, had been part of a previous, smaller group. However, neither École's principal nor myself had been involved in that group's facilitation. Focus research in planning the programme, then, centred very much on consultation with students, their parents and the teachers. These were informal conversations by phone, or brief in-person consultations at school. These short interviews were conducted to provide better context in how to best accommodate individual and family needs, as well as establish a feeling of trust. We also hoped to gain a sense of how the previous intervention had been perceived.

These consultations revealed two major themes. The first reflected an assumption inherent in the original Arc-en-ciel programme: a certain general-ised experience of war. While many of the aspects of 'the lived experience of conflict' were relevant, and while accommodations were made for sharing cultures that were 'not Canadian,' the individual facilitation plans were designed irrespective of culture, country or context and the children's experi-ences simply translated differently. Not everyone had experienced soldiers as defenders; not everyone considered their losses in the past; not everyone had losses; and not everyone had the same cultural referent to 'heaven' (or a place where their ancestors slept). These generalisations, perhaps designed in 'normalising' actual war trauma, actually translated as furthering possible feelings of stigma.

The second theme noted encounters of culture and race. Ethnically charged tensions, in the contexts of therapy, were certainly still relevant and powerful. In one instance, a parent expressed that their child had said of the previous group, 'There was nothing beautiful about the war [in the home country]. I don't want to draw a picture of all the things I don't want to see. Sometimes I felt like they only wanted me to talk about what happened so that they, the [white people], could feel better.' In another instance, a father expressed his child came home once from the group feeling he could no longer participate, and chose to subsequently and permanently withdraw: the activity had involved drawing an animal to help visualise strength in moments of vulnerability. While the parents expressed they had both understood the metaphor behind the exercise, the child's religion did not approve of representational drawings of animals. These assumptions fostered real, felt resentment in some instances where war contexts included specific cultural or racial associations, or where specific cultural referents could not accommodate the exercise at hand.

Rationale

So Arc-en-ciel 2: Saisir les étoiles was conceived, as a follow-up group for children to learn about war with/from their peers, and explore how to better, together, get along. We considered the following four ideas most appropriate in our rationale:

1   The children expressed interest to attend.
2   Parents expressed wanting to understand the daily conflicts their children experienced.
3   Facilitating the group at the school could make services accessible and friendly to families.
4   The name implied a certain space wherein a return to something familiar and being good at something – things that, especially for the children who had survived civil conflict in their countries of origin had not had opportunity to experience – could be facilitated.

To accommodate the strong intercultural context that surfaced as a result of the consultations, we designed the group to focus on collaborative projects to underpin an understanding that differences are normal, and that conflict can be bridged. For those children dealing with multiple losses, we also wanted to provide opportunity to say individual goodbyes and hellos enabling continued growth and development, as well as context for experiencing that emotional attachment does not always end in eventual loss or pain.

Contexts

The city where Saisir les étoiles was facilitated is among the largest ten cities in Canada, with a population of roughly 700,000. The leading industry of employment here is manufacturing. The province, and specifically this municipality, was declared officially and for the first time as 'have-not' status by the Canadian government in 2008 (CBC 2008; Callan/National Post 2008). Roughly one in every five inhabitants here is non-Canadian born. École is an elementary school noted within the district for its diversity: there are 42 different nationalities represented in its student population. About three-quarters of the student population (in the 2007/8 school year) were born outside of Canada. The school's mission aims to 'motivate full potential for all in a climate of respect and trust'. The group described in this chapter was held after school, in the gym and in the library at École. Participants were divided into subgroups according to age and modality preference. For the group at large, two out of every five participants were siblings. Most of the children had experienced civil conflict in central or west-central Africa, or are first-generation born after their parents fled these conflicts; a few have been Canadian-born for generations.

Resources and influences

Three main sources informed the framework for our programme. These were; the Harvard Program in Refugee Trauma (HPRT) at Massachusetts General Hospital/Harvard Medical School; the Information Centre about Asylum and Refugees at City University/King's College London (2009) and Diallo and Lafrenière's (2006) pilot project on best practices for war and torture survivors within the contexts of the Francophone Diaspora. These sources highlight the following principles:

- framework acknowledging the political contexts of the war survivor's experience
- a perspective that the person is not necessarily the root of pathology
- a belief that assimilation is a community issue
- a belief that a phenomenological approach, or placing value on each individual's story, is best.

Methodology

A more thorough discussion of these processes can be found in the first volume of *Drama as Therapy: Theatre as Living* (Jones, 1996). I summarise the key points of processes relevant to vignettes presented later in this chapter, with reference of course to Jones' volume and a select number of other sources as they have informed my (and the children's) work.

Story

The HPRT indicates that psychological states in the war-trauma story – recurring feelings of humiliation, anger, revenge/hatred and hopelessness/despair – are more distressing without psychological resolution or closure. Aspects of the trauma story are often linked to various sights, sounds, smells, places and people; with tensions often physically felt. A feeling of 'moving forward' from a war-trauma story can be difficult to achieve when the potential of being 'reminded' by any one part of it is both hard to control, and hide. Sharing and constructing an individual's story in therapy can help exteriorise the actual traumatic experience, examine specific stimuli safely, provide context in understanding lived reality of day-to-day survival and give the client a text wherein his/her voice may be heard. The act of telling a story within the group also establishes trust within the group process, and fosters insight into the participant's resilience and ability to cope.

Denborough, Freedman and White talk about their work with genocide survivors, and how retelling stories in therapy helps participants regain a sense of personal control over their lives and 'strengthen hope in contexts of hopelessness' (2007: 3). Additionally, and in congruence with feminist and post-colonial considerations discussed earlier, narrative processes in therapy help address the person outside the contexts of symptomology, and facilitate attribution of personal meaning. Van der Kolk (2003) emphasises that working through the war-trauma story, specifically in identifying a beginning, middle and end of experience, can help contextualise the individual's trauma in the past, re-orient a feeling of safety in the present and look to the future with insight. Telling a story also allows for other processes, such as projection, play, the use of symbol/metaphor and witnessing to occur.

Projection

In the first *Drama as Therapy* volume, Jones (1996, 2007) discusses projection as a core dramatherapy process wherein the self is exteriorised to a created object, thereby reflecting emotional preoccupations and providing opportunity to work out unconscious material. Actual, created objects may vary, but the basic notion of projection is that the object is used as a container: a) representative of the self; and b) for greater exploration and understanding of self/self-experience. Gerity (1999) also considers projection a technique whereby the self can be reconstructed.

Play

Jones (1996, 2005) summarises play as providing opportunity to foster resilience, cooperation, awareness of others, and broadening of expression and communication. In his work, a playful state enables the participant to harness his/her own creativity safely and towards therapeutic change. It can also facilitate moving to different levels of cognitive, emotional and interpersonal learning. Particular to trauma, the play can be a safe way to examine difficult experience and re-work stunted stages of development, through replaying episodes of actual experience, recreating alternate endings, or creating alternate realities within which to experiment. Specific to the arts therapist, play processes can be part of therapy wherein relationships themselves are recognised, formed and negotiated. Especially for a child whose attachment processes have been disrupted due to trauma, play can have an important role in helping facilitate attachments in a non-intrusive, mutually negotiated way (Harvey 1994). It further, in that all games will 'come to an end,' starts a gentle modelling for the child that not all attachment experience ends with death, loss or destruction.

Symbol and metaphor

Piaget discusses symbol as a 'deliberate illusion' (1962: 168) that can help participants 'engage with highly problematic material' (Jones 1996: 242). Jones continues to discuss that employing symbol and metaphor is a 'method of storytelling [without relying] on words' (1996: 225). For the child participant who lacks words wherein to verbalise and understand his/her experience, and especially for the child traumatised by experience where there may in fact be no words, metaphor and symbol can become important elements. They can act to contain problematic material and provide distance to reflect, sort through or inspire as the participant will intuitively allow. While it may not be necessary to verbalise or reflect upon the meaning of the metaphor, and while the meaning itself may even change over time, understanding a participant's symbolic or metaphorical intent helps facilitate sharing, meaning-making and attachment processes. These are considered essential elements of 'successful' long-term therapeutic outcome (Yalom 1995). By infusing an indirect 'other' with direct meaning, the participant is able to construct new connections and relationships with the world.

Witnessing

Jones (1996, 2007) has described that the action of witnessing can be felt as a supporting, acknowledging and holding experience. In his view, witnessing does not have to be formally designated, such as an audience sitting in a theatre; the action can occur fluidly in interaction between group participants in session, based on the material and activities at hand. Whether formal or informal, witnessing as an action can facilitate a feeling of emotional safety, understanding, and shared/mutually negotiated experience.

Vignettes

The following are a series of vignettes from the child participants. I select these as snapshots of processes that occurred within individual and collaborative group work. Names have been chosen as the children have indicated they wish to be identified.

Vignette One: R., age eight: feelings and calm-o-mètres

R., eight, is originally from the Democratic Republic of the Congo (formerly Zaire). He came to Canada unaccompanied as a preschooler, to live with his paternal aunt and uncle who had fled to Canada in 1997. R.'s aunt told us about the family with a certain amount of surprising straightforwardness: his mother and sister are no longer living, his father is in prison for political reasons, and an older brother who now resides in Belgium. R. lives with the aunt, uncle, and their six-year-old daughter. Contact with the father is 'very rarely.' R. had attended the first Arc-en-ciel group and said he had enjoyed 'eating snacks' the most. The first session with R., I noticed his perpetually furrowed eyebrows. Regardless of activity – sipping juice, cutting out a picture from a magazine, snacking on popcorn or playing tag – his eyebrows were drawn together in such a way that deep vertical creases appeared on his forehead. Attempting to initiate conversation, or sit in a chair next to him, yielded little result: he would generally respond to questions with one- or two-word responses, and if/when conversation became absent, he would move away to an adjacent chair.

Figure 14.1 shows a semi-directed exercise facilitated during the first group session. The phrase on the sheet of paper reads: 'When I am in a good mood'. The children would be able to share what they enjoyed and

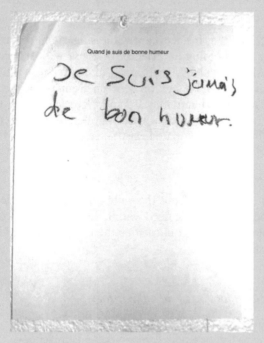

Figure 14.1 Good mood sheet (R.).

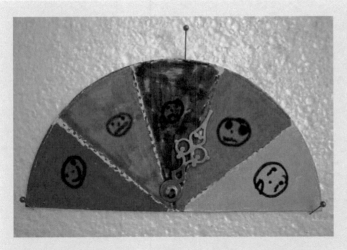

Figure 14.2 Calm-o-mètre (R.).

did not enjoy, and also see how others reacted to and coped with stress. R. wrote very quickly on his sheet the phrase, 'I am never in a good mood.'

A few sessions later, these Calm-o-mètres (Figure 14.2) were fabricated as an identification and communication tool about feelings. Feeling states could be identified, facilitating discussion about why the feeling is felt and about strategies in working towards a more neutral/positive change. The calm-o-mètre is pictured here pointing to where R. indicated he felt most of the time: 'This is when I think of things before.' What he felt during those moments was not a feeling that he could see on our list of feelings (handed out earlier during group), but described it as a time where he 'stands quiet and still'.

Vignette Two: Mathieu, age seven: Captain Cape

Mathieu, age seven, is Canadian-born, of mixed Algerian and Canadian heritage. His mother immigrated to Canada as a refugee from France in the Algerian war. During the first meeting with Mathieu, I was struck with his impressive natural physical agility. He was rather slightly built for his age, but had an incredible quickness coupled with an innate ability to focus on and anticipate movement around him. He didn't ever say much. I observed that Mathieu was sometimes teased by the older boys in the

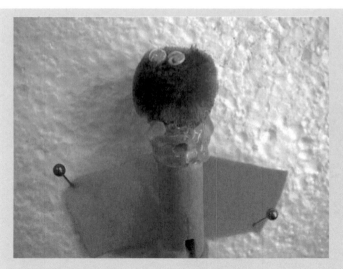

Figure 14.3 Captain Cape (Mathieu).

group, but in ways that older siblings might – holding a juice box just above his reach, making him be the 'pig' in 'pig in the middle,' telling him he had to trade his desirably-flavoured granola bar to them for something less flavourful – and that his agility, ability and coordination made him a sought-out player for their team sports. It didn't seem as though Mathieu sought out any particular initiation with these older boys, or displayed any vigilance/anxiety with or about them; but he did gravitate towards them in play.

Captain Cape (Figure 14.3) was Mathieu's creation for the session discussing resilience and coping strategies, where children made 'super characters' or characters that had 'strong' qualities in hard times. Captain Cape's superpower was his eyes: 'He can see things from far away.' Mathieu added, when a volunteer noted that Captain Cape had no arms, 'He doesn't need. He can fly.'

Vignette Three: Group collective ages six to nine

Figure 14.4 shows the banner the group of children from ages six to nine came up with, for their collaborative project. Originally the group wanted to plant real trees and flowers for École. But then some children brought up the point that they might not see everything grow until next year, and that was either too long or they would forget where to look. Others

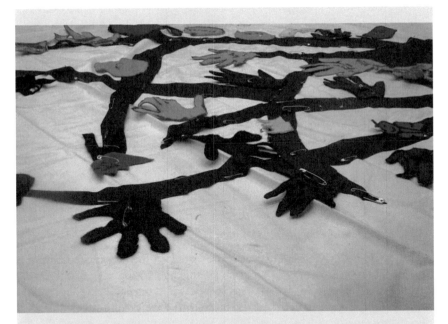

Figure 14.4 The friendship tree (collective ages six to nine).

wondered who would remember to 'feed water' through the year. Group facilitators wondered how everyone would be involved. Drawing a couple ideas to show the children different ways we could re-create trees, the idea of the friendship tree evolved: A banner of one big tree, with felt leaves that were made by tracing each child's hand, and other elements (birds, sun, grass, flowers, bugs) could be added as each child desired individually. If a child did not wish to draw anything like an animal, s/he was not obliged. The children saw this drawing and accepted it enthusiastically.

An interesting debate soon ensued, however, about the background colour for the banner: A blue sheet sparked some disagreement, as it was a hue some children associated with specific tribes/tribal conflict in their countries of origin. We did not discuss the contexts of their individual conflicts at that time, but accepted their associations as fact and redirected: Could white, instead, be OK? (As white was the background colour for the flag of Canada.) This opened up responses from other children: For some children, white was a colour of mourning; for others, it signified summer; others considered white for designated places of worship. In the end, it was acknowledged that white was not neutral for everybody – but they did all agree it could mean a new kind of growing together. So, having had dialogue, the children went forward with their project: tracing, cutting out and sewing (with assistance) hand-leaves, bugs, clouds, blades of grass and squirrels on a large white sheet. R., incidentally, drew and cut out a large sun with a pointed nose and a smile. Weeks later, the children rehearsed the banner's unveiling and presentation for the closing ceremony, where the school's principal accepted it with thanks as a gift. The parents watched in attendance, armed with cameras. This banner is still on display in École's library.

Reflections on arts processes

Projection, play, metaphor, and symbol

At many points in the group process I reflected on the interrelated nature of these processes, especially in children of this age whose play is still largely symbolic. To a certain extent, play was evident in each of the vignettes described here, as each activity – even those that were semi-directed, such as the calm-o-mètre – was designed to have value that was enjoyable, and as each child largely wanted, quite naturally, to participate. Additionally, each child was at liberty to complete the project according to his/her own design.

Captain Cape's highly developed observational powers and capacity for swift, easy movement seemed very much a projection of Mathieu's own physicality and ability to anticipate. Whether or not his response to the volunteer about having no arms or mouth reflected the fact he simply didn't, as he had put it earlier, 'like crafts' (and so maybe chose to limit his crafting to the gluing-on of 'supereyes'), it came across as a perfectly natural idea to Mathieu that his character was ill-equipped according to human standards: Captain Cape had learned to accommodate in what seemed like a matter-of-fact way, very much like Mathieu's own nature. We did not unpack the symbol of a cape as lending itself to strength, camouflage or uniform, or how it compensated for lacking a mouth or some arms (all things I assumed were important for analysis). When I commented that he had chosen the name of 'Captain Cape' without hesitation, Mathieu only said that the cape was important. Most of the children looked on with matter-of-fact understanding (one even nodded). No-one needed to unpack it; though congruent to Jones' (1996) and Yalom's (1995) discussions on group perceptions, it did seem to be a symbol that resonated. I chose to accept it as having served a purpose, and moved on.

R.'s projection by writing that he was 'never in a good mood' may have been unsurprising given his expression, but I suspect Gerity's (1999) ideas hold true here: that disclosure of this feeling in an environment where it was witnessed and accepted (Jones 1996) helped facilitate a closer examination of why that was so. A couple of sessions later, R.'s process of creating the calm-o-mètre seemed carefully reasoned and deliberate, even in the movement with which he coloured his lines. When finished, he pointed to each feeling segment with his index finger, naming the feeling each face represented and giving examples of when he might feel that way. He then turned it over and wrote his name on the back of it with big, blue, deliberate lines. It seemed the process helped facilitate a more elevated play state: as noted, during the construction of the banner, he thought of and drew the sun – a pretty optimistic symbol – and he initiated/thought of this himself.

Story and witnessing

The support of the witnessing individuals during Mathieu's discussion of Captain Cape (a nodded understanding of the importance of his symbol) lent an additional level of the witnessing process as 'holding' (Jones 1996) that was visibly felt, if not verbalised. In some ways I am not sure if I still understand how the symbol resonated within the group, but it did seem that the witnessing of his personal symbol validated his particular method of coping and strength in the face of change. Witnessing R.'s evolution in narrative was, as a therapist, personally touching. His allusion to past narratives ('when I think of things before'), although tangibly infused with loss, helped contextualise his present as being separate from the past, and reconstruct a future with meaning and insight. The cutting out and the sewing of a sun on the friendship banner reflected a movement from a perpetually no-good mood to something more worthy of dreams – a process that seemed as expressive and as heartfelt as his eyebrows.

The closing ceremonies for the groups, where parents attended and where the community was invited to view the children's artwork provided a tangible, external source of validation and belonging for the children. Watching slide shows of their work during the closing ceremony, the children spontaneously voiced the names of the individuals appearing in the photos, and clapped for the projects photographed and displayed by others. Being a part of the tangible feeling of excitement seemed contagious for each child, as I watched them point excitedly at individual contributions to the collective friendship banner on display.

Challenges and future considerations

As this was a pilot follow-up, our group was very literally a work-in-development throughout its actual facilitation. We discovered the following challenges:

- War-trauma is a current 'hot topic.' While it may attract funding, our current institutions might not attract survivors seeking services. It might thus be helpful to more closely examine the potential to make the treatment seem inappropriately exotic (and by default the participants of such a group) in service provision, as well as evaluate how best to design environments for actual service delivery. The discussion, promotion, and design of services focusing uniquely on the clinical aspects of war may contribute to feelings of exclusion and powerlessness in the group participants, indirectly perpetuating interpersonal traumas, oppressions, or other subconscious (post-colonial) tensions.

- As our point of entry with the children was (first) in partnership with the school and (second) upon consultation with the parents, it was sometimes difficult to negotiate coherent plans. As therapists, our intervention focused on encouragement, collaboration and engagement; teachers preferred curricula addressing completion of/attention to task, with more fixed learning objectives. We further focussed on process and collaboration, not 'fixing,' 'progress,' or 'results' of group. This may have proved confusing at times for the children: we obviously were at school, and therefore subject to school rules and using school-associated resources, though without aims that were 'measured' accordingly. This also blurred somewhat the idea of confidentiality: It was hard to assure parents/ caregivers of confidentiality when our first point of contact was school administration.

- The psychoeducational aspect of the group favoured projects that were largely independent of each other: this meant that every week started a new theme, or focused on a new plan. With exception to this, of course, was the collaborative project idea proposed to each subgroup, around five weeks before termination. This lack of continuity may have prevented processing and assimilation of trauma to a more complete degree.

- The contexts of this programme did not provide support options for parents or caregivers. Upon reflection, and upon more experience in working with follow-up with child war survivors, this could be helpful in the future, for two reasons: a) It helps parents establish a relationship of trust with someone in an 'authority' position/who represents a system, and trust, due to their past experiences, can be a difficult process; and b) Individual support may be helpful if talking about their child's experiences heightens the parent's own sense of personal vulnerability.

'Results' of the group and conclusion

The theme to 'Reach for the stars: how to better, together, get along' was a strong theme reflected in session content and planning – even if not evident at points throughout the journey, the outcome, specifically in the collaborative creations of the subgroups, noted a not uncertain preoccupation with varying levels about 'the meaning of' belonging. Interventions designed for both individuals and as a group helped foster self-awareness, greater understanding of others' experiences, cooperation and processes of attachment. Awareness of post-colonial and feminist frameworks also proved valuable for ensuring equity and access for each child. In review of the arts-based therapy processes presented in this chapter, witnessing was particularly key. Amongst their peers and in their classroom communities, bringing elements of the group for others to witness seemed to actively reflect support for the children as valued members. It exemplified that working together could create a positive and a visible outcome. Further, bringing various artwork that the children chose to display to the community (see Appendix for a more detailed description of the gallery exhibition) helped foster and reflect space for integration in their larger communities. The children expressed excitement about their début; the parents expressed pride for their contributing a personalised richness of heritage. The comments received by the children, parents, and community members reflected that space hoped for by Blake *et al.* (2008), wherein immigrant children and their parents can identify, participate and engage as included and valuable community citizens.

Special acknowledgments to Jaswant Guzder (Division of Social and Transcultural Psychiatry, McGill University); Mme Nicole Lauzon (Conseil scolaire du district du Centre-Sud-Ouest); Marcie Bronson (Rodman Hall); David Fancy (Brock University) and Phil Jones (benevolent editor) for their support, guidance and belief in this initiative.

Appendix

Description of the curation of the Chez soi/Home exhibit
http://www.brocku.ca/rodmanhall/exhibitions/past.php

About the work

The literal translation of Chez soi means 'at one's place,' or 'at one's home.' It is French: the child artists in this exhibit call Molière's language their own.

Chez soi/Home focuses on artwork created by child students at École. In collaboration with a community mental health agency, the children met once a week for twelve weeks to share moments and memories of family, school, community, and home. They also met to discuss how to better, together, get along. Bringing their art brut ('outsider art') to this internal space helps reflect their ideas on the need for mainstream response to, and community discourse on, how we feel we belong.

Conceived in response to the complex reality of 'citizenship' as ever-increasing numbers of individuals from diverse international backgrounds are present in and populating 'my Ontario' (the tourism slogan for the province), the goal of this project is to help the children better share their feelings of identity. These are migrant voices, who lack transitional space to link their overseas past to the North American present; these are voices from countries like Chad, the Congo, Kenya, Nigeria, Rwanda, and Togo, whose transitions in Canada have been largely without context to support their (often war-torn) circumstances; these are also second- and third-generation voices, whose transitional space has largely already been forged, and who now live with the struggle of recognising and negotiating their voices' dominance.

These children are preoccupied with personal, local, and international levels of belonging. This exhibit gives opportunity for them to express both personal stories and the hopes that they share: as individuals, as family members, as friends and as young people learning to take their space in the world. We hope these works will increase public awareness of the challenges 'the rising generation' face, drawn together by the contemporary experience of displacement, Diaspora, and relocation.

We hope you enjoy your visit.

About the group's symbol

This symbol was used to represent the group's coming together: 'Reach for the stars'.

For the banner, the children chose a tree to symbolise giving back, their ability to grow and their wish to grow together interdependently. While the colour white signified different things to different children, they all agreed that it could mean a collective new growth. They decided on a white sheet for the background cloth, because they couldn't agree on which shade of blue they liked best.

About the artists

The children are from ages six to twelve. While they like various types of cheese, orange and ivory-striped is their favourite.

Feedback from the exhibit: responses from the children and community members

The show ran for 12 days, culminating in a closing reception for the children and their families.

From a comment log, left in the room during the run of the exhibit:

- Bravo! What beautiful smiles! Thank you for sharing them with us.
- Word to the children.
- I like the calm-o-mètres. I want to make one of my own with my children.

From the curators of the exhibit and museum personnel:

- This is a first for our museum. We hope to show similar themes in the future; these are important issues to address.
- This exhibit demonstrates that mediation through art on such issues can be accomplished in a meaningful way.
- We want to address the needs and reflect the diversity of our community members more (in the future). Children need to identify and see themselves as participants in their communities. Where else is more perfect for this, than a community art gallery?

From the participant artists, visiting the exhibit (translated):

- From R.: Maybe, it's possible I can be in a good mood.
- Everyone wanted the sky to be blue (for the banner). That's true: In everyone's country the sky is blue. But we couldn't agree on the blue. Sometimes I still remember this. I wonder why.
- I liked my drawing. It was good to see it on a wall where other people could see it, and maybe like it too.
- The food they had out (for the closing reception) made me feel like it was something special.
- The food they had out (for the closing reception) made me feel like I really accomplished something.
- This was cool. I wish snacks were always this good.
- I liked the participation certificate . . . I'd never won an award before.

From the parents:

- This is really something!
- My child made that? Wow. That's really good! I am proud of him.
- This really helped me find a way to talk about something I didn't know how to, with my child.

References

Abram, J. (2007) *The Language of Winnicott: A Dictionary of Winnicott's Use of Words*, London, Karnac.

Ackroyd, J. (2000) 'Applied theatre: problems and possibilities', *Applied Theatre Researcher*, 1 www.gu.edu.au/centre/cpci/atr/journal/article1_number1.htm (accessed September 2009).

Aldridge, D. (1996) *Music Therapy Research and Practice in Medicine: From Out of the Silence*, London, Jessica Kingsley Publishers.

American Psychiatric Association (1994) *Diagnostic and Statistical Manual of Mental Disorders*, 4th edn (DSM-IV), Washington, DC, American Psychiatric Association.

American Psychiatric Association (2000) *Quick Reference to the Diagnostic Criteria from the Diagnostic and Statistical Manual of Mental Disorders*, 4th edn, revised, Washington, DC, American Psychiatric Association.

Amir, D. (1999) 'Tales from the therapy room', in J. Hibben (ed.) *Inside Music Therapy; Client Experiences*, Gilsum NH: Barcelona Publishers.

Anderson-Warren, M. and Grainger, R. (2000) *Practical Approaches to Dramatherapy: The Shield of Perseus*, London, Jessica Kingsley Publishers.

Arieti, S.A. (1980) *Creativity*, New York, Basic Books.

Arnold, R., Burke, B., James, C., Martin, D. and Martin, B. (1991) *Educating for a Change*, Toronto, Doris Marshall Institute.

Atkinson, M., Doherty, P. and Kinder, K. (2005) 'Multi-agency working: models, challenges and key factors for success', *Journal of Early Childhood Research*, 3, 1, 7–17, 17–20.

Baker, S. and McKay, E.A. (2001) 'Occupational therapists' perspectives of the needs of women in medium secure units', *British Journal of Occupational Therapy*, 64, 9, 441–448.

Bannerji, H. (2000) *The Dark Side of the Nation: Essays on Multiculturalism, Nationalism and Gender*, Toronto, Canadian Scholars' Press.

Barbarin, O. and Richter, L. (2001) *Mandela's Children: Growing Up in Post-Apartheid South Africa*, London, Routledge.

Barker, C. (1989) *Theatre Games: A New Approach to Drama Training*, Berkshire, Methuen.

Barnes, W.R., Ernst, S. and Hyde, K. (1999) *An Introduction to Groupwork*. London: Palgrave Macmillan.

Bennett, S. (1997) *Theatre Audiences: A Theory of Production and Reception*, 2nd edn, New York, Routledge.

Bion, W.R. (1967) *Second Thoughts*, London, Heinemann.

Blackwell, R.D. (2003) 'Colonialism and globalization: a group-analytic perspective', *Group Analysis*, 36, 4, 445–463.

Blackwell, D. (2005) Psychotherapy, politics, and trauma: Working with survivors of torture and organized violence, *Group Analysis*, 38, 2, 307–323.

Blake, G., Diamond, J., Foot, J., Gidley, B., Mayo, K.S. and Yarnit, M. (2008) *Community Engagement and Community Cohesion* (electronic version), York, UK, Joseph Rowntree Foundation (accessed March 2009).

Blatner, A. (2007) 'Psychodrama: Advances in theory and practice' in M. Maciel, J. Burmeister and C. Baims (eds) *Advancing Theories in Psychodrama*, London and New York, Routledge.

Boal, A. (1979) *Theatre of the Oppressed*, Finland, Pluto Press.

—— (1995) *The Rainbow of Desire: The Boal Method of Theatre and Therapy*, New York, Routledge.

Bowlby, J. (1969) *Attachment*, London, Pelican.

Bracken, P., Giller, J.E. and Summerfield, D. (1995) 'Psychological responses to war and atrocity: The limitations of current concepts', *Social Science and Medicine*, 40, 8, 1073–1083.

Bracken, P., Giller, J.E. and Summerfield, D. (1997) 'Rethinking mental health work with survivors of wartime violence and refugees', *Journal of Refugee Studies*, 10, 4, 431–442.

British Association of Dramatherapists, www.badth.org.uk.

Brook, P. (1988) *The Shifting Point*, London, Methuen.

Brown, L.K. and Lourie, K.J. (2000) 'Children and adolescents living with HIV and AIDS: a review', *Journal for Child Psychology and Psychiatry and Applied Disciplines*, 7, 5, 231–235.

Brown, L.S. (2007) 'Integrating multicultural perspectives into feminist practice', (mp3 audio recording), presentation at the International Perspectives on Feminist Perspectives on Feminist Multicultural Psychotherapy Symposium, San Francisco, www.drlaurabrown.com/ (accessed November 2008).

Bruner, E.M. (1986) 'Ethnography as narrative', in V.W. Turner and E.M. Bruner (eds) *The Anthropology of Experience*, Chicago, University of Illinois Press.

Bryman, A. (2001) *Social Research Methods*, Oxford, Oxford University Press.

Burlingame, M.G., McKenzie, K.R. and Strauss, B. (2004) 'Small group treatment: evidence for effectiveness and mechanisms of change,' in E. Lambert (ed) *Handbook of Psychotherapy and Behaviour Change*, 5th edn, New York, John Wiley and Sons.

Burman, E. (2005) 'Contemporary feminist contributions to debates around gender and sexuality: from identity to performance', *Group Analysis* 38, 1, 17–30.

Callan, E./National Post (2008) 'Ontario to get first "have-not" handout next year', November 3, Associated Press www.financialpost.com/news/story.html?id=928766 (accessed December 2008).

Canadian Association of Elizabeth Fry Societies (2000) Fact Sheets www.elizabethfry.ca/eweek08/factsht.htm (accessed December 2008).

—— (2008) www.elizabethfry.ca/eweek08/fact sht.htm (accessed December 2008).

Canadian Broadcasting Corporation (CBC) (2008) 'Ontario to receive $347M in equalization payments' Flaherty, November 22 www.cbc.ca/canada/story/2008/11/03/flaherty-ministers.html (accessed December 2008).

—— (2009) 'India Reborn: Mother India [Television series, episode 4 of 4]', Toronto, Canadian Broadcasting Corporation.

Carr, M. and Vandiver, T. (2003) 'Effects of instructional art projects on children's behavioural responses and creativity within an emergency shelter', *Journal of the American Art Therapy Association*, 20, 3, 157–162.

Casson, J. (1999) 'Evreinoff and Moreno: monodrama and psychodrama, parallel developments of hidden influences?', *Journal of the British Psychodrama Association*, 14, 1, 15–18.

—— (2003) *Dramatherapy, Psychodrama and Psychosis*, London, Routledge.

Chesner, A. (1994) 'An integrated model of dramatherapy and its application with adults with learning disabilities' in S. Jennings, A. Cattanach, S. Mitchell, A. Chesner and B. Meldrum (eds) *The Handbook of Dramatherapy*, London, Routledge.

—— (1995) *Dramatherapy for People with Learning Disabilities: A World of Difference*, London, Jessica Kingsley Publishers.

Chipman, L. (2009) 'Expanding the frame: self-portrait photography as applied to drama therapy practice', Saarbrücken, VDM Verlag Dr Müller.

Clarkson, P. and Angelo, M. (1998) 'Organisational counseling psychology: using myths and narratives as research and intervention in psychological consultancy to organizations', in P. Clarkson (ed.) *Counselling Psychology: Integrating Theory, Research and Supervised Practice*, London, Routledge.

Clinical Outcomes in Routine Evaluation (2007) CORE 10 www.coreims.co.uk (accessed September 2009).

Cohen, L., Manion, L. and Morrison, K. (2000) *Research Methods in Education*, London, Routledge Falmer.

Cohen-Cruz, J. and Schutzman, M. (1993) *Playing Boal: Theatre, Therapy, and Activism*, New York, Routledge.

Cook, A., Blaustein, M., Spinazzola, J. and van der Kolk, B. (eds) (2003) 'Complex trauma in children and adolescents', White Paper from the National Child Traumatic Stress Network. Allston, MA, The Trauma Center.

Cooper, S.A. and Bailey, N.M. (2001) 'Psychiatric disorders amongst adults with learning disabilities – prevalence and relationship to ability level', *Irish Journal of Psychological Medicine* 18, 2, 45–53.

Cosden, C. and Reynolds, D. (1982) 'Photography as therapy', *Arts in Psychotherapy*, 9, 2, 19–23.

Cossa, M., Ember, S., Grover, L. and Hazlewood, J. (1996) *Acting Out: the Workbook*, New York, Taylor and Francis.

Cox, M. (1992) *Shakespeare Comes to Broadmoor*, London, Jessica Kingsley Publishers.

Cox, M. and Theilgaard, A. (1987) *Mutative Metaphors in Psychotherapy*, London, Tavistock.

Csikszentmihalyi, M. (1992) 'Flow: the psychology of happiness' London, Rider Centre for Social Science Research.

Dadds, M. (2008) 'Perspectives on Practitioner Research, Development and Enquiry Programmes', Cranfield NCSL www.networklearning.ncsl.org.uk (accessed March 2008).

Davies, A. and Richards, E. (eds) (2002) *Music Therapy and Group Work*, London, Jessica Kingsley Publishers.

Davison, S. (2004) 'Specialist forensic mental health services', in *Criminal Behaviour and Mental Health, Special Supplement – Forensic Psychiatry, An Introduction for Medical Students*, 14, 2, London, Whurr Publishers.

Deacon, J. (2004) 'Testing boundaries: the social context of physical and relational containment in a maximum secure psychiatric hospital, *Journal of Social Work Practice*, 18, 1, 81–97.

Denborough, D. (2004) 'Stories from Robben Island. a report from a journey of healing', *The International Journal of Narrative Therapy and Community Work*, 2, 1, 19–28.

Denborough, D., Freedman, J. and White, C. (2007) *Strengthening Resistance: The Use of Narrative Practices in Responding to Genocide Survivors*, Adelaide, Dulwich Centre Publications.

Department of Health (1989) *The Children Act: Guidance and Regulations*, UK Government, Department of Health.

—— (2000) *Secure Futures for Women: Making a Difference*, London, High Security Psychiatric Services.

—— (2001) 'Valuing people: a new strategy for learning disability in the 21st century' www.archive.officialdocuments.co.uk/document/cm50/5086/5086.pdf   (accessed March 2008, September 2009, 4.9.09).

—— (2002) *Women's Mental Health: Into the Mainstream*, London, Strategic Development of Mental Health Care for Women.

—— (2005) 'Best practice guidance now I feel tall: what a patient-led NHS feels like' www.dh.gov.uk (accessed February 2008).

—— (2006) 'White Paper: our health, our care, our say: a new direction for community services' www.dh.gov.uk (accessed February 2008).

—— (2008) 'National Service Framework for Long-term Neurological Conditions: national support for local implementation' www.dh.gov.uk (accessed February 2008, March 2009).

Department of Health, South Africa (2007) *National Strategic Plan: The HIV & Aids and STI Strategic Plan for South Africa*, www.info.gov.za/otherdocs/2007/aidsplan 2007/intro.pdf (accessed November 2009).

Department of Social Development, South Africa (2005) *National Action Plan for Orphans and other Children made Vulnerable by HIV and AIDS*, www. cindi.org.za/files/Kganakga-M.pdf (accessed November 2009).

Diallo, L., and Lafrieniere, G. (2006) 'Manuel de formation sur les meilleures pratiques: Comment intervenir auprès d'une clientèle survivante de guerre, torture et violence organisée', unpublished doctoral dissertation, Ontario: Université Wilfrid Laurier.

Dintino, C. and Read Johnson, D. (1997) 'Playing with the perpetrator: gender dynamics in supervision', in S. Jennings, (ed.) *Dramatherapy: Theory and Practice 3*, London, Routledge.

Duggan, M. and Grainger, R. (1997) *Imagination, Identification and Catharsis in Theatre and Therapy*, London, Jessica Kingsley Publishers.

Emunah, R. (1994) *Acting for Real: Drama Therapy Process, Technique, and Performance*, New York, Brunner-Routledge.

Epston, D. and White, M. (1992) 'Consulting your consultants: The documentation of alternative knowledges', in *Experience, Contradiction, Narrative and Imagination: Selected Papers of David Epston and Michael White 1989–1991*, Adelaide, Dulwich Centre Publications.

Fanon, F. (2004) *The Wretched of the Earth*, New York, Grove Press.

Fitzgerald, J. (1997) 'Reclaiming the whole: self, spirit and society' *Disability and Rehabilitation*, 19, 1, 19–20.

Fletcher, R.J. (1993) 'Individual psychotherapy for persons with mental retardation' in R.J. Fletcher and A. Dosen (eds) *Mental Health Aspects of Mental Retardation*, New York, Lexington Books.

Freedman, J. and Combs, G. (1996) *Narrative Therapy: The Social Construction of Preferred Realities*, New York, Norton.

Freedman, J. and Combs, G. (2002) *Narrative Therapy With Couples . . . And a Whole Lot More! A Collection of Papers, Essays and Exercises*, Adelaide, Dulwich Centre.

Freeman, J., Epston, D. and Lobovits, D. (1997) *Playful Approaches to Serious Problems: Narrative Therapy with Children and Their Families*, New York, W.W. Norton.

Freire, P. (1970) *The Pedagogy of the Oppressed* (reprinted 2007), New York, Continuum.

Gerhardt, S. (2008) *Why Love Matters, how Affection Shapes a Baby's Brain*, New York, Routledge.

Gerity, L.A. (1999). *Creativity and The Dissociative Patient: Puppets, Narrative and Art in The Treatment of Survivors of Childhood Trauma*, London, Jessica Kingsley Publishers.

Gilroy, A. and Lee, C. (1995) *Art and Music Therapy and Research*, London, Routledge.

Gobodo-Madikizela, P. (2002) 'Remorse, forgiveness, and rehumanization: stories from South Africa', *Journal of Humanistic Psychology*, 42, 1, 7–22.

Goffman, E. (1959) *The Presentation of Self in Everyday Life*, Garden City, New York, Doubleday.

Goulet, L. and Linds, W. (2005) 'Breaking the rules of engagement: using theatre of the oppressed to foster youth leadership in anti-racism work', Conference Presentation AERA, April 12.

Grainger, R. (1999) *Arts Therapies Research: A Dramatherapist's Perspective*, London, Jessica Kingsley Publishers.

Greenspan, M. (1983) *A New Approach to Women and Therapy*, New York, McGraw-Hill.

Gross, R. (2005) *Psychology: the Science of Mind and Behaviour*, Dubai, Hodder and Stoughton.

Gunn, J. (2004) 'Introduction: what is forensic psychiatry? (S1–S5)', *Criminal Behaviour and Mental Health*, 14, 2, 1, London, Whurr.

Hadamard, J. (1945) *An Essay on the Psychology of Invention in the Mathematical Field*, New York, Dover Publishers.

Harvard Programme in Refugee Trauma www.hprt-cambridge.org/ (accessed April 2008).

Harvey, S.A. (1994). 'Dynamic play therapy: creating attachments', in B. James (ed.) *Handbook for Treatment of Attachment-Trauma in Children*, New York, Lexington.

Haugh, S. and Paul, S. (eds) (2008) *The Therapeutic Relationship*, Ross-On-Wye, PCCS Books.

Herman, J.L. (1992) *Trauma and Recovery*, New York, Basic Books.

Hewish, S. (1992) 'Geese Theatre Company', in M. Cox (ed.) *Shakespeare Comes to Broadmoor*, London, Jessica Kingsley Publishers.

Higson-Smith, C. (2002) *Supporting Communities Affected by Violence: A Casebook from South Africa*, Oxford, Oxfam GB.

Higson-Smith, C., Mulder, B. and Zondi, N. (2006) *Report on the Zakheni Arts Therapy Foundation's FireMaker Project: a Formative and Summative Evaluation*, Johannesburg, South African Institute for Traumatic Stress.

Hinshelwood, R.D. (1991) *A Dictionary of Kleinian Thought*, London, Free Association Books.

Hoffman, L. (2002) *Family Therapy. An Intimate History*, New York, W.W. Norton.

Holden, S. (1990) 'Group analytic movement psychotherapy', *Group Analysis*, 23, 1, 7–14.

Holloway, P. (1996) 'Dramatherapy in acute intervention', in S. Mitchell (ed.) *Dramatherapy: Clinical Studies*, London, Jessica Kingsley Publishers.

Holzman, L. and Mendez, R. (2003) *Psychological Investigations: A Clinician's Guide to Social Therapy*, London, Brunner-Routledge.

hooks, Bell. (1994) *Teaching to Transgress: Education as the Practice of Freedom*, New York, Routledge.

Huet, V. (1997) 'Challenging professional confidence: arts therapies and psychiatric rehabilitation', *Inscape*, 2, 1, 1–17.

Information Centre about Asylum and Refugees at City University/King's College (2009).

Jaffe, J. (2001) 'Rhythms of dialogue in infancy: coordinated timing and social development', *Society of Child Development Monographs*, 66, 2, Blackwell, Oxford.

James, J. (1996) 'Dramatherapy with people with learning disabilities', in S. Mitchell (ed.) *Dramatherapy: Clinical Studies*, London: Jessica Kingsley Publishers.

Jenkyns, M. (1996) *The Play's the Thing*, London, Routledge.

Jennings, S. (1992a) 'The nature and scope of dramatherapy', in M. Cox (ed.) *Shakespeare Comes to Broadmoor*, London, Jessica Kingsley Publishers.

—— (ed) (1992b) *Dramatherapy: Theory and Practice 2*, Routledge, London.

—— (1994) *Introduction to Dramatherapy: Theatre and Healing: Ariadne's Ball of Thread*, London, Jessica Kingsley Publishers.

—— (1997) 'Masking and unmasking: dramatherapy with offender patients', in S. Jennings (ed.) *Dramatherapy: Theory and Practice 3*, London, Routledge.

—— (2005) 'Embodiment – projection – role a developmental model for the play-therapy method', in C. Schaefer, J. McCormack and A. Ohnogi (eds), *The International Handbook of Play Therapy*, 65–75, Jason Aronson, New York.

—— (2009) *Dramatherapy and Social Theatre*, London, Routledge.

—— (2010) *Neuro-dramatic Play and Attachment*, London, Jessica Kingsley Publishers.

Jennings, S., McGinley, J.D. and Orr, M. (1997) Masking and Unmasking: Dramatherapy with offender patients. In Jennings, S. (ed.) *Dramatherapy: Theory and Practice 3*, London: Routledge.

Jiwani, Y. (2001) 'Intersecting inequalities: immigrant women of colour, violence and health care', paper presented at Vancouver, FREDA www.atira.bc.ca/Advancing-HealthCareWorkshop/mod2 (accessed March 2009).

Johnson, D. (2004). *Being in proximity to the other*, presentation at Developmental Transformations Conference, New York City.

Johnston, M. (May 1996) 'Integrating models of disability', in L. Barton and M. Oliver (eds) *Disability Studies: Past, Present and Future*, Leeds, The Disability Press.

Johnstone, E.C. (1994) *Searching for the Causes of Schizophrenia*, Oxford, Oxford University Press.

Jones, P. (1991) 'Dramatherapy: five core processes', *Dramatherapy: the Journal of the British Association of Dramatherapists*, 14, 1, 5–10.

—— (1996) *Drama As Therapy: Theatre as Living*, London, Routledge.

—— (2005) *The Arts Therapies: A Revolution in Healthcare*, London, Routledge.

—— (2007) *Drama As Therapy. Theory, Practice and Research*, London, Routledge.

Jones, P. and Dokter, D. (2008) *Supervision of Dramatherapy*, London, Routledge.

Jones, P., Moss, D., Tomlinson, P. and Welch, S. (eds) (2007) *Childhood: Services and Provision for Children*, London, Pearson.

Jung, C. (1933) *Modern Man in Search of a Soul*, London, Routledge.

Karkou, V, and Sanderson, P. (2006) *Arts Therapies: A Research Based Map of the Field*, Bodmin, Elsevier Ltd.

Kay, E., Tisdall, M., Davis, J., Hill, M. and Prout, A. (eds) (2006) *Children, Young People and Social Inclusion: Participation for What?* Bristol, Policy Press.

Kellett, M. (2005) *How to Develop Children as Researchers*, London: Paul Chapman.

Kerlinger, F.N. (1986) *Foundations of Behavioural Research*, New York, Rinehart and Winston.

Kershaw, B. (1992) *The Politics of Performance: Radical Theatre as Cultural Intervention*, New York, Routledge.

—— (2003) 'Curiosity or contempt: on spectacle, the human, and activism', *Theatre Journal*, 55, 4, 591–611.

Kilpatrick, D.G. (2005) 'Special section on complex trauma and a few thoughts about the need for more rigorous research on treatment efficacy, effectiveness, and safety', *Journal of Traumatic Stress*, 18, 5, 379–384.

Kinghorn, A. and Long, S. (2006) 'A review of IBIS HIV and AIDS work in Africa' www.positivevibes.org/02 (accessed October 2009).

Klein, M. (1963) *Envy and Gratitude and Other Works 1946–1963*, London, Vintage.

—— (1997) 'Notes on some schizoid mechanisms', in Klein *Envy and Gratitude and Other Works 1946–1963*, London, Vintage.

Lambert, M.J. (2004) *Bergin and Garfield's Handbook of Psychotherapy and Behavior Change*, New York, Wiley.

Landy, R. (1993) *Persona and Performance: The Meaning of Role in Drama, Therapy, and Everyday Life*, London, Jessica Kingsley Publishers.

—— (1994) *Drama Therapy: Concepts, Theories, and Practices*, Illinois, Charles C. Thomas.

—— (2001) *New Essays in Drama Therapy*, Illinois, Charles C. Thomas.

—— (2004) 'Research-based art: in search of a form for playing god', *Journal of Pedagogy, Pluralism and Practice*, 9, Cambridge, Mass, Lesley University, www.lesley.edu/journals/jppp/9/index.html.

—— (2006) 'Assessment through drama', in P. Taylor (ed.) *Assessment in Arts Education*, London, Heinemann.

—— (2006) 'The future of drama therapy', *Arts in Psychotherapy*, 33, 135–142.

—— (2008) 'The dramatic world view revisited: reflections on the roles taken and played by young children and adolescents', *Dramatherapy, Journal of the British Association for Dramatherapists*, 30, 2, 3–13.

—— (2009) 'Role theory and the role method of drama therapy', in R. Emunah, and D. Johnson (eds) *Current Approaches to Drama Therapy*, 2nd edn, Illinois, Charles C. Thomas.

Langley, D. (2006) *An Introduction to Dramatherapy*, Sage, London.

Latta, N. (2005) *Into The Darklands – Unveiling the Predators Among Us*, London, Harper Collins.

Macaskill, C. (1991) *Adopting or Fostering a Sexually Abused Child*, London, B. T. Batsford Ltd.

Madibbo, A. (2005) 'Immigration, race, and language: black francophones of Ontario and the challenge of intergration, racism, and language discrimination', paper presented at Toronto: Joint Centre of Excellence for Research on Immigration and Settlement.

Mahrer, A.R. (1997) 'Discovery-oriented research on how to do psychotherapy' in W. Dryden (ed.), *Research in Counselling and Psychotherapy and Practical Applications*, London, Sage.

Margai, F. and Henry, N. (2003) 'A community-based assessment of learning disabilities using environmental and contextual risk factors', *Social Science and Medicine*, 56, 1073–1085.

Martin, R. (2001) 'The performative body: phototherapy and re-enactment', *Afterimage*, 29, 17–20.

May, R. (1976) *Courage to Create*, New York, Norton.

McNeilly, G. (2006) *Group Analytic Art Therapy*, London, Jessica Kingsley Publishers.

Meldrum, B. (1994) 'A role model of dramatherapy and its application with individuals and groups', in S. Jennings, A. Cattanach, S. Mitchell, A. Chesner, and B. Meldrum (eds) *The Handbook of Dramatherapy*, London, Routledge.

Mencap (2007) 'Disablist bullying is wrecking children's lives says Mencap' www.mencap.org.uk/news.asp (accessed September 2009).

—— (2007) 'Survey' at www.mencap.org.uk (accessed September 2009).

Miedema, B., Hamilton, R. and Easley, J. (2007) 'From "invisibility" to "normalcy": coping strategies of young adults during the cancer journey', *Palliative and Supportive Care*, 5, 41–49.

Milioni, D. (2001) 'Social constructionism and dramatherapy: creating alternative discourses', *Dramatherapy*, 23, 2, 10–17.

Mindell, A. (1995) *Sitting in the Fire: Large Group Transformation Using Conflict And Diversity*, Portland, Lao Tse Press.

Mitchell, S. (ed.) (1996) *Dramatherapy: Clinical Studies*, London, Jessica Kingsley Publishers

Morgan, A. (2000) *What is Narrative Therapy? An Easy-to-read Introduction*, Adelaide, Dulwich Centre.

Morse, J. and Morgan, A. (2003) 'Group work with women who have experienced violence', *International Journal of Narrative Therapy and Community Work*, 4, 1, 37–47.

Moss, D. (2007) 'The social divisions of childhood', in P. Jones, D. Moss, P. Tomlinson and S. Welch (eds) *Childhood: Services and Provision for Children*, London, Pearson.

National Institute of Mental Health (2002) *Mental Health and Mass Violence: Evidence-based Early Psychosocial Intervention for Victims/Survivors of Mass Violence: A Workshop to Reach Consensus on Best Practices*. NIMH Publication No. 02-5138. Washington DC, US Government Printing Office.

Nitsun, M. (1996) *The Anti-Group. Destructive Forces in the Group and their Creative Potential*, London, Routledge.

Office for National Statistics (2008) 'National statistics socio-economic classification (NS-SEC)' www.ons.gov.uk/about-statistics/classifications/current/ns-sec (accessed September 2009).

Office of Public Sector Information (1989) Children Act www.opsi.gov.uk/acts/acts2004 (accessed November 2009).

—— (1995) Disability Discrimination Act www.opsi.gov.uk (accessed October 2008).

—— (2007) Mental Health Act www.opsi.gov.uk/acts/acts2007/ukpga (accessed September 2009).

Oliver, M. (1990) *The Politics of Disablement*, London, Macmillan.

Patrick, D.L. and Erickson, P. (1993) *Health Status and Health Policy: Allocating Resources to Health Care*, New York, Oxford University Press.

Payne, H. (ed.) (1993) *Handbook of Inquiry into the Arts Therapies, One River Many Currents*, London, Jessica Kingsley Publishers.

—— (2006) 'The body as container and expresser: authentic movement groups in the development of wellbeing in our bodymindspirit, in J. Corrigall, H. Payne and H. Wilkinson (eds) *Working with the Embodied Mind in Psychotherapy*, London, Routledge.

—— (2009) 'Pilot study to evaluate dance movement psychotherapy (the body mind approach) in patients with medically unexplained symptoms: participants and facilitator perceptions and a summary discussion', *Body, Movement and Dance in Psychotherapy: An International Journal for Theory, Research and Practice*, 4, 2, 77–94.

Pearson, J. (ed.) (1996) *Discovering the Self Through Drama and Movement: the Sesame Approach*, London, Jessica Kingsley Publishers.

Perry, B.D. and Azad, I. (1998) 'Post-traumatic stress states in children and adolescents', *Current Opinion in Pediatrics*, 11, 1, 121–132.

Piaget, J. (1962). *Play, Dreams, and Imitation in Childhood*, New York, Norton.

Poincaré, H. (1952) *Science and Hypothesis*, New York, Dover.

Polatajkoo, H.J., Law, M., Miller, J., Schaffer, R. and Macnab, J. (1991) 'The effect of a sensory integration programme on academic achievement, motor performance and self esteem, in children identified as learning disabled: results of a clinical trial', *Occupational Therapy Journal of Research*, 11, 1, 155–176.

Pollock, S. (2008) 'Locked in locked out: imprisoning women in the shrinking and punitive welfare state', unpublished thesis, Ontario, Wilfred Laurier University.

Prentki, T. and Selman, J. (2003) *Popular Theatre in Political Culture: Britain and Canada in Focus*, Oregon, Intellect Books.

Prigitano, G. (1989) 'Work, love and play after brain injury', *Bulletin of the Menninger Clinic*, 53, 5, 427–435.

Punamäki, R.L., Komproe, I., Qouta, S., El-Masri, M. and de Jong, J.T. (2005) 'The deterioration and mobilization effects of trauma on social support: childhood maltreatment and adulthood military violence in a Palestinian community sample', *Child Abuse and Neglect*, 29, 4, 351–373.

Radmall, B. (2001/2002) 'The dance between post-modern systemic therapy and dramatherapy', *Dramatherapy, Journal of the British Association for Dramatherapists*, 23, 3, 16–19.

Ramachandran, V.S. (2004) *A Brief Tour of Human Consciousness: From Impostor Poodles to Purple*, New York, Pi Press.

Ramsden, E., Pryor, A., Bose, S., Charles, S. and Adshead, G. (2006) 'Something dangerous: touch in forensic practice', in G. Galton (ed) *Touch: Papers, Dialogues on Touch in the Psychoanalytic Space*, London, Karnac.

Razack, S. (1998) *Looking White People in the Eye: Gender, Race, and Culture in Courtrooms and Classrooms*, Toronto, University of Toronto Press.

—— (2008) *Casting Out: The Eviction of Muslims from Western Law and Politics*, Toronto, Toronto University Press.

Read Johnson, D. (1992) 'The dramatherapist in role', in S. Jennings (ed.) *Dramatherapy: Theory and Practice 2*, London, Routledge.

—— (2005) 'Developmental transformations in the play space', in *Papers on Developmental Transformations 1985–2005*, The Institute for the Arts in Psychotherapy www.artstherapy.net.

Revell, B. (2000) *Playing with Rainbows: A National Play Program for At-risk Refugee Children*, Ottawa, YWCA of Canada.

—— (2001) *Jouons avec les arcs-en-ciel: Le program national de jeu pour des enfants à risque réfugiés*. Ottawa, YWCA du Canada.

Richards, M., Maughan, B., Hardy, R., Hall, I. and Wadsworth, M. (2001) 'Long-term affective disorder in people with mild learning disability', *British Journal of Psychiatry*, 179, 523–527.

Richter, L. (2004) 'The Impact of HIV/AIDS on the development of children', in R. Pharoah (ed.) *A Generation at Risk? HIV/AIDS, Vulnerable Children and Security in Southern Africa*, Pretoria, Institute for Security Studies.

—— (2006) *Where the Heart is? Meeting the Psychosocial Needs of Young Children in the Context of HIV/AIDS*, The Hague, The Netherlands, Bernard van Leer Foundation.

Robson, C. (2002) *Real World Research*, 2nd edn, Oxford, Blackwell.

Rosen, G.M. and Lilienfeld, S.O. (2008) 'Post-traumatic stress disorder: an empirical evaluation of core assumptions', *Clinical Psychology Review*, 28, 1, 837–868.

Roth, A. and Fonagy, P. (2005) *What Works for Whom? A Critical Review of Psychotherapy Research*, 2nd edn, London, Guildford Press.

Royal College of Psychiatrists (2004) 'Psychotherapy and learning disability,' Report Number, 116, London, Royal College of Psychiatrists.

Rushton, A. and Dance, C. (2002) *Adoption Support Services for Families in Difficulty*, London, British Association for Adoption and Fostering.

Sahhar, N. (2008) 'A therapist's perspective on psychological work within forensic settings', *DMM News*, 4, Sept 08, www.iasa-dmm.org (accessed September 2008).

Samuels, A. (2006) 'Working directly with political, cultural and social material in the therapy session', in L. Layton, N.C. Hollander and S. Gutwill (eds) *Psychoanalysis, Class and Politics: Encounters in the Clinical Setting*, Hove, Routledge.

Sandretto, S. (2008) 'Action research for social justice', Discussion Paper, Wellington, Teaching and Learning Research Initiative.

Sajnani, N. and Nadeau, D. (2006) 'Creating safer spaces for women of colour: performing the politics of possibility', *Canadian Woman Studies*, 25, 1/2, 45–52.

Sass, L.A. (2000) 'Schizophrenia, modernism, and the "creative imagination": on creativity and psychopathology', *Creativity Study Journal*, 13, 1, 55–74.

Saunders, B.E., Berliner, L. and Hanson, R.F. (eds) (2003) *Child Physical and Sexual Abuse: Guidelines for Treatment. Final Report*, Charleston, SC, National Crime Victims Research and Treatment Center.

Schaverien, J. (1992) *The Revealing Image*, London, Routledge.

—— (2000) 'The triangular relationship and the aesthetic counter transference in analytical art psychotherapy', in A. Gilroy and G. McNeilly (eds) *The Changing Shape of Art Therapy*, London, Jessica Kingsley Publishers.

Segal, H. (1982) *Introduction to the Work of Melanie Klein*, London, Hogarth Press.

Selman, J. and Prentki, T. (2003) *Popular Theatre in Political Culture*. Bristol, Intellect Books.

Shamsuddin, A.K. (2009) 'Bureaucracy in Bangladesh [letter to the editor]', *The Bangladesh Observer*, February 25, 5.

Sinason, V. (1992). *Mental Handicap and the Human Condition: New Approaches from the Tavistock*, London, Free Association Books.

Skaife, S. and Huet, V. (eds) (1998) *Art Psychotherapy Groups*, London, Routledge.

Sourkes, B. (1982) *The Deepening Shade: Psychological Aspects of Life-Threatening Illness*, Pittsburgh, University of Pittsburgh Press.

South African National Department of Health (2007) *National Strategic Plan 2007–2011*, Pretoria, Department of Health.

Spence, J. (1988) *Putting Myself in the Picture: A Political Personal and Photographic Autobiography*, Seattle, WA, The Real Comet Press.

—— (1995) *Cultural Sniping: The Art of Transgression*, London, Routledge.

Spence, J. and Martin, R. (1988) 'Phototherapy: psychic realism as a healing art?', *Ten, 8*, 30, 1, 2–10.

Spolin, V. (1998) *Improvisation for the Theatre*, New York, Northwest University Press.

Springham, N. (1998) 'The magpie's eye: patient's resistance to engagement in an art therapy group for drug and alcohol patients,' in S. Skaife and V. Huet (eds) *Art Psychotherapy Groups*, London, Routledge.

Steinberg, J. (2008) *Three Letter Plague: A Young Man's Journey through a Great Epidemic*, Jeppestown, Jonathon Ball Publishers.

Stenhouse, L. (1975) *An Introduction to Curriculum Development and Research*, London, Heinemann.

Stewart, S. and Selman, J. (2003) 'Deep listening in a feminist popular theatre project upsetting the position of audience in participatory education', *American Association for Continuing Education*, 54, 1, 7–22.

Stock Whitaker, D. (1995) *Using Groups to Help People*, London, Routledge.

Straetmans, J.M.J.A.A., Van Schrojenstein Lantman-de Valk H.M.J. Schellevis, F.G. and Dinant, G.J. (2007) 'Health problems of people with intellectual disabilities: the impact for general practice', *British Journal of General Practice*, 57, 2, 64–66.

Thomas, A. (1999) 'Remorse and reparation, a philosophical analysis', in M. Cox (ed.) *Remorse and Reparation*, London, Jessica Kingsley Publishers.

Thomas, D., O'Brien, T., Senner, A., Treadgold, C. and Young, A. (2006) 'The need for change', powerpoint presentation given at the Melbourne Cancer Conference, www.canteen.org.au/default.asp?articleid=840andmenuid=174 (accessed August 2008).

Thompson, N. (2002) 'Social movements, social justice, and social work', *British Journal of Social Work*, 32, 711–722.

Toporek, R., Gerstein, L., Roysircar, G., Fouad, N. and Israel, T. (2006) *Handbook for Social Justice in Counseling Psychology: Leadership, Vision, and Action*, Thousand Oaks, CA, Sage.

Totton, N. (2008) 'In and out of the mainstream: therapy in its political and social context', in S. Haugh and S. Paul (eds) *The Therapeutic Relationship*, Ross-On-Wye, PCCS Books.

Trevarthen, C. (2005) 'Action and emotion in development of cultural intelligence: why infants have feelings like ours', in J. Nadel and D. Muir (eds) *Emotional Development*, Oxford, Oxford University Press.

Trinh, T. Minh-ha (1989) *Woman, Native, Other (Writing Postcoloniality and Feminism)*, Indianapolis, Indiana University Press.

Tselikas-Portman, E. (ed.) (1999) *Supervision and Dramatherapy*, London: Jessica Kingsley Publishers.

United Nations (2001) *Declaration of Commitment on HIV/AIDS*, Geneva, United Nations.

University of Cape Town (2004) *Mapping Workshop Manual: Finding your Way Through*, Cape Town, University of Cape Town.

University of Exeter (2008) 'Experiences of stigma and discrimination among individuals with brain injuries', Social Neuropsychology Research Group: Headway – the Brain Injury Association, www.headway.org.uk (accessed October 2008).

van der Kolk, B.A. (2003) 'The assessment and treatment of complex PTSD', in R. van der Kolk (2003) 'The neurobiology of childhood trauma and abuse', *Child and Adolescent Psychiatric Clinics*, 12, 1, 293–317.

—— (2005) 'Developmental trauma disorder – towards a rational diagnosis for children with complex trauma histories', *Psychiatric Annals*, 12, 1, 15–28.

Vera, E.M. and Speight, S.L. (2003) 'Multicultural competence, social justice, and counseling psychology: expanding our roles', *The Counseling Psychologist*, 31, 3, 253–272.

Walker, G. (2008) 'Mind the gap', in P. Jones, D. Moss, P. Tomlinson and S. Welch (eds) *Childhood: Services and Provision for Children*, London, Pearson.

Waller, D. (1990) 'Group analysis and the arts therapies', *Group Analysis* 23, 1, 211–213.

Weiner, I. (1998) *Principles of Psychotherapy*, 2nd edn, New York, John Wiley and Sons.

Weiser, J. (1986) 'Ethical considerations in phototherapy training and practice', *Phototherapy*, 5, 12–17.

—— (1999) *PhotoTherapy Techniques: Exploring the Secrets of Personal Snapshots and Family Albums*, Vancouver, BC, PhotoTherapy Centre Publishers.

—— (2004) 'Photo therapy techniques in counseling and therapy – using ordinary snapshots and photo-interactions to help clients heal their lives', *The Canadian Art Therapy Association Journal*, 17, 1, 23–53.

Welsh Office (1995) *Welsh Health Survey*, Cardiff, Welsh Office.

West, T.C. (1999) *Wounds of the Spirit: Black Woman, Violence and Resistance Ethics*, New York, New York University Press.

Weston, S. (2004) 'Arts therapies and the brain injury pathway', unpublished paper for Sheffield Brain Injury Stakeholders Group.

White, M. (1995) *Re-Authoring Lives: Interviews and Essays*, Adelaide, Dulwich Centre.

—— (1997) *Narratives of Therapists' Lives*, Adelaide, Dulwich Centre.

—— (2004) 'Working with people who are suffering the consequences of multiple trauma: a narrative perspective', *The International Journal of Narrative Therapy and Community Work*, 1, 1, 45–76.

—— (2007) *Maps of Narrative Practice*, New York, W.W. Norton.

White, M. and Epston, D. (1990) *Narrative Means to Therapeutic Ends*, New York, Norton.

White, P. (1999) 'Ethnicity, racialzation and citizenship as diverse elements in Europe', in R. Hudson and A.M. Williams (eds) *Divided Europe: Society and Territory*, London, Sage.

Willett, J. (1964) *Brecht on Theatre*, New York, Hill and Wang.

Wink, J. (2000) *Critical Pedagogy: Notes from the Real World*, 2nd edn, New York, Longman.

Winnicott, D.W. (1971) *Playing and Reality*, London, Tavistock.

World Health Organization, (2000) 'Women and mental health', www.who.int/media-centre/factsheets/fs248/en (accessed December 2008).

—— (2004) *Promoting Mental Health: Concepts, Emerging Evidence, and Practice: Summary Report*, Geneva, World Health Organization.

Yalom, I.D. (1995) *The Theory and Practice of Group Psychotherapy*, 4th edn, New York, Basic Books.

Contacts

The following are associations or organisations who can be contacted for further information concerning dramatherapy.

The British Association of Dramatherapists www.badth.org.uk
NADT – National Association for Dramatherapists www.nadt.org
Dramatherapy Ireland Website www.dramatherapyireland.com
Dramatherapy Northern Ireland dramatherapynorthernireland.org.uk
Institute for Arts in Therapy and Education www.artspsychotherapy.org
ECARTE – The European Consortium for Arts Therapies Education.
    www.unimuenster.de/Ecarte
The South African Association of Dramatherapists www.dramatherapy.co.za
Dramatherapy in Greece and Cyprus www.dramatherapy.gr
Dramatherapy in Italy www.spid-drammaterapia.it
Dramatherapy in Korea www.dramatherapy.co.kr
Dramatherapy in Malta www.catsmalta.org.
Dramatherapy Research http://groups.yahoo.com/group/BADthResearch/
The Australia and New Zealand Art Therapy Association, which also features
    dramatherapy www.anzata.org

Index